Lecture Notes in Biomathematics

Vol. 1: P. Waltman, Deterministic Threshold Models in the Theory of Epidemics. V, 101 pages. 1974.

Vol. 2: Mathematical Problems in Biology, Victoria Conference 1973. Edited by P. van den Driessche. VI, 280 pages. 1974.

Vol. 3: D. Ludwig, Stochastic Population Theories. VI, 108 pages. 1974.

Vol. 4: Physics and Mathematics of the Nervous System. Edited by M. Conrad, W. Güttinger, and M. Dal Cin. XI, 584 pages. 1974.

Vol. 5: Mathematical Analysis of Decision Problems in Ecology. Proceedings 1973. Edited by A. Charnes and W.R. Lynn. VIII, 421 pages. 1975.

Vol. 6: H. T. Banks, Modeling and Control in the Biomedical Sciences. V. 114 pages. 1975.

Vol. 7: M.C. Mackey, Ion Transport through Biological Membranes, An Integrated Theoretical Approach. IX, 240 pages. 1975.

Vol. 8: C. DeLisi, Antigen Antibody Interactions. IV, 142 pages. 1976.

Vol. 9: N. Dubin, A Stochastic Model for Immunological Feedback in Carcinogenesis: Analysis and Approximations. XIII, 163 pages. 1976.

Vol. 10: J.J. Tyson, The Belousov-Zhabotinskii Reaktion. IX, 128 pages. 1976.

Vol. 11: Mathematical Models in Medicine. Workshop 1976. Edited by J. Berger, W. Bühler, R. Repges, and P. Tautu. XII, 281 pages. 1976.

Vol. 12: A.V. Holden, Models of the Stochastic Activity of Neurones. VII, 368 pages. 1976.

Vol. 13: Mathematical Models in Biological Discovery. Edited by D.L. Solomon and C. Walter. VI, 240 pages. 1977.

Vol. 14: L.M. Ricciardi, Diffusion Processes and Related Topics in Biology. VI, 200 pages. 1977.

Vol. 15: Th. Nagylaki, Selection in One- and Two-Locus Systems. VIII, 208 pages. 1977.

Vol. 16: G. Sampath, S.K. Srinivasan, Stochastic Models for Spike Trains of Single Neurons. VIII, 188 pages. 1977.

Vol. 17: T. Maruyama, Stochastic Problems in Population Genetics. VIII, 245 pages. 1977.

Vol. 18: Mathematics and the Life Sciences. Proceedings 1975. Edited by D.E. Matthews. VII, 385 pages. 1977.

Vol. 19: Measuring Selection in Natural Populations. Edited by F.B. Christiansen and T.M. Fenchel. XXXI, 564 pages. 1977.

Vol. 20: J.M. Cushing, Integrodifferential Equations and Delay Models in Population Dynamics. VI, 196 pages. 1977.

Vol. 21: Theoretical Approaches to Complex Systems. Proceedings 1977. Edited by R. Heim and G. Palm. VI, 244 pages. 1978.

Vol. 22: F.M. Scudo and J.R. Ziegler, The Golden Age of Theoretical Ecology: 1923–1940. XII, 490 pages. 1978.

Vol. 23: Geometrical Probability and Biological Structures: Buffon's 200th Anniversary. Proceedings 1977. Edited by R.E. Miles and J. Serra. XII, 338 pages. 1978.

Vol. 24: F.L. Bookstein, The Measurement of Biological Shape and Shape Change. VIII, 191 pages. 1978.

Vol. 25: P. Yodzis, Competition for Space and the Structure of Ecological Communities. VI, 191 pages. 1978.

Vol. 26: M.B Katz, Questions of Uniqueness and Resolution in Reconstruction from Projections. IX, 175 pages. 1978.

Vol. 27: N. MacDonald, Time Lags in Biological Models. VII, 112 pages. 1978.

Vol. 28: P.C. Fife, Mathematical Aspects of Reacting and Diffusing Systems. IV, 185 pages. 1979.

Vol. 29: Kinetic Logic – A Boolean Approach to the Analysis of Complex Regulatory Systems. Proceedings, 1977. Edited by R. Thomas. XIII, 507 pages. 1979.

Vol. 30: M. Eisen, Mathematical Models in Cell Biology and Cancer Chemotherapy. IX, 431 pages. 1979.

Vol. 31: E. Akin, The Geometry of Population Genetics. IV, 205 pages. 1979.

Vol. 32: Systems Theory in Immunology. Proceedings, 1978. Edited by G. Bruni et al. XI, 273 pages. 1979.

Vol. 33: Mathematical Modelling in Biology and Ecology. Proceedings, 1979. Edited by W.M. Getz. VIII, 355 pages. 1980.

Vol. 34: R. Collins, T.J. van der Werff, Mathematical Models of the Dynamics of the Human Eye. VII, 99 pages. 1980.

Vol. 35: U. an der Heiden, Analysis of Neural Networks. X, 159 pages. 1980.

Vol. 36: A. Wörz-Busekros, Algebras in Genetics. VI, 237 pages. 1980.

Vol. 37: T. Ohta, Evolution and Variation of Multigene Families. VIII, 131 pages. 1980.

Vol. 38: Biological Growth and Spread: Mathematical Theories and Applications. Proceedings, 1979. Edited by W. Jäger, H. Rost and P. Tautu. XI, 511 pages. 1980.

Vol. 39: Vito Volterra Symposium on Mathematical Models in Biology. Proceedings, 1979. Edited by C. Barigozzi. VI, 417 pages. 1980.

Vol. 40: Renewable Resource Management. Proceedings, 1980. Edited by T. Vincent and J. Skowronski. XII, 236 pages. 1981.

Vol. 41: Modèles Mathématiques en Biologie. Proceedings, 1978. Edited by C. Chevalet and A. Micali. XIV, 219 pages. 1981.

Vol. 42: G.W. Swan, Optimization of Human Cancer Radiotherapy. VIII, 282 pages. 1981.

Vol. 43: Mathematical Modeling on the Hearing Process. Proceedings, 1980. Edited by M.H. Holmes and L.A. Rubenfeld. V, 104 pages. 1981.

Vol. 44: Recognition of Pattern and Form. Proceedings, 1979. Edited by D.G. Albrecht. III, 226 pages. 1982.

Vol. 45: Competition and Cooperation in Neutral Nets. Proceedings, 1982. Edited by S. Amari and M.A. Arbib. XIV, 441 pages. 1982.

Vol. 46: E. Walter, Identifiability of State Space Models with applications to transformation systems. VIII, 202 pages. 1982.

Vol. 47: E. Frehland, Stochastic Transport Processes in Discrete Biological Systems. VIII, 169 pages. 1982.

Vol. 48: Tracer Kinetics and Physiologic Modeling. Proceedings, 1983. Edited by R.M. Lambrecht and A. Rescigno. VIII, 509 pages. 1983.

Vol. 49: Rhythms in Biology and Other Fields of Application. Proceedings, 1981. Edited by M. Cosnard, J. Demongeot and A. Le Breton. VII, 400 pages. 1983.

Vol. 50: D.H. Anderson, Compartmental Modeling and Tracer Kinetics. VII, 302 pages. 1983.

Vol. 51: Oscillations in Mathematical Biology. Proceedings, 1982. Edited by J.P.E. Hodgson. VI, 196 pages. 1983.

Vol. 52: Population Biology. Proceedings, 1982. Edited by H.I. Freedman and C. Strobeck. XVII, 440 pages. 1983.

Vol. 53: Evolutionary Dynamics of Genetic Diversity. Proceedings, 1983. Edited by G.S. Mani. VII, 312 pages. 1984.

Vol. 54: Mathematical Ecology. Proceedings, 1982. Edited by S.A. Levin and T.G. Hallam. XII, 513 pages. 1984.

Vol. 55: Modelling of Patterns in Space and Time. Proceedings, 1983. Edited by W. Jäger and J.D. Murray. VIII, 405 pages. 1984.

Vol. 56: H.W. Hethcote, J.A. Yorke, Gonorrhea Transmission Dynamics and Control. IX, 105 pages. 1984.

Vol. 57: Mathematics in Biology and Medicine. Proceedings, 1983. Edited by V. Capasso, E. Grosso and S.L. Paveri-Fontana. XVIII, 524 pages. 1985.

ctd. on inside back cover

Lecture Notes in Biomathematics

Managing Editor: S. Levin

70

Stochastic Methods in Biology

Proceedings of a Workshop held in Nagoya, Japan July 8–12 1985

Edited by M. Kimura, G. Kallianpur and T. Hida

Springer-Verlag

Editors

Motoo Kimura
National Institute of Genetics
Yata 1, 111 Mishima, Shizuoka-ken
411 Japan

Gopinath Kallianpur
Center for Stochastic Processes
Department of Statistics, University of North Carolina
Chapel Hill, NC 27514, USA

Takeyuki Hida
Department of Mathematics, Faculty of Science, Nagoya University
Chikusa-ku, Nagoya, 464 Japan

Mathematics Subject Classification (1980): 60-XX, 92-XX

ISBN-13: 978-3-540-17648-0 e-ISBN-13: 978-3-642-46599-4
DOI: 10.1007/978-3-642-46599-4

2146/3140-543210

Preface

The use of probabilistic methods in the biological sciences has been so well established by now that mathematical biology is regarded by many as a distinct discipline with its own repertoire of techniques. The purpose of the Workshop on stochastic methods in biology held at Nagoya University during the week of July 8-12, 1985, was to enable biologists and probabilists from Japan and the U.S. to discuss the latest developments in their respective fields and to exchange ideas on the applicability of the more recent developments in stochastic process theory to problems in biology.

Eighteen papers were presented at the Workshop and have been grouped under the following headings:

I. Population genetics (five papers)
II. Measure valued diffusion processes related to population genetics (three papers)
III. Neurophysiology (two papers)
IV. Fluctuation in living cells (two papers)
V. Mathematical methods related to other problems in biology, epidemiology, population dynamics, etc. (six papers)

An important feature of the Workshop and one of the reasons for organizing it has been the fact that the theory of stochastic differential equations (SDE's) has found a rich source of new problems in the fields of population genetics and neurobiology. This is especially so for the relatively new and growing area of infinite dimensional, i.e., measure-valued or distribution-valued SDE's. The papers in II and III and some of the papers in the remaining categories represent these areas. Papers [3], [4], [6] and [14] discuss other applications of stochastic processes, the last mentioned being the only one devoted to epidemiology. Included in the volume are also articles ([14]-[17]) of a general methodological character that have been motivated by diverse problems in biology and physics. Finally, the papers [1] and [2] as well as earlier work of the authors has provided the stimulus for [3],[4],[5] and others. The motivation for [12] comes from [11].

An enthusiastic and major participant in the Workshop and indeed one who helped us with his constant encouragement and advice was Professor Kiyosi Itô. Professor Itô's pioneering work in infinite dimensional SDE's has been the foundation on which most of the later work in this area is based. Although he himself did not contribute an article to these Proceedings, the pervasive influence of his ideas on the stochastic theory developed by the other participants will be evident to any reader of this volume. It is our great pleasure to dedicate this volume to Professor Itô.

We would like to express our gratitude to our colleagues, Professors A. Shimizu and H. Oodaira for assistance with the editorial work. Our thanks are also due to the officials of Nagoya University for making their facilities available for the Workshop. The meeting was held under the auspices of the joint Japan-USA program of the National Science Foundation and the Japan Society for the Promotion of Science.

November 4, 1986 M.K., G.K., T.H.

CONTENTS

I. POPULATION GENETICS

A STOCHASTIC MODEL OF COMPENSATORY NEUTRAL EVOLUTION

Motoo Kimura
National Institute of Genetics,
Mishima, 411 Japan

INTRODUCTION

The main aim of this paper is to develop population dynamics of 'compensatory neutral mutations' which are individually deleterious but restore the normal fitness in combination. I shall make use of the diffusion equation method and investigate the problem: how long does it take for such a pair of compensatory mutations to become fixed in a finite population under mutational pressure in the course of evolution.

Before I go into the main problem involving two dimensional diffusion process, I would like to discuss briefly a similar, but much simpler problem involving one dimensional diffusion, namely, I shall consider the problem: how long does it take for a mutant allele at a single locus to become fixed in a finite population under continued mutation pressure. This will serve as a preliminary to treat the more difficult problem of our main interest.

AVERAGE TIME UNTIL FIXATION UNDER MUTATION PRESSURE AT A SINGLE LOCUS

Let us consider a particular locus, and denote the normal, wild-type allele by A. We assume that A mutates irreversibly to its allele A' at the rate v per generation. In reality, the mutant allele A' is not usually a single entity (particularly at the molecular level) but a set of mutant alleles, but, we designate them collectively as A'. Let 1 + s and 1 + h be respectively the relative fitnesses of mutant homozygote (A'A') and heterozygote (A'A), taking the fitness of wild-type homozygote (AA) as unity.

We assume a random mating, diploid population of effective size N_e; roughly speaking, N_e is equal to the number of breeding individuals in one generation (For more details, see Crow and Kimura, 1970; Kimura and Ohta, 1971; Kimura, 1983).

Let p be the frequency of mutant allele $\underline{A}'$ in the population and denote by u(p, t) the probability that $\underline{A}'$ becomes fixed in the population by time t (or the t-th generation), given that its initial frequency (at time t = 0) is p. Then, u(p, t) satisfies the following Kolmogorov backward equation

$$\frac{\partial u(p,t)}{\partial t} = \frac{1}{2}V_{\delta p}\frac{\partial^2 u(p,t)}{\partial p^2} + M_{\delta p}\frac{\partial u(p,t)}{\partial p}, \tag{1}$$

where

$$M_{\delta p} = p(1-p)[sp + h(1-2p)] + v(1-p) \tag{2}$$

and

$$V_{\delta p} = p(1-p)/(2N_e). \tag{3}$$

In these expressions, $M_{\delta p}$ represents the mean change of p per generation due to mutation and natural selection, and we assume that the selection coefficients are small (i.e. $|s| \ll 1$, $|h| \ll 1$).

Let $\bar{T}(p)$ be the average time until fixation of the mutant allele, given that its initial frequency is p, so that

$$\bar{T}(p) = \int_0^\infty t\frac{\partial u(p,t)}{\partial t}dt. \tag{4}$$

Then, it can be shown (see Kimura, 1980) that $\bar{T}(p)$ satisfies the ordinary differential equation

$$\frac{1}{2}V_{\delta p}\frac{d^2\bar{T}(p)}{dp^2} + M_{\delta p}\frac{d\bar{T}(p)}{dp} + 1 = 0, \tag{5}$$

where the appropriate boundary conditions are

$$\bar{T}'(0) = \text{finite} \tag{6a}$$

and

$$\bar{T}(1) = 0. \tag{6b}$$

Note that if the population is finite in size, the mutant allele (even when it is deleterious) becomes fixed in the population under irreversible mutation. In other words,

$$u(p,\infty) = 1,$$

although the time required for such fixation may be exceedingly long if the mutant is definitely deleterious.

The solution of equation (5) with coefficients given by (2) and (3), and with boundary conditions (6a) and (6b) is

$$\bar{T}(p) = 4N_e y(p), \tag{7}$$

where

$$y(p) = \int_p^1 e^{-B(\eta)} \eta^{-V} d\eta \int_0^\eta \frac{e^{B(\xi)} \xi^{V-1}}{1 - \xi} d\xi, \tag{8}$$

in which

$$B(\xi) = (S/2)\xi^2 + H\xi(1 - \xi), \tag{9}$$

$S = 4N_e s$, $H = 4N_e h$, and $V = 4N_e v$ (Kimura, 1980). Note that $y(p)$ depends on the products $N_e s$, $N_e h$, and $N_e v$, but not on N_e, s, h, and v separately.

In what follows we shall be concerned with the fixation time for a slightly deleterious mutant. Particularly, for the purpose of comparing the single locus case with the two-locus case to be studied in the next section, we consider the semi-dominant deleterious mutation so that

$$h = -s' \quad \text{and} \quad s = -2s', \tag{10}$$

where s' ($\geqq 0$) is the selection coefficient against <u>A</u>'. For this case, $B(\xi)$ of formula (9) reduces to

$$B(\xi) = -S'\xi \tag{11}$$

where $S' = 4N_e s'$. An equivalent case has been studied by Li and Nei (1977), in which their p and s correspond to our $1 - p$ and $-s'$. We shall also restrict our consideration to the case $p = 0$. In other words, we shall investigate the average number of generations until fixation of the mutant allele, starting from a population consisting exclusively of the wild-type allele (see Fig. 1). Under these restrictions, formula (7) reduces to

$$\bar{T}(0) = 4N_e \int_0^1 e^{S'\eta} \eta^{-V} d\eta \int_0^\eta e^{-S'\xi} \xi^{V-1}(1 - \xi)^{-1} d\xi, \tag{12}$$

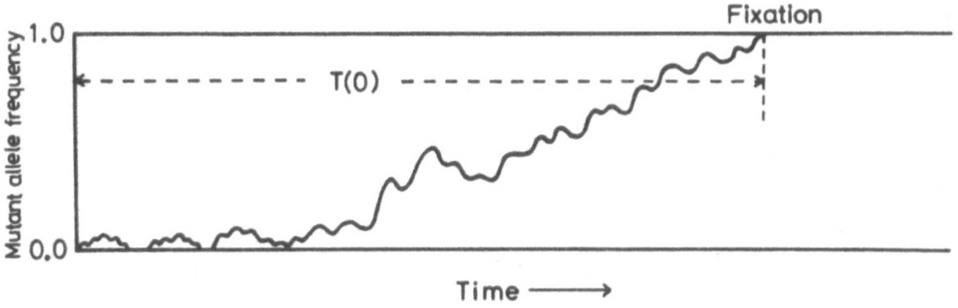

Fig. 1. A diagram illustrating the process of mutant fixation under continued irreversible mutation pressure. T(0) stands for the length of time for the mutant allele $\underline{A}'$ to become fixed in the population, starting from the state in which the population is free of $\underline{A}'$, and $\bar{T}(0)$ is the average of T(0).

where $S' = 4N_e s'$ and $V = 4N_e v$. For a selectively neutral mutant ($S' = 0$), the formula is much simplified: if $V = 4N_e v \neq 1$, we have

$$\bar{T}(0) = \frac{4N_e}{V-1}\int_0^1 \frac{1-\xi^{V-1}}{1-\xi}\,d\xi = \frac{4N_e}{V-1}\,[\gamma + \psi(V)] \qquad (13)$$

(Kimura, 1980), where $\psi(\cdot)$ stands for the digamma function and $\gamma = 0.577\cdots$. If, on the other hand, $4N_e v = 1$, we have $\bar{T}(0) = 4N_e(\pi^2/6) \approx 6.58N_e$.

An interesting special case occurs when $V = 2$ or $2N_e v = 1$. In this case we have $\bar{T}(0) = 4N_e$. In other words, it takes on the average four times the effective population size for a neutral mutant allele to become fixed under continued irreversible mutation pressure, with the rate such that one mutant gene is fed into the population in each generation if the population consists exclusively of the wild type allele (assuming that N_e is equal to the actual population size).

In Fig. 2, the average time until fixation $\bar{T}(0)$ is illustrated for various values of $4N_e s'$ ranging from 0 to 12 (abscissa) assuming $2N_e v = 1$. The solid curve in this figure represents the theoretical results obtained by numerical integration of Equation (12) for V = 2, while dots represent the corresponding results obtained by Monte Carlo simulation experiments.

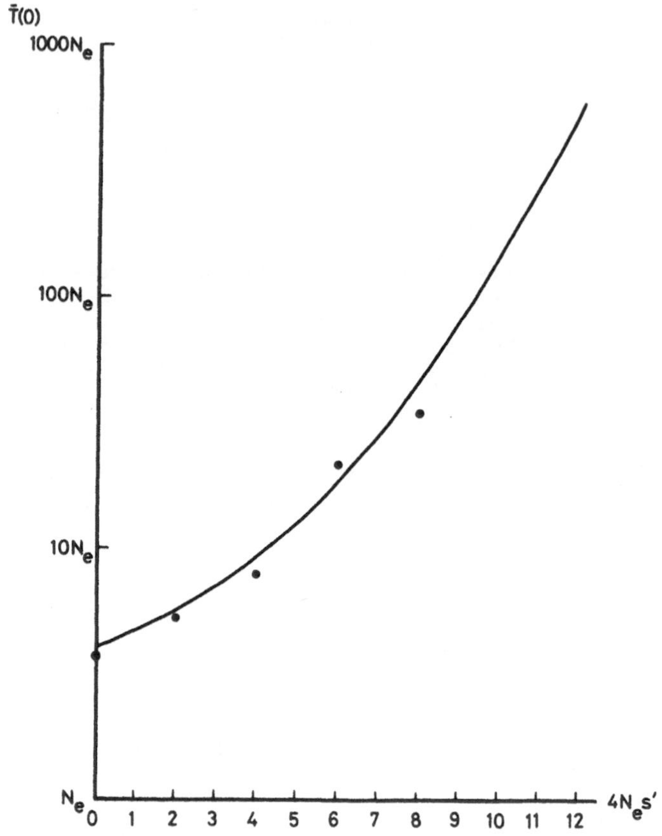

Fig. 2. Relationship between $\bar{T}(0)$ and $4N_e s'$, where $\bar{T}(0)$ is the average time until fixation of the mutant allele starting from $p = 0$, N_e is the effective population size and s' is selective disadvantage. It is assumed that $2N_e v = 1$, where v is the mutation rate for deleterious allele ($\underline{A} \rightarrow \underline{A}'$). The solid curve represents the analytical result based on the diffusion model and dots represent the results of Monte Carlo simulation experiments. For details, see text.

The experiments were performed using an improved version of PSV (pseudo-sampling variable) method: It differs from the original PSV method (Kimura, 1980) in that it incorporates a correction for low frequency classes, namely, if, at any generation, one of the alleles happens to be represented in the population less than five times, a Poisson random variable is used to sample that allele. Each dot represents the average of 50 replicate trials assuming 100 diploid breeding individuals ($N_e = 100$) and the mutation rate $v = 0.005$ so that one mutation on the average is assumed to occur in each generation ($2N_ev = 1$) when the population consists exclusively of the wild type allele. The agreement between the analytical and experimental results is satisfactory. These results show that deleterious mutations are unlikely to be incorporated into the species in the course of evolution unless $4N_es'$ is small, say, less than ten. In other words, if $4N_es'$ is larger than 10, the average time taken for fixation under mutation pressure is so enormously long that we can practically disregard such an event. For example, if $4N_es' = 13$, it takes more than a thousand times the effective population size. This means that, if $N_e = 10^5$ and if the generation span is one year, it takes more than 10^8 years for the incorporation of such a mutant, which is too long to be of practical significance in evolution.

MUTATION AT TWO LOCI WITH COMPENSATORY INTERACTION IN FITNESS

I shall now consider a more interesting case involving two loci (or sites) in which mutations are individually deleterious but becomes harmless (i.e. selectively neutral) in combination. Let A' be the mutant allele which is produced irreversibly at the rate v per generation from its wild type allele A at the first locus (or site). Likewise, let B' be the mutant allele at the second locus (or site) produced at the same rate v from its allele B. We denote by s' the selection coefficient against the single mutant (A'B or AB'), and assume that the double mutant A'B' has the same fitness as the wild type AB (Table 1). To simplify the treatment, we disregard dominance at each locus, so that we adopt the scheme of genic selection or haploid selection model. As to the effective population size, we again denote by N_e the effective size, assuming a random mating, diploid population. Since the selection model is haploid, we can just as well consider a haploid population consisting of $2N_e$ breeding individuals.

As to recombination between the two loci (or sites), I shall consider two extreme situations, namely, (i) the case of free recombination between loci, and (ii) that of complete linkage.

Table 1. Table of fitness of four gene combinations at two loci.

	$\underline{A}$	$\underline{A}'$
$\underline{B}$	1	1 - s'
$\underline{B}'$	1 - s'	1

As we shall see subsequently, these two cases give quite different results.

(i) Case of free recombination between loci

We assume independent assortment of alleles between the two loci. Let $\bar{T} = \bar{T}(p, q)$ be the average time until joint fixation of $\underline{A}'$ and $\underline{B}'$ under continued mutation pressure, given that the initial frequencies of $\underline{A}'$ and $\underline{B}'$ are p and q respectively. Then, $\bar{T}(p, q)$ satisfies the equation,

$$\frac{1}{2}V_{\delta p}\frac{\partial^2 \bar{T}}{\partial p^2} + \frac{1}{2}V_{\delta q}\frac{\partial^2 \bar{T}}{\partial q^2} + M_{\delta p}\frac{\partial \bar{T}}{\partial p} + M_{\delta q}\frac{\partial \bar{T}}{\partial q} + 1 = 0, \tag{14}$$

where

$$V_{\delta p} = p(1 - p)/(2N_e),\ V_{\delta q} = q(1 - q)/(2N_e),$$

$$M_{\delta p} = -s'p(1 - p)(1 - 2q) + v(1 - p)$$

and

$$M_{\delta q} = -s'q(1 - q)(1 - 2p) + v(1 - q).$$

The appropriate boundary conditions are

$$\bar{T}(1, q) = \bar{T}_1(q),\ \bar{T}(p, 1) = \bar{T}_1(p),$$

$$\lim_{p\to 0}\frac{\partial}{\partial p}\bar{T}(p, q) = \text{finite, and } \lim_{q\to 0}\frac{\partial}{\partial q}\bar{T}(p, q) = \text{finite},$$

where

$$\bar{T}_1(x) = 4N_e\int_x^1 e^{-S'\eta}\,\eta^{-V}\,d\eta\int_0^\eta e^{S'\xi}\,\xi^{V-1}\,(1-\xi)^{-1}d\xi. \tag{15}$$

Note that if $\underline{A}'$ is fixed in the population, mutant $\underline{B}'$ becomes more advantageous than $\underline{B}$. Similarly, if $\underline{B}'$ is fixed in the population, $\underline{A}'$

becomes more advantageous than A. I have not been able to obtain the analytical solution of the partial differential equation (14), but I applied a numerical method to obtain the values of $\bar{T}(0, 0)$ for some sets of parameter values. More specifically, I used the method of approximating a partial differential equation by a finite difference equation and then applying Gauss-Seidel iteration procedure (see, e.g., Ortega and Poole, 1981) to obtain the numerical solutions on $n \times n$ square meshes that cover the domain ($0 \leqq p \leqq 1$, $0 \leqq q \leqq 1$), where I usually assumed $n = 10$.

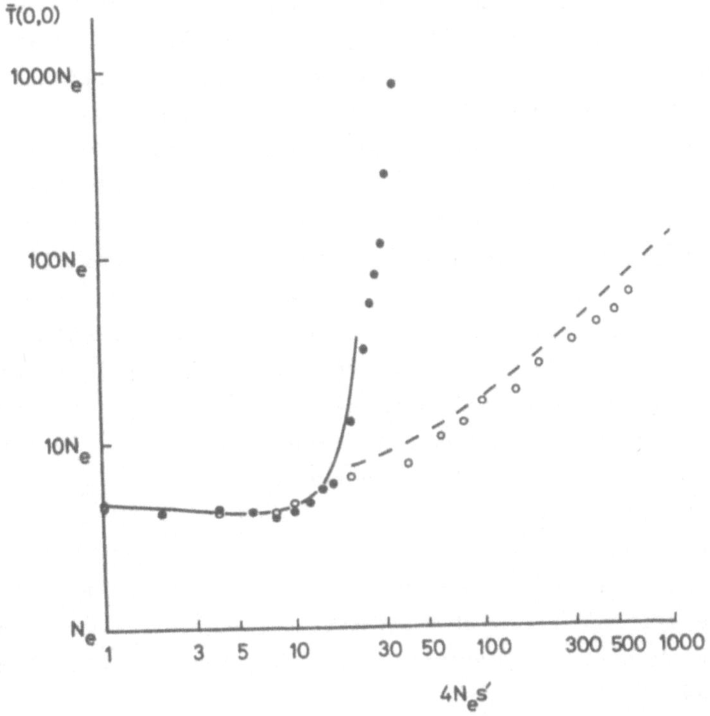

Fig. 3. Relationship between $\bar{T}(0, 0)$, the average time until joint fixation at two loci (with time expressed as multiples of N_e), and $4N_es'$ (N_e = effective population size, s' = the selection coefficient against the single mutants), assuming $2N_ev = 1$ (v = mutation rate per locus). For details, see text.

The solid curve in Fig. 3 illustrates the relationship between $\bar{T}(0, 0)$ and $4N_e s'$ thus obtained assuming $2N_e v = 1$. For $4N_e s' = 0$ (neutral mutations), it takes about $5.1N_e$ generations until joint fixation of mutants starting from $p = q = 0$, i.e., when the initial population consists exclusively of wild type alleles at both loci. I owe the following analytical demonstration which leads to the same result to Dr. G. Watterson (personal communication): If $2N_e v = 1$ (i.e. $\theta = 2$ in Watterson, 1983), the mean time for the $\underline{A}'$ allele to fix is $E(T_{A'}) = 4N_e$. Also, according to Table 5 of Watterson, 1983, $E(T_{A'}|\underline{A}'$ fixes before $\underline{B}') = 2.9N_e$. But, by symmetry between $\underline{A}'$ and $\underline{B}'$, $E(T_{A'}) = (1/2)E(T_{A'}|\underline{A}'$ fixes before $\underline{B}') + (1/2)E(T_{A'}|\underline{A}'$ fixes after $\underline{B}')$. Thus $E(T_{A'}|\underline{A}'$ fixes after $\underline{B}') = 2E(T_{A'}) - E(T_{A'}|\underline{A}'$ fixes before $\underline{B}') = 2 \times 4N_e - 2.9N_e = 5.1N_e$. For slightly deleterious mutations in the range $0 < 4N_e s' \leqq 10$, the joint fixation time is slightly shorter than this. For $4N_e s' = 10$, for example, I obtained $\bar{T}(0, 0) \approx 4.5N_e$ by numerical method. For larger values of $4N_e s'$ the fixation time quickly grows to become very large. The result that, for a region of s' with very small values, mutant alleles with more deleterious effect shorten the fixation time was rather unexpected, and error in numerical solution was suspected. However, the same result was obtained by extensive simulation experiments so this must be a valid result. Two types of Monte Carlo experiments were performed, one which made use of the improved PSV (pseudo-sampling variable) method, the other which used the standard method of faithfully sampling $2N_e$ gametes in each generation. In Fig. 3, the results obtained by using the standard type simulation method are plotted with solid dots. Each dot represents the average of 50 replicate trials, assuming $N_e = 100$ and $v = 0.005$ so that $2N_e v = 1$. From these results it appears that for compensatory mutations with enough deleterious effect so that $4N_e s' > 40$, the average time until joint fixation is so enormously long that they are unlikely to be incorporated in the species in evolution.

(ii) Case of complete linkage between loci

Since we assume no crossing-over between the two loci (or sites) in this case, we may treat four genotypes as if they were four alleles at a single locus. Furthermore we may lump $\underline{A'B}$ and $\underline{AB}'$ together because of equal fitnesses and denote their frequencies collectively as p_1 (See Table 2). Let us denote the frequency of the double mutant $\underline{A'B}'$ by p_2, and that of the wild type by p_0 $(= 1 - p_1 - p_2)$.

Table 2. Assignment of fitness and frequency parameters for 4 genotypes under complete linkage between the two loci.

Genotype	AB	A'B or AB'	A'B'
Fitness	1	1 - s'	1
Frequency	p_0	p_1	p_2

For a full treatment of the process of fixation of A'B', we must consider simultaneously the behavior of the single mutants as well as that of the double mutant. Thus, let $u = u(p_1, p_2; t)$ be the probability that the double mutant A'B' becomes fixed in the population by the t-th generation given that the initial frequencies of the single and the double mutants are p_1 and p_2 respectively. Then u satisfies the equation

$$\frac{\partial u}{\partial t} = \frac{p_2(1-p_2)}{4N_e}\frac{\partial^2 u}{\partial p_2^2} - \frac{p_1 p_2}{2N_e}\frac{\partial^2 u}{\partial p_2 \partial p_1}$$

$$+ \frac{p_1(1-p_1)}{4N_e}\frac{\partial^2 u}{\partial p_1^2} + M_{\delta p_2}\frac{\partial u}{\partial p_2} + M_{\delta p_1}\frac{\partial u}{\partial p_1}, \qquad (16)$$

where

$$M_{\delta p_2} = vp_1 + s'p_1p_2 \qquad (17a)$$

and

$$M_{\delta p_1} = 2vp_0 - s'p_1(1-p_1) - vp_1. \qquad (17b)$$

The analytical solution of equation (16) appears to be very difficult to obtain, but for the biologically interesting case in which

$$s' \gg v > 0, \qquad (18)$$

we may apply the following shortcut approximation. It is reasonable to assume that in this case single mutants, because of their selective disadvantage, remain in low frequencies throughout the process and that the quasi-equilibrium

$$M_{\delta p_1} = 0 \tag{19}$$

holds approximately. Then, if we disregard the second order term p_1^2, we have

$$2v(1 - p_1 - p_2) - s'p_1 - vp_1 = 0. \tag{20}$$

This gives

$$p_1 = \frac{2v}{s' + 3v}(1 - p_2), \tag{21}$$

and therefore we have

$$M_{\delta p_2} = (v + s'p_2)\frac{2v}{s' + 3v}(1 - p_2) \tag{22}$$

from (17a). Under the assumption of quasi-equilibrium of p_1, it is only necessary to consider the process of change of p_2. Writing p for p_2, let us denote by u(p; t) the probability that A'B' becomes fixed in the population by the t-th generation given that its frequency is p at time 0. Then, we can apply equation (1) with the mean and the variance of change per generation given by

$$M_{\delta p} = \frac{2s'v}{s' + 3v}p(1 - p) + \frac{2v^2}{s' + 3v}(1 - p) \tag{23}$$

and

$$V_{\delta p} = p(1 - p)/(2N_e). \tag{24}$$

Formally, this corresponds to the case of an advantageous mutant at a single locus with selection coefficient

$$s_1 = \frac{2s'v}{s' + 3v} \tag{25a}$$

and the mutation rate

$$v_1 = \frac{2v^2}{s' + 3v}. \tag{25b}$$

Note that these are very small quantities particularly when s' is very much larger than v. Then the average time until fixation of the double mutant A'B' starting from the population consisting exclusively of the wild type (AB) is given by (7) by putting p = 0 and assuming

$S = 8N_es_1 = 4AB/(B + 3A)$, $H = S/2$, and $V = 4N_ev_1 = 2A^2/(B + 3A)$, in which $A = 4N_ev$ and $B = 4N_es'$.

In figure 3, the average fixation time computed by this approximation method is plotted as a function of $4N_es'$ (≥ 20) with a broken line. In order to check the validity of this approximation, Monte Carlo simulation experiments were performed, and the results are plotted by open circles. Each circle is the average of 50 replicate trials assuming 250 breeding individuals ($N_e = 250$) with mutation rate $v = 0.002$ so that $2N_ev = 1$. The agreement between the approximate treatment and the results of simulation experiments is satisfactory, although there is a possibility that the approximation method slightly over-estimates the true value. Fig. 4 illustrates an example of sample paths drawn from the simulation experiments in order to explain the meaning of the quasi-equilibrium assumed.

These results, when compared with the results obtained in the previous subsection, bring to light a remarkable point that the average fixation time is very much shorter under complete linkage than with free recombination when the deleterious effect of single mutants is large such that $4N_es' > 20$. Indeed, the difference between these two cases grows very rapidly as $4N_es'$ becomes larger. For example, when $4N_es' = 30$, the mean fixation time is about $8N_e$ generations under complete linkage, whereas it is over $100N_e$ generations under free recombination (still assuming the mutation rate so that $2N_ev = 1$).

The remarkable effect of very tight linkage in reducing the fixation time of the compensatory deleterious mutants is evident from the fact that, even for $4N_es' = 400$, the average fixation time under complete linkage is about $50N_e$, which is only 10 times as long as the selectively neutral case. This means that if this model of compensatory effect in fitness is realistic, deleterious mutants such that $4N_es' = 400$ still have an ample chance to participate in evolution by random drift under continued mutation pressure.

I shall now discuss the implication of such a finding in the context of considering the mechanism of molecular evolution.

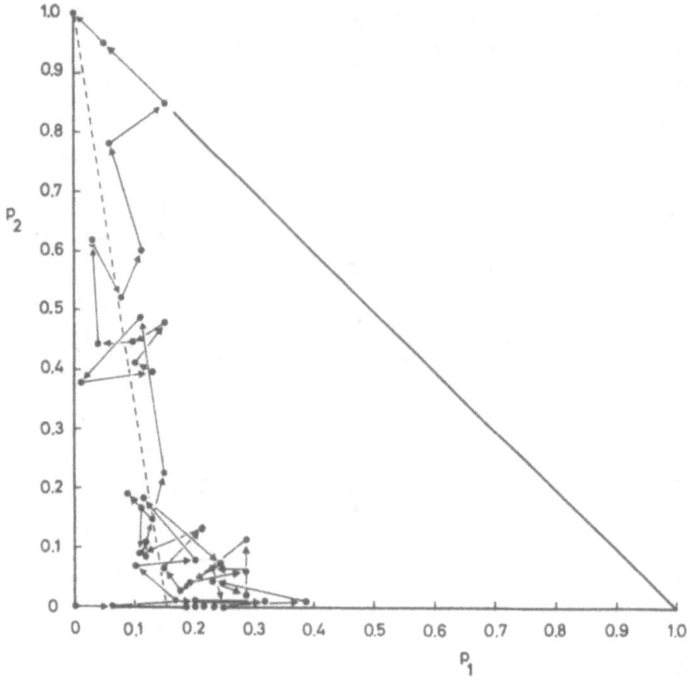

Fig. 4. An example of a sample path obtained from the Monte Carlo simulation experiments as illustrated with intervals of 5 generations. Parameter values are $N_e = 50$, $s' = 0.1$ and $v = 0.01$ so that $2N_e v = 1$ and $4N_e s' = 20$. The broken line represents the quasi-equilibrium or "moving equilibrium" computed by using Equation (21). In this figure, the abscissa (p_1) represents the frequency of single mutants (A'B or AB'), while the ordinate (p_2) represents the frequency of the double mutant (A'B').

DISCUSSION

The problem of whether evolution can proceed through an intermediate deleterious state has often been debated in the literature of evolution. Usually the issue is settled by claiming that the presumed deleterious state is misconceived, and that it is in fact advantageous or at least neutral.

The present model of "compensatory neutral evolution" is rather unusual in that a marked deleterious intermediate state can easily be overcome by mutational pressure and random drift under complete linkage. Probably the most appropriate circumstance to which this model applies is the coupled substitutions of amino acids within molecules, which Ohta (1973, 1974) referred to in relation to her hypothesis that very slightly deleterious as well as neutral mutations play an important role in molecular evolution. Wyckoff (1968), in his comparison of rat and bovine pancreatic ribonucleases, noted that "a number of changes are paired." For example, in bovine RNase, amino acid positions 57 and 79 are occupied respectively by valine and methionine, while in rat RNase, these positions are occupied by isoleucine and leucine. What is important is that these two amino acid sites are close to each other in the three-dimensionally folded structure, although they are relatively far apart in the linear sequence.

A similar example was found by Tsukihara et al. (1982) in their study of [2Fe-2S] ferredoxins isolated from various plants and algae. According to them, in Equisetum (horsetail) species, when two duplicated genes (I and II) of this protein are compared in terms of amino acid sequence, a change from threonine to arginine at position 25 correlates with change from arginine to glutamine at position 42 in the molecule. Again, these two amino acid positions are close each other in the three-dimensionally folded structure.

That such physical proximity of sites within a folded protein is the basis of fitness interaction is strongly suggested by mutation studies of Yanofsky et al. (1964) on tryptophan synthetase A protein. For example, position 210 in the wild type protein is occupied by glycine, but, if this is replaced by glutamic acid by mutation, the enzyme becomes nonfunctional. However, if a further change occurs at position 174, changing tyrosine of the wild type to cysteine, the activity of the enzyme is recovered, although a mutation (Tyr → Cys) at the second position alone causes loss of function. By extensive reversion studies of this sort, these authors came to the conclusion that the interacting amino acid sites (as in positions 210 and 174) are close to each other in the folded protein.

Now, we can envisage two sites A and B assumed in our model in the previous section as representing two amino acid sites within a protein (see Fig. 5). These two codon positions, being in the same cistron, must be very tightly linked, approximating the complete linkage model studied in the previous section. I conclude that compensatory neutral mutations may play an important role in molecular evolution.

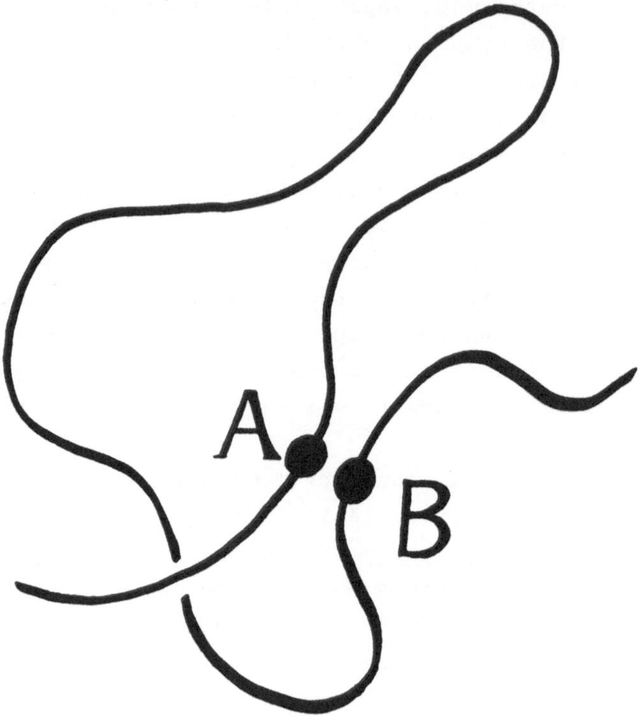

Fig. 5. A diagram illustrating two interacting amino acid sites (A and B) within a folded protein whose evolutionary pattern may conform to the model of "compensatory neutral evolution."

SUMMARY

Using the diffusion equation method, I investigate the average time until fixation of a mutant gene or genes in a finite population under continued (irreversible) mutation pressure. I mainly consider the situation in which the initial population consists exclusively of the wild type allele (or alleles). I denote by v the mutation rate per locus per generation.

The treatment for the single locus case (with a pair of alleles A and A') is straightforward. It is shown that for a slightly deleterious mutant the average time taken for fixation is too long to be of practical significance in evolution unless $4N_e s' < 10$, where

N_e is the effective population size and s' is the selection coefficient against the mutant allele (A').

The main aim of this paper is to investigate the two locus case. I assume a pair of alleles A and A' at the first locus, and B and B' at the second locus, and investigate the situation in which mutations are individually deleterious but become harmless (i.e., selectively neutral) in combination. Such mutations may be termed 'compensatory neutral mutations.' I assign relative fitnesses 1, 1 - s', 1 - s' and 1 respectively to AB, A'B, AB' and A'B'. Two extreme cases, i.e., (i) free recombination, and, (ii) complete linkage between the loci are considered. Assuming $2N_ev = 1$, where v is the mutation rate per locus, the following results are obtained. (i) In the case of free recombination, the average time until fixation ($\bar{T}$) is about $5N_e$ generations for neutral mutations (s' = 0). For slightly deleterious mutations in the range $0 < 4N_es' \leqq 10$, $\bar{T}$ is slightly shorter but not very much (e.g. $\bar{T} = 4.5N_e$ for $4N_es' = 10$). If $4N_es'$ is much larger, the fixation time quickly becomes very large, and for mutations with $4N_es' > 40$, $\bar{T}$ becomes so enormously large that such mutations are unlikely to play a part in evolution. (ii) In the case of complete linkage, single mutations with much larger deleterious effects are allowed to participate in "compensatory neutral evolution," namely, joint fixation of the selectively neutral double mutant (A'B') occurs without having to wait an unrealistically long time. In fact, even for $4N_es' = 400$, the average fixation time is only 10 times as long as the completely neutral case. The bearing of this finding on molecular evolution is discussed with special reference to coupled substitutions at interacting amino acid (or nucleotide) sites within a folded protein (or RNA) molecule. It is concluded that compensatory neutral mutations may play an important role in molecular evolution.

REFERENCES

Crow, J. F. and Kimura, M. (1970) An Introduction to Population Genetics Theory. Harper and Row, New York.

Kimura, M. (1980) Average time until fixation of a mutant allele in a finite population under continued mutation pressure: Studies by analytical, numerical and pseudo-sampling methods. Proc. Natl. Acad. Sci. USA 77: 522-526.

Kimura, M. (1983) The Neutral Theory of Molecular Evolution. Cambridge University Press, Cambridge.

Kimura, M. and Ohta, T. (1971) Theoretical Aspects of Population Genetics. Princeton University Press, Princeton.

Li, W.-H. and Nei, M. (1977) Persistence of common alleles in two related populations or species. Genetics 86: 901-914.

Ohta, T. (1973) Slightly deleterious mutant substitutions in evolution. Nature, Lond. 246: 96-98.

Ohta, T. (1974) Mutational pressure as the main cause of molecular evolution and polymorphism. Nature, Lond. 252: 351-354.

Ortega, J. M. and Poole, Jr., W. G. (1981) An Introduction to Numerical Methods for Differential Equations. Pitman Pub., Marshfield, Mass.

Tsukihara, T., Kobayashi, M., Nakamura, M., Katsube, Y., Fukuyama, K., Hase, T., Wada, K., Matsubara, H. (1982) Structure-function relationship of [2Fe-2S] Ferredoxins and design of a model molecule. BioSystems 15: 243-257.

Watterson, G. A. (1983) On the time for gene silencing at duplicate loci. Genetics 105: 745-766.

Wyckoff, H. W. (1968) Discussion. Brookhaven Symp. Biol. 21: 252-257.

Yanofsky, C., Horn, V. and Thorpe, D. (1964) Protein structure relationships revealed by mutational analysis. Science 146: 1593-1594.

SOME MODELS FOR TREATING EVOLUTION OF MULTIGENE FAMILIES AND OTHER REPETITIVE DNA SEQUENCES

Tomoko Ohta
National Institute of Genetics
Mishima, 411 Japan

INTRODUCTION

During the last several years, molecular biology has undergone a second round of remarkable development. This has brought a number of new findings regarding the genetic organization of higher organisms, as distinct from that of lower organisms. One such discovery is the prevalence of multigene families and other repetitive sequences. For about ten years, I have been studying the evolution of multigene families from the standpoint of population genetics. Recently, I extended the analyses to treat repetitive DNA sequences that are dispersed in genomes. Repetitive sequences are characterized by concerted evolution, i.e., gene copies belonging to a family of repeating elements do not evolve independently, but evolve as a set through various molecular interaction mechanisms such as unequal crossing-over, gene conversion and duplicative transposition. By incorporating such interaction mechanisms, the population genetics model of an evolving multigene family becomes very complicated. In this paper, I shall review models and analyses on repetitive gene families.

MODEL OF GENE CONVERSION FOR MULTIGENE FAMILIES

The analyses use the identity coefficient that is defined as the probability of identity of genes or DNA segments belonging to the multigene family. In the following, I shall review a most simple model of intrachromosomal gene conversion.

Let us assume a random mating population of effective size, N. Each genome of the population contains a multigene family of n tandemly arranged copies. In one generation, the family undergoes gene conversion, interchromosomal recombination at meiosis, mutation and random sampling of gametes at reproduction. Let λ_c be the rate at which a gene is converted by the remaining (n - 1) genes on the same chromosome (intrachromosomal conversion) in one generation (Ohta 1982). Let v be the mutation rate per unit whose identity is compared per generation under the infinite allele model (Kimura and Crow 1964). Recombination at meiosis is assumed always to be equal, and let β be the rate per generation between adjacent units. All evolutionary forces are assumed to be weak, i.e., v, λ_c, β and 1/N << 1.

It is possible to formulate the process of concerted evolution by using three identity coefficients; f is the probability of identity of two randomly chosen allelic genes, C_1 is the identity coefficient of genes at different loci on one chromosome, and C_2 is that of genes at different loci of two chromosomes randomly chosen from the population. Then it can be shown that the change of the three identity coefficients in one generation (from (t - 1)-th to t-th generation), is expressed by the following transition equations (Ohta 1982, 1983a, b; Nagylaki 1984).

$$C_t = \underset{\sim}{A} C_{t-1} + \underset{\sim}{b} \tag{1}$$

where

$$\underset{\sim}{A} = (1-2v)\begin{bmatrix} 1-\frac{1}{2N}-(n-1)\alpha_c & 0 & (n-1)\alpha_c \\ 0 & 1-\alpha_c-\frac{(n+1)}{3}\beta & \frac{(n+1)}{3}\beta \\ \alpha_c & \frac{1}{2N} & 1-\alpha_c-\frac{1}{2N} \end{bmatrix} \tag{2}$$

and

$$\underset{\sim}{b} = \left(\frac{1}{2N}, \alpha_c, 0\right), \tag{3}$$

with

$$\alpha_c = 2\lambda_c/(n-1).$$

By using the above transition equation, it is possible to predict the identity of gene copies of the multigene family under various sets of parameter values. Also interesting is the measure of the diversity of gene copies. It can be simply defined as one minus the identity coefficient. Let us call this the diversity coefficient.

The above theory can also be used to predict approximately the time for spreading of a single gene copy into the multigene families forming the total population. Let ξ_{max} be the maximum eigenvalue of the matrix $\underset{\sim}{A}$ when mutation is excluded ($v = 0$). Then the approximate time until fixation of a single copy becomes (Ohta 1983b, Nagylaki 1984),

$$T = \frac{2}{1 - \xi_{max}} . \tag{4}$$

Table 1 gives several interesting numerical examples of diversity coefficients at equilibrium and time until fixation of a single copy. The mutation rate, v, is chosen as 10^{-8}, a value close to the maximum rate of nucleotide or amino acid substitution per year (Kimura 1983). When the conversion rate, λ_c, is extremely large compared to the other parameters, the gene copies of the multigene family are expected to be uniform. See cases (1) - (3) of Table 1. This is particularly so when linkage is tight, i.e., the meiotic recombination rate (β) is low. In such cases, the allelic diversity ($1 - f$) is almost equal to the nonallelic ($1 - C_2$), but the coefficient within the chromosome ($1 - C_1$) is lower than the other two. By lowering the conversion rate, the diversity coefficients increase, and allelic and nonallelic coefficients become very different. Here the nonallelic ones become more equal whether they are measured within or between chromosomes. Cases (4) - (6) show such a result. Diversity coefficients also depend on the copy number, n, increasing for larger values of n. The time until fixation is longer for a gene family with more diverse members (see Tab. 1). This is because, during such a long course of spreading, the gene copy will accumulate many mutations.

The case of no interchromosomal recombination ($\beta = 0$), has been mathematically studied by Shimizu (this volume). He has shown that the stationary distribution of the diffusion process with respect to the chromosomal types becomes the same as in the infinite allele mutation and random drift model of Kimura and Crow (1964), by replacing their parameter, 4Nv, with v/λ. As a related problem, I would like to mention that my extensive Monte Carlo experiments have shown

Table 1 Diversity coefficients at equilibrium and time until fixation of a single gene copy.

λ_c	$(n-1)\beta$	n	1-f	$1-C_1$	$1-C_2$	T in units of 10^5 gns.
0.01	0.01	100	.0061	.0058	.0061	6.19
0.01	0.001	100	.0012	.0008	.0012	1.12
0.001	0.001	100	.0068	.0066	.0069	6.92
0.0001	0.001	100	.0266	.0318	.0320	32.95
0.00001	0.001	100	.0336	.1168	.1168	131.94
0.000001	0.001	100	.0198	.5062	.5062	1024.36
0.00001	0.001	50	.0179	.0616	.0616	65.41
0.00001	0.001	200	.0602	.2090	.2090	265.00

Other parameters: $N = 10^4$, $v = 10^{-8}$.

that the Ewens' sampling theory (Ewens 1972) successfully predicts the actual number of different alleles contained in a single multigene family (Ohta 1986a).

MODEL OF DUPLICATIVE TRANSPOSITION

The changes of identity coefficients by duplicative transposition can be similarly calculated as those by gene conversion. By duplicative transposition, a unit moves to a new and different chromosomal site. Since we are mainly concerned with higher organisms, I shall present here the case where different chromosomal sites freely recombine at meiosis.

In addition to identity coefficients, one needs the probability of identity of chromosomal sites. Let us define allelism, F, as the probability that a random copy of a genome finds a homologous copy at the same chromosomal site of another genome of the population. Let λ_t be the rate at which a unit duplicatively transposes in one generation. For simplicity, let us assume that duplicative transposition is always accompanied by deletion of another unit belonging to the same genome. Therefore, the copy number, n, per genome remains unchanged. Random drift and mutation are assumed to be the same as before.

Under free recombination, the two identity coefficients, C_1 and C_2 become the same, and we denote them by C. Then the transitional equations of allelism (F) and two identity coefficients (f and C) become as follows (Ohta 1985, 1986b).

$$F_{t+1} = (1 - 2\lambda_t)F_t + \frac{1}{2N}(1 - F_t) \qquad (5)$$

$$f_{t+1} = (1 - 2v)f_t + \frac{1}{2NF_t}(1 - f_t) \qquad (6)$$

and

$$C_{t+1} = (1 - 2v)C_t + \alpha_t F_t'(f_t - C_t) + \frac{\alpha_t}{4N}(1 - C_t), \qquad (7)$$

where $\alpha_t = 2\lambda_t/(n - 1)$ and $F_t' = (n - F_t)nF_t/\{n(n - F_t) + 2n\lambda_t F_t\}$. At equilibrium, when $2N\lambda_t >> 1$, F is close to zero, so we often expect that f is close to unity. In such cases, we have,

$$\hat{F} = \frac{1}{1 + 4N\lambda_t} \qquad (8)$$

$$\hat{f} = \frac{1}{1 + 4N\hat{F}v} \qquad (9)$$

and

$$\hat{C} \approx \frac{1}{1 + 4Nv/\{\alpha_t(1 + 4N\hat{F})\}}, \qquad (10)$$

where a hat over F, f and C denotes equilibrium values. The above formula (10) suggests that C is often very small, as $\hat{C}$ is roughly $1/(1 + 4Nnv)$ when $2N\lambda_t \gg 1$, as noted by Slatkin (1985) and Brookfield (1986).

DISCUSSION

The models reviewed here are the simplest ones so far studied. Let us examine some extensions of these models. The process of unequal crossing-over is more difficult to formulate, but an approximate analysis is given in Ohta (1980). The difficulty arises because, through the shift of chromosomal positions by unequal crossing-over, the identity of units between the two chromosomes becomes ambiguous.

As to the model of gene conversion, Nagylaki and Barton (1986) have performed a more exact analysis incorporating the effect of interchromosomal recombination as function of chromosomal distance. Nagylaki (1984b) also studied the case where conversion occurs between the units belonging to two chromosomes. I have formulated a model in which both gene conversion and duplicative transposition occur, and in addition, some fraction of these interactions take place between the units belonging to two genomes, i.e., the mixed model (Ohta 1985). I have also extended the analysis to include subdivided structure and correlation between identity and chromosomal distance, in order to apply the theory to the immunoglobulin gene family (Ohta 1984).

From the mathematical standpoint, Shimizu (1985) has analysed the case of no interchromosomal recombination by regarding the concerted evolution as a measure-valued diffusion process. Kaplan and Hudson (1986) have formulated the conversion model in terms of the infinite site model.

All these analyses treat equilibrium state in the sense of constant copy number per genome. However, from the biological point of view, non-equilibrium theory is more interesting. For multigene families with functionally diverse gene copies such as those of immunoglobulin, the origin of gene families has the most significant meaning for the evolution of complexity of higher organisms. I have just started to study the case where gene copy number is increasing by incorporating natural selection (Ohta 1986c). The model can not be analytically solved and I have resorted to extensive Monte Carlo studies. Also necessary are the analyses on an expanding family of transposons. The rate of duplicative transposition is considered to be fairly high, and expansion of some families of transposons seems to be quite rapid in evolution. I have studied one such model, and shown that the rate of approach to equilibrium of identity coefficient of genes at different chromosomal sites is extremely low when the copy number gets large (Ohta 1986b). In any case, more general and exact formulation of the non-equilibrium models awaits future investigation.

SUMMARY

The evolution of multigene families and other repetitive DNA sequences is characterized by concerted evolution. Two very simple models of concerted evolution are reviewed. In the first, intrachromosomal unbiased gene conversion is treated, and in the second, duplicative transposition is studied under the assumption of free recombination between any two different chromosomal sites. Various extensions of these models are discussed.

I thank Dr. Kenichi Aoki for his useful suggestions to improve the presentation.

REFERENCES

Brookfield, J. F. Y. (1986) A model for DNA sequence evolution within transposable element family. Genetics 112: 393-407.

Ewens, W. (1972) The sampling theory of selectively neutral alleles. Theor. Pop. Biol. 3: 87-112.

Kaplan, N. M. and Hudson, R. R. (1986) On the divergence of genes in multigene families. Theor. Pop. Biol. (in press).

Kimura, M. (1983) The Neutral Theory of Molecular Evolution. Cambridge Univ. Press, Cambridge.

Kimura, M. and Crow, J. F. (1964) The number of alleles that can be maintained in a finite population. Genetics 49: 725-738.

Nagylaki, T. (1984a) The evolution of multigene families under intrachromosomal gene conversion. Genetics 106: 529-548.

Nagylaki, T. (1984b) Evolution of multigene families under inter-chromosomal gene conversion. Proc. Natl. Acad. Sci. USA 81: 3796-3800.

Nagylaki, T. and Barton, N. (1986) Intrachromosomal gene conversion, linkage, and the evolution of multigene families. Theor. Pop. Biol. Theor. Pop. Biol. 29: 407-437.

Ohta, T. (1980) Evolution and Variation of Multigene Families. Lecture Notes in Biomathematics, Vol. 37, Springer-Verlag, Berlin, New York.

Ohta, T. (1982) Allelic and non-allelic homology of a supergene family. Proc. Natl. Acad. Sci. USA 79: 3251-3254.

Ohta, T. (1983a) On the evolution of multigene families. Theor. Pop. Biol. 23: 216-240.

Ohta, T. (1983b) Time until fixation of a mutant belonging to a multigene family. Genet. Res., Camb. 41: 47-55.

Ohta, T. (1984) Population genetics theory of concerted evolution and its application to the immunoglobulin V gene tree. J. Mol. Evol. 20: 274-280.

Ohta, T. (1985) A model of duplicative transposition and gene conversion for repetitive DNA families. Genetics 110: 513-524.

Ohta, T. (1986a) Actual number of alleles contained in a multigene family. Genet. Res. (in press).

Ohta, T. (1986b) Population genetics of an expanding family of mobile genetic elements. Genetics 113: 145-159.

Ohta, T. (1986c) A model of evolution for accumulating genetic information. J. Theor. Biol. (in press).

A GENEALOGICAL DESCRIPTION OF THE INFINITELY-MANY NEUTRAL ALLELES MODEL

P. J. Donnelly
Department of Statistical Science
University College London
London WC1E 6BT
ENGLAND

S. Tavaré
Department of Mathematics
University of Utah
Salt Lake City, UT 84112
U.S.A.

1. INTRODUCTION

Kingman [8], [9] introduced the coalescent as a means of describing the genealogy of samples taken from a large evolving haploid population. The coalescent partitions a sample of genes into equivalence classes with respect to an ancestral population some time t into the past; genes in the same equivalence class in the sample have the same ancestors. As t increases the equivalence classes coalesce until, sufficiently far in the past, all individuals in the sample are equivalent, being descended from a common ancestor.

Watterson [11] showed that the effects of mutation in the genealogy could be allowed for explicity by constructing a process with two different types of equivalence classes. Specifically, consider a sample of n genes chosen at reference time 0. Genes i and j are in the same "old" equivalence class at time $-t$ if i and j share a common ancestor at time $-t$, and no mutation has occurred in the line of descent from that ancestor to i and j between time 0 and time $-t$. On the other hand, i and j might be descended from a common ancestor at time $-s$ $(> -t)$, that ancestor being a new mutant. If no further mutation occurs in the line of descent to i and j, then we say that i and j are in the same "new" equivalence class. Each new equivalence class contains genes of identical type, and with the infinitely-many alleles assumption that each mutation leads to a novel allelic type, distinct new equivalence classes have distinct types.

Donnelly and Tavare [3] observed that keeping track of the new equivalence classes in order of their appearance leads to a direct way of studying questions involving the ages of alleles and the age ordering in samples.

In this paper, we will focus on an age-ordered genealogical description of the infinitely-many neutral alleles diffusion model from which the samples were taken. After a brief review of the stochastic structure of the age-ordered sample coalescent, we construct a Markov process which keeps track of the allele frequencies in the (infinite) population and the order of their occurrence by mutation. In the final section, we use this population frequency process to give a unified treatment of several aspects of neutral mutation theory.

2. A COALESCENT WITH AGES

We will need later the basic properties of the sample coalescent with ages. The necessary results are taken, with minor changes of notation, from [3]. This process is a continuous-time Markov chain $\{A_t, t \geq 0\}$ in which a typical state can be represented as a collection $(\xi_1, \ldots, \xi_k; \eta_1, \ldots, \eta_\ell)$ of equivalence classes in which $\xi_1, \ldots, \xi_k$ denote old classes, and $\eta_1, \ldots, \eta_\ell$ represent new classes, those genes in class η_r having arisen by mutation after (that is, further into the past!) those in class η_s if $r < s$. Let $\mathcal{E}_n^*$ be the collection of such ordered equivalence relations. Initially, each individual is in his own old equivalence class, and there are no new classes. For sufficiently large t, all individuals in the sample are in new classes, since the sample must comprise only mutants with respect to sufficiently remote generations.

One of the attractive features of these coalescents is that the process changes state through one of only two possible mechanisms: either two old equivalence classes coalesce to form a single (old) class, or an old class becomes the oldest of the new classes. In each case, the number of old classes decreases by exactly one, and the times between such changes depend only on the number of old classes then present, and not on the detailed structure of the current configuration.

Let $\{D_t, t \geq 0; D_0 = n\}$ be a pure death process on $\{n, n-1, \ldots, 0\}$ with death rate $k(k+\theta-1)/2$ from state k, where $\theta > 0$ is the scaled mutation parameter. Let $\{\mathcal{A}_k, k = n, \ldots, 0\}$ be a discrete-time Markov chain on $\mathcal{E}_n^*$, independent of the death process. $\mathcal{A}_k$ is an element of $\mathcal{E}_n^*$ having k old equivalence classes, and the transition probabilities are given by

$$P(\mathcal{A}_{k-1}=(\xi_1,\dots,\xi_{i-1},\xi_i,\dots,\xi_k;\xi_i,\eta_1,\dots,\eta_\ell)\mid \mathcal{A}_k=(\xi_1,\dots,\xi_k;\eta_1,\dots,\eta_\ell)) = \theta/k(k+\theta-1). \tag{2.1a}$$

$$P(\mathcal{A}_{k-1}=(\xi_1,\dots,\xi_i\cup\xi_j,\dots,\xi_k;\eta_1,\dots,\eta_\ell)\mid \mathcal{A}_k=(\xi_1,\dots,\xi_k;\eta_1,\dots,\eta_\ell)) = 2/k(k+\theta-1), \tag{2.1b}$$

for $k = 1,\dots,n;\ 1 \leq i < j \leq k$. Here $\xi_i \cup \xi_j$ denotes the union of the two old equivalence classes ξ_i and ξ_j. The marginal distribution of $_k$ is obtained from [3], equation (3.2):

$$P(\mathcal{A}_k=(\xi_1,\dots,\xi_k;\eta_1,\dots,\eta_\ell)) = \frac{\Gamma(k+\theta)(n-k)!k!\theta^\ell\lambda_1!\lambda_2!\dots\lambda_k!\mu_1!\dots\mu_\ell!}{n!\Gamma(n+\theta)(\mu_1+\dots+\mu_\ell)(\mu_2+\dots+\mu_\ell)\dots(\mu_{\ell-1}+\mu_\ell)\mu_\ell}, \tag{2.2}$$

where λ_i is the number of genes in ξ_i and μ_i is the number of genes in η_i. Finally, we have

$$A_t = \mathcal{A}_{D_t}, \quad t \geq 0. \tag{2.3}$$

The results (2.2) and (2.3) provide a detailed description of age-ordered samples from the infinitely-many neutral alleles model. A number of further applications are given in [3]. We turn now to the corresponding population structure.

3. THE POPULATION FREQUENCY PROCESS

If we are not particularly interested in which genes in our sample belong to which equivalence classes, but rather in the numbers of genes in those classes, we obtain another Markov process $\{M_t, t\geq 0\}$ whose structure follows immediately from (2.1)-(2.3). Its jump chain, $\mathcal{M}_k$, consists of collections of integers of the form $(\lambda_1,\dots,\lambda_k;\mu_1,\dots,\mu_\ell)$ giving the numbers of individuals in each of the equivalence classes of $\mathcal{A}_k$, and

$$P(\mathcal{M}_k=(\lambda_1,\dots,\lambda_k;\mu_1,\dots,\mu_\ell)) = \frac{\Gamma(k+\theta)(n-k)!k!\theta^\ell}{\Gamma(n+\theta)\alpha_1!\alpha_2!\dots\alpha_n!\mu_\ell(\mu_\ell+\mu_{\ell-1})\dots(\mu_\ell+\dots+\mu_1)} \tag{3.1}$$

where $\alpha_i = \#\{j:\lambda_j=i\}$. See [11] equation (3.3.1) for the corresponding result where age ordering is ignored.

In order to describe the population structure that corresponds, as it were, to samples of size $n = \infty$, we will need the following notation. Let $\mathbb{N}_0 = \{0,1,\ldots,\infty\}$, let Δ be the collection of sequences $\{x_1, x_2, \ldots\}$ satisfying

$$x_i \geq 0, \ \sum_{i=1}^{\infty} x_i \leq 1,$$

and Δ^1 the subset of Δ comprising those sequences with sum 1. Let $S = \mathbb{N}_0 \times \Delta$. Fix $k \geq 1$, and let V_k be a random variable having the beta density f_k given by

$$f_k(x) = \frac{\Gamma(k+\theta)x^{k-1}(1-x)^{\theta-1}}{\Gamma(\theta)(k-1)!}, \ x \in (0,1).$$

Let $(U_1,\ldots,U_k)$ be a random k-vector having a uniform distribution on the simplex $\{(u_1,\ldots,u_k); u_i \geq 0, \ u_1+u_2+\ldots+u_k = 1\}$ (i.e. density proportional to Lebesgue measure on the simplex), and let Z_1, $Z_2, \ldots$ be independent identically distributed random variables with density f given by

$$f(x) = \theta(1-x)^{\theta-1}, \ x \in (0,1), \tag{3.2}$$

and take $\{U_i\}$, V_k and $\{Z_j\}$ mutually independent. Finally, define the random vector $\underset{\sim}{F}^{(k)}$ by

$$\begin{aligned} \underset{\sim}{F}^{(k)} = \ & (V_k U_1, V_k U_2, \ldots, V_k U_k, (1-V_k)Z_1, \\ & (1-V_k)(1-Z_1)Z_2, (1-V_k)(1-Z_1)(1-Z_2)Z_3, \ldots) . \end{aligned} \tag{3.3}$$

When $k = 0$, put

$$\underset{\sim}{F}^{(0)} = (Z_1, (1-Z_1)Z_2, (1-Z_1)(1-Z_2)Z_3, \ldots). \tag{3.4}$$

Remark: These definitions are for fixed but arbitrary k. The $\{Z_i\}$ and $\{U_j\}$ that appear in (3.2) and (3.3) should perhaps be written $\{Z_i^{(k)}\}$, $\{U_j^{(k)}\}$ to emphasise that they vary with k. We are only interested in distributional properties, and so will continue to suppress the dependence on k.

One can view $\underset{\sim}{F}^{(k)}$ as a random point in Δ^1; we will use it to construct a sequence $\{\nu_k, k = 0,1, \ldots\}$ of probability measures on S as follows. ν_k concentrates on $\{k\} \times \Delta^1$, and for any Borel subset A of Δ

$$\nu_k(\{k\} \times A) = P(\underset{\sim}{F}^{(k)} \in A), \; k = 0,1, \ldots \tag{3.5}$$

Our key result, which has close affinities with the work of Griffiths [6] is the following theorem.

Theorem:

(i) There is a discrete time Markov chain $\{\mathfrak{M}_k, k = 0,1,\ldots\}$ on S such that $\mathfrak{M}_k$ has distribution ν_k, and

$$P(\mathfrak{M}_{k-1} = (k-1; x_1, \ldots, x_{i-1}, x_{i+1}, \ldots, x_k, x_i, y_1, y_2, \ldots)$$
$$| \mathfrak{M}_k = (k; x_1, \ldots, x_k, y_1, y_2, \ldots,)) = \frac{\theta}{k(k+\theta-1)},$$

$$P(\mathfrak{M}_{k-1} = (k-1; x_1, \ldots, x_i + x_j, \ldots x_k, y_1, y_2, \ldots)$$
$$| \mathfrak{M}_k = (k; x_1, \ldots, x_k, y_1, y_2, \ldots)) = \frac{2}{k(k+\theta-1)},$$

for $k = 1,2,\ldots$; $1 \leq i < j \leq k$.

(ii) Let $\{D_t\}$ be a pure death process with death rate $k(k+\theta-1)/2$ from state k, starting at infinity, and independent of $\{\mathfrak{M}_k\}$. Then the process $\{M_t, t \geq 0\}$ defined by

$$M_0 = (\infty; 0,0,\ldots), M_t = \mathfrak{M}_{D_t}, \; t > 0$$

is a Markov process on S.

Proof. (i) We need to check the consistency of the finite dimensional distributions of $\{\mathfrak{M}_k\}$. This follows after some lengthy but straightforward calculations using the structure (3.3) of the ν_k's . To establish (ii), we can use an argument similar to that of [9], p. 244.

The process $\{M_t, t \geq 0\}$ may be thought of as a genealogical representation of the infinitely-many neutral alleles diffusion model;

cf. Ethier and Kurtz [4]. Our explicit recognition of the age-ordering of novel alleles leads to a variety of interesting results which we will exploit in the final expository section.

4. APPLICATIONS

(a) Limit distributions

As $t \to \infty$, $D_t \to 0$ a.s., and so $M_t \Rightarrow \nu_0$, defined by (3.4) and (3.5). Eventually, then, the population comprises only new lines of descent, and it follows that at stationarity the frequencies of the oldest, next oldest ,..., alleles in the infinitely-many neutral alleles diffusion model have the representation Z_1, $(1-Z_1)Z_2$, $(1-Z_1)(1-Z_2)Z_3, \ldots$ where the Z_i's are independent and identically distributed r.v.'s with density (3.2). The decreasing order statistics of such a random vector have the Poisson-Dirichlet distribution with parameter θ (cf. [7] and [10]), which distribution is well-known to be the stationary measure of the infinitely-many neutral alleles diffusion model (cf. [4]). The Poisson-Dirichlet distribution is an intractable object to handle explicitly; as well as giving the age ordering of the population frequencies, our approach mitigates some of these difficulties. Donnelly [2] gives a number of interconnections between the distribution ν_0, and the properties of samples taken from such a distribution, exploiting more fully the consequences of size-biased sampling.

(b) K-allele models

Many of the fundamental results about the infinitely-many neutral alleles process were discovered by taking suitable limits in a K-allele model with symmetric mutation, as $K \to \infty$. Here we observe that the fundamental structure of K-allele models with scaled mutation rates $\varepsilon_{ij} \equiv \varepsilon_j$ from alleles of type i to type j (cf. Griffiths [5]) can be recovered from the frequency process $\{M_t, t > 0\}$. The idea is to construct the K allele model from a realisation of $\{M_t, t>0\}$, as in [1]. Lines of descent are initiated by mutations, but now the (age-ordered) classes do not have distinct allelic types. Define $\theta = \varepsilon_1 + \ldots + \varepsilon_K$, and $p_j = \varepsilon_j/\theta$, $j = 1,2,\ldots,K$. Fix $t > 0$, and suppose that the number of old classes, D_t, of M_t is equal to $k > 0$. The relative frequencies of the new classes, normalised to have sum 1, have distribution ν_0 (cf. (3.3) and

(3.4)). Allelic labels $1,2,\ldots,K$ are given to each class frequency by labelling each independently, assigning label j with probability p_j, $j = 1,\ldots,K$. Recall from [7] and [10] that the points Z_1, $(1-Z_1)Z_2,\ldots$ in (3.4) are an enumeration of the points of a non-homogeneous Poisson process with mean measure density $\theta e^{-x}/x$, normalised to have sum 1. It follows that the collections of points $\mathcal{P}_j$, say, of frequencies which are labelled j may be viewed as the (normalised) points of K independent non-homogeneous Poisson processes with mean measure density $p_j \theta e^{-x}/x = \varepsilon_j e^{-x}/x$, $j = 1,\ldots,K$. It can be shown that the total frequencies of new classes labelled j have jointly a K-dimensional Dirichlet distribution, with parameters $\varepsilon_1,\ldots,\varepsilon_K$. Thus when $D_t = k$, the frequencies $X_1,\ldots,X_k$ of old classes, and the frequencies $Y_1,Y_2,\ldots,Y_K$ of alleles of types $1,\ldots,K$ that arose by mutations in $(0,t)$ have the structure

$$
\begin{aligned}
(X_1,\ldots,X_k,\ Y_1,\ldots,Y_K) &\overset{d}{=} \\
&(U_1V_k,\ldots,U_kV_k,(1-V_k)D_1,\ldots,(1-V_k)D_K),
\end{aligned}
\tag{4.1}
$$

where $(D_1,\ldots,D_K)$ have the Dirichlet distribution with parameters $\varepsilon_1,\ldots,\varepsilon_K$, independent of $(U_1,\ldots,U_k)$, and V_k (cf. (3.1)). The structure exhibited by (4.1) was found by different means by Griffiths [5] and it leads immediately to an explicit representation for the transition density of the K-allele diffusion process.

(c) A Population Coalescent

The process $\{M_t,\ t > 0\}$ is closely related to an age-ordered coalescent via a modification of Kingman's paint box scheme. Fix $t > 0$, and assume that $D_t = k$, and $\mathfrak{M}_k = (k;x_1,x_2,\ldots)$. Define a sequence of independent and identically distributed random variables $\tau_1,\tau_2,\ldots$, with

$$P(\tau_1 = r) = x_r, r = 1,2,\ldots . \tag{4.2}$$

We can then define a labelled equivalence relation $\mathcal{R}$ on $\mathbb{N}$ as follows. We say that genes i and j are equivalent, in an equivalence class labelled 0, if $\tau_i = \tau_j < k$, while genes i and j are in the equivalence class labelled r if $\xi_i = \xi_j = k + r, r = 1,2,\ldots$. There are thus k equivalence classes labelled 0 (corresponding to the old classes in the introduction) and age-ordered new equivalence classes in which a class with label r is older than a class with label s if $r < s$. Note that by the structure of the measure ν_k, each class is a.s. infinite.

We conclude with a brief discussion of how this process is related to the sample coalescent of section 1. One obtains from $\mathcal{R}$ an equivalence relation in $\mathcal{E}_n^*$ by restricting attention to the labels assigned to genes $1,2,\ldots,n$. This relation, $\mathcal{A}^n$ say, will have some number $m(\leq k)$ of old equivalence classes, and a number $\ell\ (\geq 0)$ of new equivalence classes, age ordered in the natural way. It can then be shown that

$$P(\mathcal{A}^n = (\xi_1,\ldots,\xi_m;\eta_1,\ldots,\eta_\ell) \mid D_t = k) = \frac{k!\,\Gamma(k+\theta)\,\theta^\ell \lambda_1!\ldots\lambda_m!\,\mu_1!\ldots\mu_\ell!}{(k-m)!\,\Gamma(n+k+\theta)\,\mu_\ell(\mu_\ell+\mu_{\ell-1})\ldots(\mu_\ell+\ldots+\mu_1)} \tag{4.3}$$

where λ_i is the number of genes in class ξ_i, and μ_i the number of genes in class η_i This result should be compared to that in (2.2), the difference arising from the fact that the number of old classes m in $\mathcal{A}^n$ may be less than the number of old classes k in $\mathcal{R}$.

ACNOWLEDGEMENT

The authors were supported in part by National Science Foundation grants DMS 85-01763 and DMS 86-08857.

REFERENCES

[1] Donnelly, P. J.(1986) Dual processes in population genetics. In Stochastic Spatial Processes. Ed. P. Tautu. Springer Lecture Notes in Mathematics, in press.

[2] Donnelly, P. J.(1986) Partition structures, Polya urns, the Ewens sampling formula and the ages of alleles. Theor. Popn. Biol., in press.

[3] Donnelly, P. J., Tavare S.(1986) The ages of alleles and a coalescent. Adv. Appl. Prob., 18, 1-19.

[4] Ethier S. N., Kurtz, T.G.(1981) The infinitely-many-neutral-alleles diffusion model. Adv. Appl. Prob. 13, 439-452.

[5] Griffiths, R. C.(1979) A transition density expansion for a multiallele diffusion model. Adv. Appl. Prob., 11, 310-325.

[6] Griffiths, R. C.(1980) Lines of descent in the diffusion approximation of neutral Wright-Fisher models. Theor. Popn. Biol., 17, 37-50.

[7] Kingman, J. F. C.(1975) Random discrete distributions, J. Roy. Statist. Soc., B, 37, 1-22.

[8] Kingman J. F. C.(1982) On the genealogy of large populations. J. Appl. Prob.,19A, 27-43.

[9] Kingman, J. F. C.(1982) The coalescent. Stoch. Proc. Appln., 13, 235-248.

[10] Patil, G. P., Taillie, C.(1977) Diversity as a concept and its implications for random communities. Bull. Internat. Stat. Inst., 47, 497-515.

[11] Watterson, G. A.(1984) Lines of descent and a coalescent. Theor. Popn. Biol., 26, 77-92.

EQUILIBRIUM MEASURES OF THE STEPPING STONE MODEL WITH SELECTION IN POPULATION GENETICS

S. Itatsu

Department of Mathematics, Faculty of Science

Shizuoka University, Ohya Shizuoka

Summary. Let X be a countable set and N be a positive integer. X is a collection of colonies. Consider the process of gene frequencies of an allele A_1, which is subjected to the following changes:(a) mutation occurs from A_1 into A_2 and from A_2 into A_1 with mutation rates u and v, respectively, (b) for any colonies x and z the genes migrate from z to x with migration rates λ_{xz}, (c) selection occurs in each colony x, where A_1 and A_2 have relative fitness $1 + s_x/2$, $1 - s_x/2$ respectively, and (d) after having reproduced an infinite numbers of offsprings, N individuals are sampled at random within each colony. The process is called the stepping stone model. The process is a Markov chain with state space describing gene frequencies at colonies. Possible values of gene frequencies at each colony are $0, 1/(2N), \cdots, (2N)/(2N)$. We say the process is ergodic if the distribution of the process at the n-th time converges to the unique equilibrium measure independently of the initial distribution as $n \to \infty$. It is shown that if $s_x \geq 0$ for all x in X or $s_x \leq 0$ for all x in X, and $u + v \leq 1$ and $u, v > 0$, the process is ergodic, but assuming $u > 0$ and $v = 0$ and $X = Z^d$ the d-dimensional lattice, then there exists a constant $s_1 < 2$ such that the process is ergodic if $\sup_{x \in X} s_x < s_1$ and is not ergodic if $\inf_{x \in X} s_x > s_1$. The latter fact shows that under the condition $u > 0 = v$, the process has a nontrivial equilibrium measure, if s_x is large enough. Assume $X = Z^1$

and consider the case that sign of s_x is different between $x \geq 0$ and $x < 0$. Some monotonicity properties concerning the equilibrium measure and related estimates are obtained under the condition that the process is ergodic.

1. Introduction.

The stepping stone model has been proposed by M. Kimura [4] to describe the evolution of a genetical population with mating and geographical structures. It has been investigated and developed by M. Kimura and G. H. Weiss [5], G. H. Weiss and M. Kimura [11], W. Fleming and C. -H. Su [1], S. Sawyer [10], T. Nagylaki [8], [9], and others.

We will discuss the time evolution of the distribution of gene frequencies and describe the ergodic properties of the model by using a Markov chain.

Our formulation of the model is given as follows. Let X be a discrete countable set and set $S = \{0, 1/(2N), \cdots, (2N)/(2N)\}^X$ where N is a positive integer. We consider a Markov process $M = \{S, p(n) = \{p_x(n) ; x \in X\}, n \geq 0, P_\nu\}$ with state space S and with probability law P_ν given as an initial measure ν on S.

Let u, v be nonnegative constants with $0 \leq u, v \leq 1$ and s_x be constants with $-2 < s_x < 2 (x \in X)$. Let $\Lambda = (\lambda_{xz})_{x,z \in X}$ be a stochastic matrix, that is, Λ satisfies $\lambda_{xz} \geq 0$ and $\sum_z \lambda_{xz} = 1$. Define an operation H from S to $[0, 1]^X$ by

(1) $H(p)_x =$

$$(1 + s_x/2)[(1-u-v)\sum_z \lambda_{xz} p_z + v]/[s_x\{(1-u-v)\sum_z \lambda_{xz} p_z + v\} + 1 - s_x/2]$$

for each element $p = \{p_x\}_{x \in X}$ of S. The transition probability

$$Q(p, A) = P_\nu(p(n+1) \in A ; p(n) = p)$$

is expressed in the form

$$Q(p, A) = \prod_{x \in Y} \binom{2N}{k_x} (H(p)_x)^{k_x} (1 - H(p)_x)^{2N-k_x}$$

for the cylindrical set $A = \{p = \{p_x\}_{x \in X} \in S \ ; \ p_x = k_x/(2N),\ x \in Y\}$ given by a finite subset Y of X. The Markov process above is called the stepping stone model. Our aims are to state some ergodic properties for the model(Theorems 1-3), and also to give the non-ergodic case and the case in which s_x are different between sites x.

We shall explain the genetical meaning of the model. The set X is the collection of colonies each of which contains exactly N individuals. Each colony is to contain 2N genes. Regard $p_x(n)$ as the frequency of an allele A_1 in the colony x at the n-th generation. The distribution of frequencies changes from p(n) to p(n+1) in the following manner. First mutation occurs from A_1 into another allele A_2 and from A_2 into A_1 with mutation rates u and v, respectively. Second, for any colonies x and z the genes migrate from z to x with migration rates λ_{xz}. Third, selection occurs in each colony x, where A_1 and A_2 have relative fitness $1 + s_x/2$ and $1 - s_x/2$ respectively. Finally having reproduced an infinite numbers of offsprings, N individuals are sampled at random within each colony.

2. Ergodic properties.

We say that a probability measure μ on S is an equilibrium measure of M if $\mu Q = \mu$ holds and that M is ergodic if there exists an equilibrium measure μ uniquely such that $\lim_{n \to \infty} \nu Q^n = \mu$ holds independently of the initial probability measure ν on S. Then the following results hold.

Theorem 1. Assume $s_x \geq 0$ for all x in X, or $s_x \leq 0$ for all x in X. If $u + v \leq 1$ and $u, v > 0$, then M is ergodic.

Theorem 2. Assume there exists a constant k with $k < 1$ such that

(2) $$\sup_{x\in X} (1+s_x/2)(1-s_x/2)|1-u-v|(1 + s_x(1/2-u))^{-2} \leq k,$$

$$\sup_{x\in X} (1+s_x/2)(1-s_x/2)|1-u-v|(1 - s_x(1/2-v))^{-2} \leq k.$$

Then M is ergodic.

If the sign of s_x is different in x, M does not satisfy the assumption of Theorem 1, but satisfies the assumption of Theorem 2, if $u + v \neq 1$ and s_x is uniformly small enough in x.

Theorem 3. 1) Assume $u > 0$ and $v = 0$, then there exists s_1 $(2u(2-u)^{-1} \leq s_1 \leq 2)$such that M is ergodic and $\delta_0 = \lim_{n\to\infty} \nu Q^n$ if $\sup_{x\in X} s_x < s_1$, and M is not ergodic if $\inf_{x\in X} s_x > s_1$.
2) Assume $u = 0$ and $v > 0$, then there exists $s_2(-2 \leq s_2 \leq -2v(2-v)^{-1})$ such that M is ergodic and $\delta_1 = \lim_{n\to\infty} \nu Q^n$ if $\inf_{x\in X} s_x > s_2$, and M is not ergodic if $\sup_{x\in X} s_x < s_2$.

Remark 1. In the above theorem δ_0 and δ_1 are equilibrium measures for 1) and 2) respectively, where δ_0, δ_1 are probability measures of pointmass on $p \equiv 0$, $p \equiv 1$, respectively.

We give the case in which M is not ergodic. Let $X = Z^d$ the d-dimensional lattice and suppose Λ is homogeneous, that is, $\lambda_{xz} = \lambda_{x-z,0}$. The following example shows the existence of the non-ergodic case.

Example 1. Let $\lambda_{xz} = m$ if $|x-z| = 1$, $\lambda_{xz} = 1 - 2dm$ if $x = z$, and

$\lambda_{xz} = 0$ otherwise, where m is a constant with $0 < m \leq 1/(2d)$. If M satisfies the assumption of Theorem 3, then $s_1 < 2$, $s_2 > -2$.

Let us consider $X = Z^1$ and the sign of s_x is different between $x \geq 0$ and $x < 0$.

Example 2. Assume Λ is homogeneous, $1-u-v \geq 0$, u, v > 0, and $s_x = s$ if $x \geq 0$, $s_x = -s$ if $x < 0$, where s is a constant with $0 \leq s < 2$. Assume

(3) $$(1-s/2)(1+s/2)(1-u-v)\max\{(1-s(1/2-u))^{-2},\ (1-s(1/2-v))^{-2}\} < 1.$$

Then the assumption (2) holds. Therefore M is ergodic, and the equilibrium measure μ satisfies

$$E_\mu p_x \leq E_\mu p_y \qquad \text{for } x \leq y.$$

We shall show in section 5 the estimate of orders of $E_\mu p_x$ as x tends to infinity.

3. Discrete time spin systems.

The spin systems are necessary for the proof of the results of section 2. We shall explain the spin systems in this section(c.f. R. Holley [2], Liggett, T. M. [6], [7]). Let W be a countable set. We consider a discrete time Markov process η_n on state space $T = \{0, 1\}^W$. Let $\rho_x(\eta)$ be a function on $W \times T$ and $0 \leq \rho_x(\eta) \leq 1$. We say η_n is a spin system corresponding to $\rho_x(\eta)$ if it is a Markoc process on T with a transition probability

(4) $$P_\eta[\eta_1(x) = 1\ ;\ x \in Y] = \prod_{x \in Y} \rho_x(\eta) \qquad \text{for finite subset Y of W.}$$

We say the spin system corresponding to ρ is attractive if ρ satisfies

(5) $\rho_x(\eta) \leq \rho_x(\zeta)$ for $\eta \leq \zeta$ (that is, $\eta(x) \leq \zeta(x)$, $x \in W$).

We have the following

Lemma 1. Let there be spin systems η_n^1, η_n^2 on T corresponding to $\rho_x^1(\eta)$, $\rho_x^2(\eta)$. Assume $\rho_x^1(\eta) \leq \rho_x^2(\zeta)$ for $\eta \leq \zeta$.

Then there exists a spin system $\gamma_n = (\eta_n, \zeta_n)$ on T such that η_n and ζ_n have the same law as η_n^1 and η_n^2, respectively, if $\eta_0 = \eta_0^1$ and $\zeta_0 = \eta_0^2$ and that

$$\eta_n \leq \zeta_n \quad n \geq 0, \text{ if } \eta_0 \leq \zeta_0.$$

Proof. Define the probability law of γ_n by

$$P_{(\eta,\zeta)}[\gamma_1(x) = (1, 1)] = \rho_x^1(\eta),$$

$$P_{(\eta,\zeta)}[\gamma_1(x) = (0, 1)] = \rho_x^2(\zeta) - \rho_x^1(\eta),$$

$$P_{(\eta,\zeta)}[\gamma_1(x) = (0, 0)] = 1 - \rho_x^2(\zeta).$$

and define

$$P_{(\eta,\zeta)}[\gamma_1(x) = (k_x, j_x),\ x \in Y] = \prod_{x \in Y} P_{(\eta,\zeta)}[\gamma_1(x) = (k_x, j_x)]$$

for $k_x, j_x = 0, 1 (x \in W)$, where Y is a finite subset of W. Then $P_{(\eta,\zeta)}$ satisfies the Markov transition probability on $T \times T$ and clearly has the properties of the Lemma. Q.E.D.

Lemma 2. Let $\rho_x^1(\eta)$, $\rho_x^2(\eta)$ be functions on $W \times T$ with $0 \leq \rho_x^j(\eta) \leq 1$ $(j = 1, 2)$. Assume that

(6) $\rho_x^1(\eta) \leq \rho_x^1(\zeta)$ for $\eta \leq \zeta$, $x \in W$, or

(7) $\rho_x^1(\eta) \geq \rho_x^1(\zeta)$ for $\eta \leq \zeta$, $x \in W$,

and that

(8) $\quad |\rho_x^{\,1}(\eta) - \rho_x^{\,1}(\zeta)| \le \rho_x^{\,2}(\xi) \qquad$ for $|\eta - \zeta| \le \xi$.

Then there exists a spin system $\gamma_n = (\eta_n, \zeta_n, \xi_n)$ on $T \times T \times T$ such that

$$|\eta_n - \zeta_n| \le \xi_n \quad n \ge 0, \text{ if } |\eta_0 - \zeta_0| \le \xi_0,$$

and η_n, ζ_n, ξ_n have the same probability law as the spin systems corresponding to ρ^1, ρ^1, ρ^2, respectively.

Remark 2. Under the assumption of Lemma 2 if the spin system corresponding to ρ^2 is ergodic and has the equilibrium measure δ_0, then the spin system corresponding to ρ^1 is ergodic.

Proof. Assume (6). Put $T_0 = \{(\eta, \zeta, \xi) \in T^3 ; \eta \le \zeta, |\eta-\zeta| \le \xi\}$. For $(\eta, \zeta, \xi) \in T_0$, the values of $(\eta, \zeta, \xi)(x)$ are the elements $a_1 = (0, 0, 0)$, $a_2 = (0, 0, 1)$, $a_3 = (0, 1, 1)$, $a_4 = (1, 1, 0)$, $a_5 = (1, 1, 1)$. Define the transition probability on T_0 as follows: Set

$$P_{(\eta,\zeta,\xi)}[(\eta, \zeta, \xi)_1(x) = r_x, \; x \in Y] = \prod_{x \in Y} P_{(\eta,\zeta,\xi)}[(\eta, \zeta, \xi)_1(x) = r_x]$$

for $r_x = a_1, \cdots, a_5$ $(x \in Y)$. Put $p_j = P_{(\eta,\zeta,\xi)}[(\eta, \zeta, \xi)_1(x) = a_j]$, $j = 1, \cdots, 5$, then it is necessary and sufficient for the condition of γ_n in Lemma 2 that $p_1 + p_2 = 1 - \rho_x^{\,1}(\zeta)$, $p_3 = \rho_x^{\,1}(\zeta) - \rho_x^{\,1}(\eta)$, $p_4 + p_5 = \rho_x^{\,1}(\eta)$, $p_1 + p_4 = 1 - \rho_x^{\,2}(\xi)$, and $0 \le p_j \le 1$. Put $q = p_5$, then the above relations become $0 \le q \le \rho_x^{\,2}(\xi) - \rho_x^{\,1}(\zeta) + \rho_x^{\,1}(\eta)$, $q \le \rho_x^{\,1}(\eta)$, $q \ge \rho_x^{\,2}(\xi) + \rho_x^{\,1}(\eta) - 1$. Therefore define q by

$$q = \rho_x^{\,1}(\eta) \wedge (\rho_x^{\,2}(\xi) - \rho_x^{\,1}(\zeta) + \rho_x^{1}(\eta)),$$

then the above condition is satisfied by the assumption of Lemma. If assumption (7) is made in place of (6), the discussion is the same as with assumption (6). Q.E.D.

Lemma 3. Let $\rho_x^1(\eta)$, $\rho_x^2(\eta)$, $\rho_x^3(\eta)$ be functions on $W \times T$ with $0 \leqq \rho_x^j(\eta) \leqq 1$ $(j = 1, 2, 3)$. Assume that

$$\rho_x^1(\eta) \leqq \rho_x^2(\zeta) \qquad \text{for } \eta \leqq \zeta,\ x \in W.$$

1) Assume that

$$|\rho_x^2(\eta) - \rho_x^1(\zeta)| \leqq \rho_x^3(\xi) \qquad \text{for } |\eta-\zeta| \leqq \xi.$$

Then there exists a spin system $\gamma_n = (\eta_n, \zeta_n, \xi_n)$ on $T \times T \times T$ such that

$$|\eta_n - \zeta_n| \leqq \xi_n \qquad n \geqq 0, \text{ if } |\eta_0 - \zeta_0| \leqq \xi_0,$$

and η_n, ζ_n, ξ_n have the same probability law as the spin systems corresponding to ρ^1, ρ^2, ρ^3, respectively.

2) Assume that

$$\rho_x^3(\xi) \leqq \rho_x^2(\zeta) - \rho_x^1(\eta) \qquad \text{for } \xi \leqq \zeta-\eta.$$

Then there exists a spin system $\gamma_n = (\eta_n, \zeta_n, \xi_n)$ on $T \times T \times T$ such that

$$\xi_n \leqq \zeta_n - \eta_n \qquad n \geqq 0, \text{ if } \xi_0 \leqq \zeta_0 - \eta_0,$$

and η_n, ζ_n, ξ_n have the same probability law as the spin systems corresponding to ρ^1, ρ^2, ρ^3, respectively.

Proof. 1) is proved by the same way in Lemma 2. We will show 2).

Put $T_0 = \{(\eta, \zeta, \xi) \in T^3 ; \eta \leq \zeta, \xi \leq \zeta-\eta\}$. For $(\eta, \zeta, \xi) \in T_0$, the values of $(\eta, \zeta, \xi)(x)$ are the elements $a_1 = (0, 0, 0)$, $a_2 = (0, 1, 0)$, $a_3 = (0, 1, 1)$, $a_4 = (1, 1, 0)$. Define transition probability on T_0 as in Lemma 2. Put $p_j = P_{(\eta,\zeta,\xi)}[(\eta, \zeta, \xi)_1(x) = a_j]$, $j = 1, \cdots, 4$, and let $p_1 = 1 - \rho_x^2(\zeta)$, $p_2 = \rho_x^2(\zeta) - \rho_x^1(\eta) - \rho_x^3(\xi)$, $p_3 = \rho_x^3(\xi)$, $p_4 = \rho_x^1(\eta)$, then the condition $0 \leq p_j \leq 1$, $j = 1, \cdots, 4$ is satisfied by the assumption of the Lemma. Q.E.D.

Let us consider the stepping stone model M defined in section 1 and let W be $\{1, 2, \cdots, 2N\} \times X$ in this section. Put

(9) $$\rho_{(j,x)}(\eta) = H(\textstyle\sum_{k=1}^{2N} \eta(k, \cdot)/(2N))_x, \quad \eta \in T, \ (j, x) \in W.$$

Then the spin system $\eta_n = \{\eta_n(j, x)\}$ corresponding to $\{\rho_{(j,x)}(\eta)\}$ is defined. Let $\xi_n(x) = \sum_{j=1}^{2N} \eta_n(j, x)/(2N)$, then $\{\xi_n ; n \geq 0\}$ is a Markov process which is equivalent to $\{p(n) ; n \geq 0\}$ in probability law, if $\xi_0 = p(0)$. We say η_n is the spin system corresponding to M in this relation. If $\{\eta_n ; n \geq 0\}$ is ergodic, then $\{p(n) ; n \geq 0\}$ is ergodic. Conversely, assume η_n is attractive, let $\nu_0 = \lim_{n \to \infty} \delta_0 Q_0^n$, $\nu_1 = \lim_{n \to \infty} \delta_1 Q_0^n$, where Q_0 is the transition probability of η_n. By [7], η_n is ergodic if and only if $\nu_0 = \nu_1$. If η_n is not ergodic, then $\nu_0 \neq \nu_1$, and there exist $x_1, \cdots, x_L \in X$, and integers $k_1, \cdots, k_L \geq 0$ such that

$$\lim_{n \to \infty} E_{\delta_0} \prod_{i=1}^{L} (\sum_j \eta_n(j, x_i)/(2N))^{k_i} \lneqq \lim_{n \to \infty} E_{\delta_1} \prod_{i=1}^{L} (\sum_j \eta_n(j, x_i)/(2N))^{k_i}.$$

This implies

$$\lim_{n\to\infty} E_{\delta_0} \prod_{i=1}^{L} p_{x_i}(n)^{k_i} \lneq \lim_{n\to\infty} E_{\delta_1} \prod_{i=1}^{L} p_{x_i}(n)^{k_i}.$$

Therefore $\{p(n)\ ;\ n \geq 0\}$ is not ergodic.

4. Proof of Theorems 1 - 3.

By section 3, given M, there exists a spin system η_n corresponding to M, in which the function $\rho_{(j,x)}$ determines the transition probability, where

(10) $\rho_{(j,x)}(\eta) =$

$$(1+s_x/2)[(1-u-v)\textstyle\sum_{k,z}\lambda_{xz}\eta(k,z)/(2N) + v]$$

$$/[s_x\{(1-u-v)\textstyle\sum_{k,z}\lambda_{xz}\eta(k,z)/(2N) + v\} + 1 - s_x/2].$$

Proof of Theorem 1. Assume $s_x \leq 0$ for all x in X. By (10)

$$\rho_{(j,x)}(\eta) = c_x + \sum_{n=1}^{\infty} b_x\, a_x^{\,n-1}(\textstyle\sum_{k,z}\lambda_{xz}\eta(k,\ z)/(2N))^n,$$

where $a_x = -\ s_x(1-u-v)/\{1 - s_x(1/2-v)\}$, $b_x =$

$(1+s_x/2)(1-s_x/2)(1-u-v)/\{1 - s_x(1/2-v)\}$, $c_x = (1+s_x/2)v/\{1 - s_x(1/2-v)\}$.

Therefore for finite subset A of W,

$$\prod_{w\in A} \rho_w(\eta) = \textstyle\sum_B c(A,\ B) \displaystyle\prod_{w\in B} \eta(w),$$

where the sum of the right side is over the finite subset B of W, and c(A, B) are nonnegative constants such that

$$\textstyle\sum_B c(A,\ B) = \displaystyle\prod_{(j,x)\in A} (1+s_x/2)(1-u)/\{1 + s_x(1/2-u)\} \leq (1-u)^{|A|}.$$

By the definition of transition probability of η_n

$$E_\nu \prod_{w\in A} \eta_{n+1}(w) = E_\nu \prod_{w\in A} \rho_w(\eta_n) = \sum_B c(A, B) E_\nu \prod_{w\in B} \eta_n(w).$$

Put $r_n(A) = E_\nu \prod_{w\in A} \eta_n(w)$, then it satisfies

$$r_{n+1}(A) = \sum_B c(A, B) r_n(B), \quad r_n(\emptyset) = 1.$$

In the case $u > 0$, by the relation of $c(A, B)$, the above recursive equation has a solution with a unique limit as n tends to ∞. Therefore η_n is ergodic, that is, M is ergodic.

In the case $s_x \geq 0$ for all x in X, by using $p_x'(n) = 1 - p_x(n)$ and taking $u' = v$, $v' = u$, $s_x' = - s_x$ in place of u, v, s_x, respectively, the discussion is the same as in the case $s_x \leq 0$ for all x in X.

<u>Proof of Theorem 2.</u> Define the stochastic matrix K on W by $K((k,x),(j,z)) = \lambda_{xz}/(2N)$, then by (10) the transition function of the spin system corresponding to M is given by

$\rho_{(k,x)}(\eta) = F_x(K\eta(k,x))$, where F_x are functions from $[0, 1]$ into $[0, 1]$ defined by

$$F_x(\xi) = [(1+s_x/2)(1-u-v)\xi + (1+s_x/2)v]/[s_x(1-u-v)\xi + 1 - s_x(1/2-v)].$$

Differentiation of this equation gives

$$(d/d\xi)F_x(\xi) = (1+s_x/2)(1-s_x/2)(1-u-v)/[s_x(1-u-v)\xi + 1 - s_x(1/2-v)]^2,$$

and (2) is equivalent to $|(d/d\xi)F_x(\xi)| \leq k$. Put $\rho^1_{(j,x)}(\eta) = \rho_{(j,x)}(\eta)$, $\rho^2_{(j,x)}(\eta) = kK\eta(j,x)$. Then the assumption in Lemma 2 is satisfied.

The spin system corresponding to ρ^2 is ergodic, and has the equilibrium measure δ_0. Therefore by Remark 2 the spin system corresponding to ρ^1 is ergodic and M is ergodic. Q.E.D.

Proof of Theorem 3. By $u+v \leq 1$, for any constants σ_1, σ_2 $(-2 < \sigma_1 < \sigma_2 < 2)$ define $\rho^1_{(j,x)}(\eta)$, $\rho^2_{(j,x)}(\eta)$ by (10) as $s_x = \sigma_1$, $s_x = \sigma_2$, respectively, then the spin system η_n^j corresponding to ρ^j $(j = 1, 2)$ is attractive. They satisfy the assumption in Lemma 1. In case 1) by $v = 0$, if η_n^2 is ergodic, then δ_0 is the unique equilibrium measure of η_n^2, η_n^2 converges to 0 in law, and η_n^1 converges to 0 in law also. Therefore there exists s_1 such that this process η_n^1 with $s_x = \sigma_1$ is ergodic and η_n^1 converges to 0 in law if $\sigma_1 < s_1$ and it is not ergodic if $\sigma_1 > s_1$. By the same way for the spin system η_n defined by (10) we can show that it is ergodic and it converges to 0 if $\sup_{x \in X} s_x < s_1$ and it is not ergodic if $\inf_{x \in X} s_x > s_1$. By Theorem 2 it is ergodic if $\sup_{x \in X} s_x < 2u(2-u)^{-1}$, and $u > 0$. Therefore $s_1 \geq 2u(2-u)^{-1}$ and 1) holds. 2) is proved by using $\eta_n^{j\prime} = 1 - \eta_n^j$ instead of η_n^j.

5. Examples.

Now consider $X = Z^d$, by which we shall mean the d-dimensional lattice. Let η_n be a spin system on $\{0, 1\}^Z$ corresponding to $\rho_x(\eta)$ given by

$$\rho_x(\eta) = (1 - \vartheta)(\eta(x-1) + \eta(x+1) - \eta(x-1)\eta(x+1)).$$

By [7] we have the following

Lemma 4. If ϑ is small enough, then η_n has an equilibrium measure not identical to δ_0.

Proof of Example 1. Let η_n^1 be the spin system corresponding to $\rho_{(j,x)}^1(\eta)$ given by

$$\rho_{(j,x)}^1(\eta) = (1-\vartheta)(\eta(j,x-1) + \eta(j,x+1) - \eta(j,x-1)\eta(j,x+1)),$$

$j = 1, \cdots, 2N$, $x \in X$. By Lemma 4 we can choose constant ϑ such that η_n^1 is not ergodic. In the case $d = 1$,under the assumption of Theorem 3-1) let η_n^2 and $\rho_{(j,x)}^2(\eta)$ be the spin system and its transition function corresponding to M. Under the assumption of Example 1, suppose $s_x = s$ is large enough, then

$$\rho_{(j,x)}^2(\eta) \geq (1-\vartheta)\{1 - \prod_{j=1}^{2N} (1-\eta(j, x+1))(1-\eta(j, x-1))\}.$$

This implies $\rho_{(j,x)}^1(\eta) \leq \rho_{(j,x)}^2(\eta)$ $(j = 1, \cdots, 2N, x \in X)$. By Lemma 1 η_n^2 is not ergodic and M is not ergodic. $s_1 < 2$ of Example 1 is proved in the case $d = 1$. In the case $d > 1$, define the map π_d from Z^d into Z^1 by $\pi_d(x_1, \cdots, x_d) = x_1 + \cdots + x_d$, and define the spin system η_n^0 on $\{0, 1\}^{Z^d}$ by $\eta_n^0(x_1, \cdots, x_d) = \eta_n(\pi_d(x_1, \cdots, x_d))$. η_n^0 has the transition function

$$\rho_{(x_1, \cdots, x_d)}^0(\eta) = (1-\vartheta)(\eta(x_1 + \cdots + x_d - 1) + \eta(x_1 + \cdots + x_d + 1)$$
$$- \eta(x_1 + \cdots + x_d - 1)\eta(x_1 + \cdots + x_d + 1)).$$

Then it is proved by the result of the case $d = 1$ that the spin system

η_n^0 is not ergodic if ϑ is small enough. Therefore $s_1 < 2$ is proved in the case $d > 1$ by using η_n^0 in place of η_n of the case $d = 1$. $s_2 > -2$ is similarly proved under the assumption of Theorem 3-2).

We shall show the following

Theorem 4. Suppose M satisfies the assumption of Example 2. Let μ be the equilibrium measure of M and put

$$u(x) = E_\mu p_x.$$

Then u(x) satisfies

$$(11) \quad \frac{c_1}{2\pi}\int_0^{2\pi} \frac{e^{-ix\vartheta}}{1 - k_1\psi(e^{i\vartheta})} d\vartheta \leq u(x) - u(x-1) \leq \frac{c_2}{2\pi}\int_0^{2\pi} \frac{e^{-ix\vartheta}}{1 - k_2\psi(e^{i\vartheta})} d\vartheta,$$

where $\psi(e^{i\vartheta}) = \sum_{x\in Z} \lambda_{x0}\, e^{ix\vartheta}$, and c_1, c_2, k_1, k_2 are constants such that

$k_1 = (1-s/2)(1+s/2)(1-u-v)\min\{(1 + s(1/2-u))^{-2}, (1 + s(1/2-v))^{-2}\}$,

$k_2 = (1-s/2)(1+s/2)(1-u-v)\max\{(1 - s(1/2-u))^{-2}, (1 - s(1/2-v))^{-2}\}$,

$c_1 = 2su(1-u)/\{1 - s^2(1/2-u)^2\}$ if $u \leq v$ and

$c_1 = 2sv(1-v)/\{1 - s^2(1/2-v)^2\}$ if $u > v$,

$c_2 = s/2$ if $u \leq 1/2$, $v \leq 1/2$, $c_2 = 2su(1-u)/\{1 - s^2(1/2-u)^2\}$ if $u > 1/2$, and $c_2 = 2sv(1-v)/\{1 - s^2(1/2-v)^2\}$ if $v > 1/2$.

Example 2 follows from the fact that the left side of inequality (11) is nonnegative. Theorem 4 implies the following results.

Assume $\lambda_{xz} = m$ if $|x-z| = 1$, $\lambda_{xz} = 1 - 2m$ if $x = z$, and $\lambda_{xz} = 0$ otherwise, where m is constant with $0 < m \leq 1/2$. Let

$$\alpha_j = [1 - k_j(1 - 2m) - \{(1 - k_j(1 - 4m))(1-k_j)\}^{1/2}]/(2k_jm),$$

$(j = 1, 2)$ then the inequality (11) becomes

$$c_1\alpha_1^{|x|}/(1 - k_1(1-2m+2m\alpha_1)) \leqq u(x) - u(x-1) \leqq c_2\alpha_2^{|x|}/(1 - k_2(1-2m+2m\alpha_2)).$$

Proof of Theorem 4. Let $X = Z$ and put $W = \{1, \cdots, 2N\} \times X$, define a shift T_x on $\{0, 1\}^W$ $(x \in X)$ by $T_x\eta(j,z) = \eta(j,z+x)$. Let η_n^2 and $\rho_{(j,x)}^2$ be the spin system and its transition function corresponding to M. Put $\rho_{(j,x)}^1(\eta) = \rho_{(j,x-1)}^2(T_1\eta)$. Then $\eta_n^1 = T_{-1}\eta_n^2$ is the spin system corresponding to $\rho_{(j,x)}^1(\eta)$. By assumption Λ is homogeneous $\rho_{(j,x-1)}^2(T_1\eta) = F_{x-1}(K\eta(j,x))$. By definition of k_1, k_2, c_1, c_2

$$c_1 + k_1K\eta(j,x) \leqq F_x(K\eta(j,x)) - F_{x-1}(K\eta(j,x)) \leqq c_2 + k_2K\eta(j,x)$$

if $x = 0$, and

$$k_1K\eta(j,x) \leqq F_x(K\eta(j,x)) - F_{x-1}(K\eta(j,x)) \leqq k_2K\eta(j,x)$$

if $x \neq 0$. Therefore let $\rho_{(j,x)}^3(\eta) = \min\{c_2 + k_2K\eta(j,x), 1\}$ if $x = 0$ and $\rho_{(j,x)}^3(\eta) = k_2K\eta(j,x)$ if $x \neq 0$. Then ρ^1, ρ^2, ρ^3 satisfy the assumption of Lemma 3-1). Let η_n^3 be the spin system corresponding to ρ^3. Then we have for any initial measure ν on $\{0, 1\}^W$

$$E_\nu\eta_n^2(j,x) - E_\nu\eta_n^1(j,x) \leqq E_\nu\eta_n^3(j,x).$$

As n tends to ∞, we get the inequality of the right side of (11). As to the left side of (11) the proof is similar. Q.E.D.

We shall present another example whch is not ergodic and has s_x different in x.

Example 3. Assume $v = 0$, $u > 0$. Λ is defined as $\lambda_{xz} = m$ if $z = x+1$, $\lambda_{xz} = 1 - m$ if $x = z$, $\lambda_{xz} = 0$ otherwise$(0 < m < 1)$. Let s be a constant with $0 < s < 2$ and define $s_x = s$ if $x \geqq 0$ and $s_x = -s$ if $x < 0$. Then if s is near enough to 2, M is not ergodic.

This is proved as follows. Let $Z_+ = \{x \in Z ; x \geqq 0\}$ and define

$$\rho_x(\eta) = (1 - \vartheta)(\eta(x) + \eta(x+1) - \eta(x)\eta(x+1)), \eta \in \{0, 1\}^{Z_+}, x \in Z_+.$$

Then if ϑ is small enough, the spin system η_n corresponding to $\rho_x(\eta)$ has a nontrivial equilibrium measure. By using η_n the discussion is the same as in the Example 1.

References

[1] Fleming, W. and Su, C. -H., Some one-dimensional migration models in population Genetics theory, Theoret. Population Biology 5(1974), 431-449.

[2] Holley, R., An ergodic theorem for interacting systems with attractive interactions. Z. Wahrscheinlichkeittheorie und Verw. Gebiete 24(1972), 325-334.

[3] Itatsu, S., Ergodic properties of the equilibrium measure of the stepping stone model in population genetics, Nagoya Math. J. 83(1981), 37-51.

[4] Kimura, M., "Stepping stone" model of population, Annual Report of the National Institute of Genetics, Japan 3(1953), 63-65.

[5] Kimura, M. and Weiss, G. H., The stepping stone model of population structure and the decrese of genetic correlation with distance, Genetics, 49(1964), 561-576.

[6] Liggett, T. M., The stochastic evolution of infinite systems of interacting particles. Springer Lecture notes in Mathematics 598 (1977), 187-248.

[7] ____, Attractive nearest neighbor spin systems on the integers, Ann. Prob. 4(1978), 629-636.

[8] Nagylaki, T., Random genetic drift in a cline, Proc. Natl. Acad. Sci. USA 75(1978), 423-426.

[9] ____, The geographical structure of populations, Studies in Mathematical Biology II. (1978), 588-624, The Mathematical Association of America, Washington.

[10] Sawyer, S., Results for the stepping stone model for migration in population genetics, Ann. Probability 4(1976), 699-728.

[11] Weiss, G. H. and Kimura, M., A mathematical analysis of the stepping stone model of genetics correlation, J. Appl. Prob., 2(1965), 129-149.

ASYMPTOTIC PROPERTIES FOR KIMURA'S DIFFUSION MODEL WITH ALTRUISTIC ALLELE

Yukio Ogura
Department of Mathematics
Saga University, 840 Saga, Japan

and

Norio Shimakura
Department of Mathematics
Kyoto University, 606 Kyoto, Japan

Summary. We study the diffusion model for a random mating diploid species in population genetics admitting intergroup selection, which was recently proposed by M. Kimura. We first enumerate the stationary distributions for the relative gene frequencies of the altruistic allele and inspect their stability. According to the regions of the parameters, we divide the model into seven cases. In the three of them, there are only 'trivial' stationary distributions, i.e. the relative gene frequency is equal to zero with probability one or equal to one. But in the other four cases, we can find one or infinitely many stationary distributions with density functions. Under a mild assumption, we also show that, for any initial distribution, the distribution of the gene frequencies goes to one of the stationary distributions as time goes to infinity. We next study how the data affect the distribution of the gene frequencies. Actually, the moment sequence of the distribution depends on the data monotonically. As a result, we verify one of the main results of M. Kimura, which gives a criterion for predominance of the altruistic allele or the other allele by a simple index $D = c/m - 4Ns$.

1. Introduction

Recently, M. Kimura proposed a diffusion model of intergroup selection in population genetics, with special regards on an altruistic allele (see [3], [4] and [5]). Later, one of the present authors proved the existence and uniqueness of the solutions (see [9]). Also recently, T. Shiga [8] gave those for a class of non-linear equations including the present model as well as the multi-dimensional ones.

The next target of our study is the asymptotic properties of the solution. Actually, in the previous paper [7], we studied (i) the existence and the number of stationary solutions, (ii) the stability of the stationary solutions and (iii) monotone dependence of a stationary solution on the parameters. The object of this article is to review the results in [7] first, and then give some further results on these subjects.

The contents of this article are as follows. In Section 2, we restate the mathematical description of the model and enumerate its stationary solutions following [7]. In Section 3, we review the results in [7] on the stability of the stationary solutions and advance them a little. More precisely, we remove the restriction on the initial distribution for the cases (d) and (e) (see Section 2 for the classification of the model), and also obtain the stability theorem for the case (g). In the last Section 4, we give the monotone dependence of the moment sequence of the solution on the parameters (Theorem 2), and improve a little the result in [7] on Kimura's property (Theorem 3).

2. The model and stationary solutions

The derivation and analysis of the present Kimura's diffusion model from the point of view of the theory of population genetics are given in [3], [4] and [5]. So, we will not step into them again in this article.

The mathematical description of the model is as follows. Let $\mathcal{M}$ be the space of all finite measures on $[0,1]$ with weak topology, and $\mathcal{P}$ the closed subset of $\mathcal{M}$ consisting of all probability measures on $[0,1]$. Let also $C[0,1]$ ($C^2[0,1]$) be the space of all continuous functions on $[0,1]$ (resp. twice continuously differentiable functions on a neighbourhood of $[0,1]$). For $U \in \mathcal{M}$ and $f \in C[0,1]$, we denote $\langle f,U\rangle = \int_{[0,1]} f(x)U(dx)$. Further, we set $\psi_n(x) = x^n$, $n \in Z_+$, where Z_+ stands for the set of all non-negative integers. Notice that a sequence $(U_k)_{k=1}^{\infty}$ in $\mathcal{M}$ converges to a $U \in \mathcal{M}$ if and only if $\lim_{k\to\infty}\langle\psi_n,U_k\rangle = \langle\psi_n,U\rangle$ for all $n \in Z_+$.

Now let (N,v',v,s,m,c) be a hexad of real numbers satisfying

$$N > 0,\ v' \geq 0,\ v \geq 0,\ s > 0,\ m > 0 \ \text{ and } \ c \geq 0, \tag{2.1}$$

whose components represent the effective population size of the group, the rates of mutation in both directions, the rate of individual selection, that of migration and that of intergroup competetion, respectively. Except in Theorem A below, we assume

$$c \leq m + v. \tag{2.2}$$

We next define a second order differential operator

$$\mathcal{D}_y f(x) = \frac{x(1-x)}{4N} f''(x) + \{v'(1-x)-vx-sx(1-x)+m(y-x)\}f'(x), \; x \in (0,1) \tag{2.3}$$

on $C^2[0,1]$, where f' and f'' stand for the first and the second derivatives of f, respectively. Now our basic problem is as follows.

Problem (K) or the diffusion model of Kimura Given a hexad (N,v',v,s,m,c) and a $\Phi \in \mathcal{P}$, find a $\mathcal{P}$-valued continuous function $U(t)$ in $t \in [0,\infty)$ satisfying

$$\frac{d}{dt}\langle f,U(t)\rangle = \langle \mathcal{D}_{\langle\psi_1,U(t)\rangle} f + c(\psi_1-\langle\psi_1,U(t)\rangle)f, U(t)\rangle, \; t \in (0,\infty),$$
$$f \in C^2[0,1], \tag{2.4}$$

$$U(0) = U(0+) = \Phi. \tag{2.5}$$

For the above Problem (K), the next existence and uniqueness theorem is obtained.

Theorem A([7], [8] and [9]). Under the assumption (2.1), Problem (K) has a unique solution $U(t)$.

In order to state an alternative of Problem (K), we need a difference operator

$$(\mathcal{G}_y \gamma)_n = ns\gamma_{n+1} + n(\frac{n-1}{4N}+v'+my)\gamma_{n-1} - n(\frac{n-1}{4N}+v'+v+s+m)\gamma_n, \; n \in \mathbf{N} \tag{2.6}$$

on the space of all real sequences $(\gamma_n)_{n=0}^{\infty}$.

Moment equation problem (M) Given a hexad (N,v',v,s,m,c) and a $\Phi \in \mathcal{P}$, find a sequence-valued function $M(t) = (M_n(t))_{n=0}^{\infty}$ in $t \in [0,\infty)$ satisfying

$$\frac{d}{dt}M_n(t) = (\mathcal{G}_{M_1(t)}M(t))_n + c(M_{n+1}(t) - M_1(t)M_n(t)),$$
$$n \in \mathbf{N},\; t \in (0,\infty), \tag{2.7}$$

$$M_n(0) = M_n(0+) = \langle\psi_n,\Phi\rangle, \quad n \in Z_+, \tag{2.8}$$

and the condition

for each $t \in [0,\infty)$, $M_0(t) = 1$ *and the sequence* $(M_n(t))_{n=0}^{\infty}$ *is completely monotone, i.e.,* $\sum_{p=0}^{n}(-1)^p\binom{n}{p}M_{k+p}(t) \geq 0$, $k,n \in Z_+$. (2.9)

Notice that Problems (K) and (M) are equivalent through the relation $M_n(t) = \langle\psi_n, U(t)\rangle$, $n \in Z_+$, where $U(t)$ and $(M_n(t))_{n=0}^{\infty}$ are the solutions of Problems (K) and (M) respectively (see [7] for details).

We next proceed to the stationary problem.

Stationary problem (SK) Given a hexad (N,v',v,s,m,c), find a $U \in \mathcal{P}$ satisfying

$$\langle \mathcal{D}_{\langle\psi_1,U\rangle}f + c(\psi_1 - \langle\psi_1,U\rangle)f, U\rangle = 0, \quad f \in C^2[0,1]. \tag{2.10}$$

Stationary moment equation problem (SM) Given a hexad (N,v',v,s,m,c), find a completely monotone sequence $M = (M_n)_{n=0}^{\infty}$ with $M_0 = 1$ which satisfies the equation

$$(\mathcal{G}_{M_1}M)_n + c(M_{n+1} - M_1M_n) = 0, \quad n \in \mathbf{N}. \tag{2.11}$$

Notice again that Problems (SK) and (SM) are equivalent through the relation $M_n = \langle\psi_n, U\rangle$, $n \in Z_+$, where U and $(M_n)_{n=0}^{\infty}$ are the solutions of Problems (SK) and (SM) respectively.

For each $x \in [0,1]$, define the delta measure $\delta_x \in \mathcal{P}$ by

$$\langle f, \delta_x\rangle = f(x), \quad f \in C[0,1].$$

Then it follows from (2.11) that δ_0 (δ_1) is a solution of Problem (SK) if and only if $v' = 0$ (resp. $v = 0$). Any other solution U of Problem (SK) has a density function $u \in L^1([0,1])$; $U(dx) = u(x)dx$. We call the density u as well as the solution U itself a stationary L^1-solution (see [7]).

Set

$$\lambda_n = ns + c, \quad \mu_n = n\left(\frac{n-1}{4N} + v' + my\right),$$
$$\nu_n = n\left(\frac{n-1}{4N} + v' + v + s + m\right) + cy, \tag{2.12}$$

$$a_n(y) = \mu_n/\lambda_n, \quad b_n(y) = \nu_n/\lambda_n, \quad n \in \mathbf{N}. \tag{2.13}$$

Then, for each $n \in \mathbf{N}$, the continued fraction

$$F_n(y) = \frac{a_n(y)}{b_n(y)} - \frac{a_{n+1}(y)}{b_{n+1}(y)} - \dots \tag{2.14}$$

converges in power series sense at $y \in [0,1]$ and belongs to $C^1[0,1]$

(see [7] for details). Further, it is clear that the sequence

$$\gamma_0^{(y)} = 1,\ \gamma_n^{(y)} = \prod_{k=1}^{n} F_k(y),\ n \in \mathbf{N} \tag{2.15}$$

satisfies the equation

$$(\mathcal{G}_y \gamma^{(y)})_n + c(\gamma_{n+1} - y\gamma_n) = 0,\quad n \in \mathbf{N}. \tag{2.16}$$

Comparing (2.11) and (2.16), we can easily see that the solution $\gamma^{(y)} = (\gamma_n^{(y)})_{n=0}^{\infty}$ given by (2.15) satisfies the equation (2.11) if and only if $y = \gamma_1^{(y)} = F_1(y)$. We actually have the following lemma, where we set $F(y) = F_1(y)$, $y \in [0,1]$.

Lemma A([7;Lemma 1.1]) 1) Let U be a solution of Problem (SK). Then $\overline{x} = \langle \psi_1, U\rangle$ solves the equation

$$y = F(y),\ y \in [0,1]. \tag{2.17}$$

2) For each solution $\overline{x}$ of (2.17), there exists a unique solution U of Problem (SK) such that $\overline{x} = \langle \psi_1, U\rangle$. Further, $\overline{x} \in (0,1)$ if and only if U is a stationary L^1-solution.
3) Unless $v' = v = c - 4Nsm = 0$, the equation (2.17) has at most one solution $\overline{x}$ in $(0,1)$. Further, it satisfies (if it exists) the inequality $F'(\overline{x}) < 1$.

Lemma A together with some supplementary arguments implies the following theorem, where the names of the cases are in accordance with those in [7].

Theorem B ([7; Theorem 2]) Assume that the hexad (N,v',v,s,m,c) satisfies (2.1) and (2.2).
1) Suppose that $v' > 0$ and $v > 0$ (case (a)). Then Problem (SK) has a unique solution. It is a stationary L^1-solution.
2) Suppose that $v' = 0$ and $v > 0$. (i) If $F'(0) \le 1$ (case (b)), then Problem (SK) has a unique solution δ_0. (ii) If $F'(0) > 1$ (case (d)), then Problem (SK) has exactly two solutions; δ_0 and an L^1-solution U.
3) Suppose that $v' > 0$ and $v = 0$. (i) If $F'(1) \le 1$ (case (c)), then Problem (SK) has a unique solution δ_1. (ii) If $F'(1) > 1$ (case (e)), then Problem (SK) has exactly two solutions; δ_1 and an L^1-solution U.
4) Suppose that $v' = v = 0$. (i) If $c \ne 4Nsm$ (case (f)), then Problem (SK) has exactly two solutions; δ_0 and δ_1. (ii) If $c = 4Nsm$ (case (g)), then Problem (SK) has infinitely many solutions. More precisely, for each $y \in [0,1]$, there corresponds a unique solution U_y such that

$\langle\psi_1, U_y\rangle = y$. $U_0 = \delta_0$, $U_1 = \delta_1$ and U_y is an L^1-solution for every $y \in (0,1)$.

Remark 1 We can give an explicit formula of $F'(0)$ ($F'(1)$) in the case of $v' = 0$ (resp. $v = 0$) in terms of Kummer's confluent hypergeometric series;

$$ {}_1F_1(\alpha,\gamma;t) = \sum_{n=0}^{\infty} \frac{\Gamma(\alpha+n)\Gamma(\gamma)t^n}{\Gamma(\alpha)\Gamma(\gamma+n)n!}. $$

In fact, if $v' = 0$, then

$$ F'(0) = \frac{m}{v+m}\, {}_1F_1((c/s)+1, 4N(v+m)+1; -4Ns)/{}_1F_1(c/s, 4N(v+m); -4Ns), $$

and if $v = 0$, then

$$ F'(1) = 1 - {}_1F_1(c/s, 4N(v'+m); 4Ns) + \frac{m}{v'+m}\, {}_1F_1((c/s)+1, 4N(v'+m)+1; 4Ns) $$

(see [7; § B (9) and (10)]).

Remark 2 In the case (g), the solution U_y, $y \in (0,1)$ has the density

$$ u_y(x) = \frac{\Gamma(4Nm)}{\Gamma(4Nmy)\Gamma(4Nm(1-y))}\, x^{4Nmy-1}(1-x)^{4Nm(1-y)-1} \tag{2.18} $$

(see [7; § 1 (10)]).

3. Stability of the stationary solutions

In this section, we inspect the stability of the stationary solutions given in § 2.

Let $\mathcal{P}_* = \mathcal{P}_*(v,m,N)$ be the set of all $\Phi \in \mathcal{P}$ such that

$$ \liminf_{n\to\infty} n^{\beta}\langle\psi_n, \Phi\rangle > 0 \quad \text{for some } \beta < 4N(v+m), \tag{3.1} $$

and $\mathcal{P}^*$ be the set of all $\Phi \in \mathcal{P}$ such that

$$ \limsup_{n\to\infty} n^{\varepsilon}\langle\psi_n, \Phi\rangle < \infty \quad \text{for some } \varepsilon > 0. \tag{3.2} $$

In the previous paper [7], we obtained the following theorem, where $U(t) = U(t;\Phi)$ stands for the solution of Problem (K), U is the stationary L^1-solution given by Theorem B and the convergence is the weak one in the space $\mathcal{M}$.

Theorem C ([7;Theorem 3]) Assume that the hexad (N,v',v,s,m,c) satisfies (2.1) and (2.2).

1) Suppose that $c \le m$, $v' > 0$ and $v > 0$. Then $\lim_{t\to\infty} U(t;\Phi) = U$ for all $\Phi \in \mathcal{P}$.

2) Suppose that $c \le m$, $v' = 0$ and $v > 0$. (i) If $F'(0) \le 1$, then

$\lim_{t\to\infty} U(t;\Phi) = \delta_0$ for all $\Phi \in \mathcal{P}$. (ii) If $F'(0) > 1$, then $\lim_{t\to\infty} U(t;\Phi) = U$ for all $\Phi \in \mathcal{P}_*$.

3) Suppose that $c \le m$, $v' > 0$ and $v = 0$. (i) If $F'(1) \le 1$, then $\lim_{t\to\infty} U(t;\Phi) = \delta_1$ for all $\Phi \in \mathcal{P}$. (ii) If $F'(1) > 1$, then $\lim_{t\to\infty} U(t;\Phi) = U$ for all $\Phi \in \mathcal{P}^*$.

4) Suppose that $v' = v = 0$. (i) If $c < 4Nsm$, then $\lim_{t\to\infty} U(t;\Phi) = \delta_0$ for all $\Phi \ne \delta_1$, $\Phi \in \mathcal{P}$. (ii) If $c > 4Nsm$, then $\lim_{t\to\infty} U(t;\Phi) = \delta_1$ for all $\Phi \ne \delta_0$, $\Phi \in \mathcal{P}$.

As in [7], we set

$$P = 4Nv',\ Q = 4Nv,\ S = 4Ns,\ M = 4Nm,\ C = 4Nc. \tag{3.3}$$

Also we need the following subsets of $\mathcal{P}$;

$$\mathcal{P}_\eta = \{\Phi \in \mathcal{P}: \int_{[0,1]} e^{Sx}\Phi(dx) = {}_1F_1(M\eta, M; S)\},\quad \eta \in (0,1),$$

$$\mathcal{P}_0 = \{\delta_0\},\quad \mathcal{P}_1 = \{\delta_1\}.$$

The following theorem improves the assertions in Theorem C 2) (ii) and 3) (iii) and gives the answer for the case (g) where we could not discuss in our previous paper [7].

<u>Theorem 1</u> Assume that the hexad (N,v',v,s,m,c) satisfies (2.1).

1) Suppose that $c \le m$, $v' = 0$, $v > 0$ and $F'(0) > 1$ (case (d)). Then

$$\lim_{t\to\infty} U(t;\Phi) = U,\quad \Phi \in \mathcal{P},\ \Phi \ne \delta_0. \tag{3.4}$$

2) Suppose that $c \le m$, $v' > 0$, $v = 0$ and $F'(1) > 1$ (case (e)). Then

$$\lim_{t\to\infty} U(t;\Phi) = U,\quad \Phi \in \mathcal{P},\ \Phi \ne \delta_1. \tag{3.5}$$

3) Suppose that $v' = v = c - 4Nsm = 0$ (case (g)) and $4Ns \le 2$. Then, for each $\eta \in [0,1]$,

$$\lim_{t\to\infty} U(t;\Phi) = U_\eta,\quad \Phi \in \mathcal{P}_\eta. \tag{3.6}$$

For the proof of Theorem 1, we need the following

<u>Lemma 3.1.</u> For each $y \in (0,1)$ and $z \in [-1,1]$, the equation

$$\begin{aligned} &\frac{d}{dt}\langle f, U(t)\rangle = \langle \mathcal{D}_y f, U(t)\rangle + cz\langle f, U(t)\rangle,\quad t > 0,\\ &\langle f, U(0)\rangle = \langle f, U(0+)\rangle = \langle f, \Phi\rangle,\qquad f \in C^2[0,1] \end{aligned} \tag{3.7}$$

has a unique solution $U(t) = U_{y,z}(t) = U_{y,z}(t;\Phi) \in \mathcal{M}$. It satisfies

$$\liminf_{n\to\infty} n^{Q+M(1-y)}\langle\psi_n, U_{y,z}(t)\rangle > 0, \quad y \in (0,1),\ t > 0, \tag{3.8}$$

$$\limsup_{n\to\infty} n^{Q+M(1-y)}\langle\psi_n, U_{y,z}(t)\rangle < \infty, \quad y \in (0,1),\ t > 0. \tag{3.9}$$

Proof. We first note that our operator $\mathcal{D}_y$ is a diffusion operator. The corresponding scale function $s_y(x)$ and the speed measure function $m_y(x)$ are given by

$$\begin{aligned} s_y(x) &= \int_{1/2}^{x} w^{-p}(1-w)^{-q}e^{Sw}dw, && x \in (0,1), \\ m_y(x) &= 4N\int_{1/2}^{x} w^{p-1}(1-w)^{q-1}e^{-Sw}dw, && x \in (0,1) \end{aligned} \tag{3.10}$$

respectively, where

$$p = p_y = P + My, \quad q = q_y = Q + M(1 - y).$$

Hence the boundaries 0 and 1 are regular or 'entrance and non-exit' in Feller's sense for all $y \in (0,1)$. We set the reflecting boundary condition on the boundary whenever it is regular.

Now let $p(t,x,w) = p_y(t,x,w)$, $t > 0$, x, $w \in (0,1)$ be the elementary solution of the diffusion equation

$$\frac{\partial u(t,x)}{\partial t} = \mathcal{D}_y u(t,x), \quad t > 0,\ x \in (0,1) \tag{3.11}$$

(see [6]). Then the function

$$u(t,x) = u_y(t,x) = \int_{[0,1]} p_y(t,x,w)\Phi(dw), \quad t > 0,\ x \in (0,1) \tag{3.12}$$

satisfies (3.11) with the initial and the boundary conditions

$$\lim_{t\downarrow 0}\int_0^1 f(x)u(t,x)dm_y(x) = \langle f,\Phi\rangle, \quad f \in C[0,1],$$

$$\lim_{x\to\ell,\, x\in(0,1)} du(t,x)/ds_y(x) = 0,$$

where $\ell = 0$ or $\ell = 1$ (if it is regular). Hence, due to the symmetry of $\mathcal{D}_y$ on the space $L^2([0,1],dm_y)$ (see [7; Proof of Lemma 3.1]), it follows that the measure $U_{y,z}(t) \in \mathcal{M}$ defined by

$$\langle f, U_{y,z}(t)\rangle = e^{czt}\int_0^1\int_{[0,1]} f(x)p_y(t,x,w)\Phi(dw)dm_y(x), \quad f \in C[0,1] \tag{3.13}$$

solves (3.7).

In order to show the uniqueness, take a solution $U_{y,z}(t)$ of (3.7) and let

$$\gamma_n^{y,z} = \int_0^\infty e^{-(\alpha-cz)t}\langle\psi_n, U_{y,z}(t)\rangle dt, \quad n \in Z_+, \ \alpha > cz. \tag{3.14}$$

Then the sequence $\gamma^{y,z} = (\gamma_n^{y,z})_{n=0}^\infty$ is bounded in $n \in Z_+$ and satisfies

$$(\mathcal{G}_y \gamma^{y,z})_n - (\alpha-cz)\gamma_n^{y,z} = -\langle\psi_n, \Phi\rangle, \quad n \in Z_+. \tag{3.15}$$

But a bounded solution of (3.15) is unique by the same arguments as in [7; Proof of Lemma 3.1]. Hence, due to the uniqueness theorem for Laplace transforms, the sequence $(\langle\psi_n, U_{y,z}(t)\rangle)_{n=0}^\infty$ is uniquely determined through (3.14). This implies the uniqueness of the solution of (3.7).

Turning to the proof of (3.8) and (3.9), we note that, for each $t > 0$, there exists a $K = K(t) > 0$ such that

$$1/K \le p_y(t,x,w) \le K, \quad x, w \in [0,1].$$

Hence it follows from (3.10) and (3.13) that

$$K^{-1}e^{-S_{4N}}\frac{\Gamma(n+p)\Gamma(q)}{\Gamma(n+p+q)} \le \langle\psi_n, U_{y,z}(t)\rangle \le Ke^{S_{4N}}\frac{\Gamma(n+p)\Gamma(q)}{\Gamma(n+p+q)}.$$

This with the well known formula $\lim_{n\to\infty} n^{-a}\Gamma(n+a)/\Gamma(n) = 1$ implies (3.8) and (3.9). q.e.d.

Lemma 3.2. Let $U(t) = U(t;\Phi)$ be the solution of Problem (K). Suppose further that

$$y_1 \le \langle\psi_1, U(t)\rangle \ (y_2 \ge \langle\psi_1, U(t)\rangle), \quad t \in [0,t_o] \tag{3.16}$$

for some $y_1 \in (0,1)$ (resp. $y_2 \in (0,1)$) and $t_o > 0$. Then it holds that

$$\langle\psi_n, U_{y_1,-1}(t)\rangle \le \langle\psi_n, U(t)\rangle \ (\text{resp. } \langle\psi_n, U_{y_2,1}(t)\rangle \ge \langle\psi_n, U(t)\rangle),$$
$$n \in Z_+, \ t \in [0,t_o]. \tag{3.17}$$

Proof. Let (B_t, P) be a standard Brownian motion and

$$\beta_y(x) = v'(1-x) - vx - sx(1-x) + m(y-x).$$

Then the stochastic differential equations (SDE's)

$$dX(t) = \sqrt{X(t)(1-X(t))/2N}\, dB_t + \beta_y(X(t))dt, \quad X(0) = x, \tag{3.18}$$

$$dX(t) = \sqrt{X(t)(1-X(t))/2N}\, dB_t + \beta_{\langle\psi_1, U(t)\rangle}(X(t))dt, \quad X(0) = x \tag{3.19}$$

have unique strong solutions $X_y^x(t)$ and $X^x(t)$ in $[0,1]$, respectively (see [1; Chap. IV] e.g.). Further, as in [8], we have the expressions

$$\langle f, U_{y,z}(t)\rangle = \int_{[0,1]} (Ef(X_y^x(t)))e^{czt}\Phi(dx), \tag{3.20}$$

$$\langle f, U(t)\rangle = \int_{[0,1]} (Ef(X^x(t))\exp\{c\int_0^t (X^x(s)-\langle\psi_1, U(s)\rangle)ds\})\Phi(dx). \tag{3.21}$$

By the way, (3.16) implies

$$\beta_{y_1}(x) \le \beta_{\langle\psi_1,U(t)\rangle}(x) \text{ (resp. } \beta_{y_2}(x) \ge \beta_{\langle\psi_1,U(t)\rangle}(x)),$$
$$x \in [0,1],\ t \in [0,t_o].$$

Hence, due to the comparison theorem for SDE's (see [1; Chap. VI] e.g.), we have

$$X_{y_1}^x(t) \le X^x(t) \text{ (resp. } X_{y_2}^x(t) \ge X^x(t)), \quad t \in [0,t_o], \text{ a.s.}(P). \tag{3.22}$$

Since the function $\psi_n(x) = x^n$ is non-decreasing in $x \in [0,1]$ for all $n \in Z_+$, this implies

$$\psi_n(X_{y_1}^x(t))e^{-ct} \le \psi_n(X^x(t))\exp\{c\int_0^t (X^x(s)-\langle\psi_1,U(s)\rangle)ds\}$$

$$\text{(resp. } \psi_n(X_{y_2}^x(t))e^{ct} \ge \psi_n(X^x(t))\exp\{c\int_0^t (X^x(s)-\langle\psi_1,U(s)\rangle)ds\})$$
$$t \in [0,t_o], \quad \text{a.s.}(P). \tag{3.23}$$

This with (3.20) and (3.21) proves (3.17). q.e.d.

<u>Proof of Theorem 1 1) and 2)</u> 1) Suppose that $c \le m$, $v' = 0$, $v > 0$, $F'(0) > 1$, $\Phi \in \mathcal{P}$ and $\Phi \ne \delta_0$. Noting that $\langle\psi_1,\Phi\rangle \in (0,1]$ and that $\langle\psi_1,U(t)\rangle$ is continuous in $t \in [0,\infty)$, we have (3.16) for some $y_1 \in (0,1)$ and $t_o > 0$. Hence we obtain (3.17), which with (3.8) implies $U(t_o) \in \mathcal{P}_*$. Now, by virtue of the relation

$$U(t;\Phi) = U(t-t_o;U(t_o;\Phi)), \quad t \ge t_o, \tag{3.24}$$

the desired (3.4) follows from Theorem C 2) (ii).

The proof of Part 2) is the same and will be omitted. q.e.d.

We now turn to the proof of Part 3). Assume that $P = Q = C\text{-}SM = 0$ and, let $M(t) = (M_n(t))_{n=0}^{\infty}$ be the solution of Problem (M). We set

$$D_n(t) = (n-1+M)M_n(t) - (n-1+M\overline{x}(t))M_{n-1}(t), \ n \in \mathbf{N}, \tag{3.25}$$

where $\overline{x}(t) = M_1(t)$. Notice that $D_1(t) = 0$ automatically. Further, it follows from (2.7) that

$$4N\ dM_n(t)/dt = SD_{n+1}(t) - nD_n(t), \quad n \in \mathbb{N}. \tag{3.26}$$

For a $\rho > 0$, let

$$E(t) = \sum_{n=1}^{\infty} \frac{1}{n!}\rho^n D_{n+1}^2(t), \quad t \geq 0. \tag{3.27}$$

Lemma 3.3. Assume that $P = Q = C - SM = 0$ (case (g)). Suppose further that $S \leq 2$. Then it holds that

$$4N \frac{d}{dt}E(t) \leq -\alpha E(t), \quad t > 0, \tag{3.28}$$

for an appropriate choice of $\rho > 0$ and $\alpha > 0$.

Proof. Step 1 It follows from (3.26) that

$$4N\ dD_{n+1}(t)/dt = S(n+M)D_{n+2}(t) + n(n+M\bar{x}(t))D_n(t) - SMM_n(t)D_2(t)$$
$$- \{(n+1)(n+M) + S(n+M\bar{x}(t))\}D_{n+1}(t), \quad n \in \mathbb{N}. \tag{3.29}$$

This with (3.27) implies

$$4N\ dE(t)/dt + 2\sum_{n=1}^{\infty} \frac{\rho^n}{n!}\{(n+1)(n+M) + S(n+M\bar{x}(t))\}D_{n+1}^2(t)$$
$$= F_1(t) + F_2(t) + F_3(t), \tag{3.30}$$

where

$$F_1(t) = 2S\sum_{n=1}^{\infty} \frac{\rho^n}{n!}(n+M)D_{n+1}(t)D_{n+2}(t),$$
$$F_2(t) = 2\sum_{n=2}^{\infty} \frac{\rho^n}{n!}n(n+M\bar{x}(t))D_n(t)D_{n+1}(t), \tag{3.31}$$
$$F_3(t) = -2SMD_2(t)\sum_{n=1}^{\infty} \frac{\rho^n}{n!}M_n(t)D_{n+1}(t).$$

Step 2 Set $\rho = S$. It suffices for (3.28) to find a positive $(A_n)_{n=1}^{\infty}$ such that

$$F_1(t) + F_2(t) + F_3(t) \leq \sum_{n=1}^{\infty} \frac{S^n}{n!}A_n D_{n+1}^2(t) \tag{3.32}$$

and

$$2\{(n+1)(n+M) + S(n+M\bar{x}(t))\} - A_n \geq \alpha, \quad n \in \mathbb{N}. \tag{3.33}$$

Due to the inequality $2D_{n+1}D_{n+2} \leq D_{n+1}^2 + D_{n+2}^2$, it follows from (3.31) that

$$F_1(t) \leq S\sum_{n=1}^{\infty} \frac{S^n}{n!}(n+M)D_{n+1}^2(t) + \sum_{n=2}^{\infty} \frac{S^n}{n!}n(n-1+M)D_{n+1}^2(t),$$

$$F_2(t) \le S\sum_{n=1}^{\infty}\frac{S^n}{n!}(n+1+M\bar{x}(t))D_{n+1}^2(t) + \sum_{n=2}^{\infty}\frac{S^n}{n!}n(n+M\bar{x}(t))D_{n+1}^2(t).$$

Further, using the inequality $-2D_2M_nD_{n+1} \le \bar{x}D_2^2 + \bar{x}D_{n+1}^2$, we have

$$F_3(t) \le -2SMD_2^2(t)\bar{x}(t) + SM\sum_{n=2}^{\infty}\frac{S^n}{n!}\bar{x}(t)D_2^2(t) + SM\sum_{n=2}^{\infty}\frac{S^n}{n!}\bar{x}(t)D_{n+1}^2(t)$$

$$= M\bar{x}(t)(e^S-1-3S)SD_2^2(t) + SM\bar{x}(t)\sum_{n=2}^{\infty}\frac{S^n}{n!}D_{n+1}^2(t).$$

Thus, for (3.32), we may choose $(A_n)_{n=1}^{\infty}$ as

$$A_1 = S(3+M) + M\bar{x}(t)(e^S-1-2S)$$

$$A_n = S(2n+1+M+2M\bar{x}(t)) + 2n^2 - n + nM(1+\bar{x}(t)), \quad n = 2,3,\ldots$$

Now the left hand side of (3.33) with $n = 1$ is reduced to

$$2\{2(1+M) + S(1+M\bar{x}(t))\} - A_1 = (4-S)(M+1) + (4S+1-e^S)M\bar{x}(t). \qquad (3.34)$$

Since $4S + 1 - e^S > 0$ for $0 < S \le 2$, the right hand side of (3.34) is greater than 2. Similarly, for $n \ge 2$, we have

$$2\{(n+1)(n+M) + S(n+M\bar{x}(t))\} - A_n \ge 4 + (2-S)(1+M) \ge 4. \qquad (3.35)$$

Thus we obtain (3.33) with $\alpha = 2$, proving (3.28). q.e.d.

<u>Proof of Theorem 1 3)</u> Assume that $P = Q = C - SM = 0$ and $S \le 2$. Let further $\Phi \in \mathcal{P}_\eta$. Then, by Lemma 3.3, we have (3.28), which implies

$$|D_{n+1}(t)| \le \rho^{-n/2}(n!E(0))^{1/2}e^{-\alpha t/8N}, \quad t \ge 0. \qquad (3.36)$$

It then follows from (3.26) that the function $f(t) = dM_n(t)/dt$ is absolutely integrable over $[0,\infty)$. Thus there exist the limits

$$M_n = \lim_{t\to\infty} M_n(t) = M_n(0) + \int_0^{\infty}(dM_n(t)/dt)dt, \quad n \in \mathbf{N}.$$

Since $\lim_{t\to\infty}D_{n+1}(t) = 0$, (3.25) implies

$$M_{n+1} = \frac{n+M\bar{x}}{n+M}M_n, \quad n \in \mathbf{N},$$

where $\bar{x} = M_1$. Hence we have

$$M_n = \langle\psi_n, U_{\bar{x}}\rangle, \quad n \in Z_+,$$

where U_y, $y \in (0,1)$ are those given in Remark 2. But we know that $U_{\bar{x}} \in \mathcal{P}_\eta$ by [7; Remark to Theorem 3]. Thus we have $\bar{x} = \eta$, and obtain (3.6). q.e.d.

4. Monotone dependence on parameters

In the sequel, we assume that $c \le m$. Let $U(t) = U(t;\Phi)$ be the solution of Problem (K), U the stationary L^1-solution of Problem (SK) and $M(t) = (M_n(t))_{n=0}^{\infty}$, $M = (M_n)_{n=0}^{\infty}$ their moment sequences, respectively. In our previous paper [7], we have determined the sign of the derivatives of M_n with respect to the parameters N, v', v, s, m and c and obtained an asymptotic result ensuring Kimura's property (see [7; Theorems 4 and 5]). In this article, we study the monotone dependence of $M_n(t)$ on the parameters and give a slight improvement of the previous asymptotic result.

Let ξ be one of the parameters $\{N,v',v,s,m,c\}$. When we consider $U(t;\Phi)$ as a function of ξ, the rest of parameters being fixed, we denote it by $U(t;\Phi;\xi)$.

Theorem 2 Assume that $c \le m$ ($\xi_2 = c_2 \le m$ if $\xi = c$).

1) Let $\xi = v'$ or c and $\xi_1 < \xi_2$. Then

$$\langle\psi_n, U(t;\Phi;\xi_1)\rangle \le \langle\psi_n, U(t;\Phi;\xi_2)\rangle, \quad t \ge 0, \quad n \in \mathbf{N}. \tag{4.1}$$

2) Let $\xi = N$, v, s or m and $\xi_1 < \xi_2$. Then

$$\langle\psi_n, U(t;\Phi;\xi_1)\rangle \ge \langle\psi_n, U(t;\Phi;\xi_2)\rangle, \quad t \ge 0, \quad n \in \mathbf{N}. \tag{4.2}$$

Theorem 3 (Kimura's property) Assume that $c \le m$.

1) Fix the parameters $\{N,v,s,m,c\}$ so that $D = (c/m) - 4Ns < 0$. Suppose further that $\Phi \in \mathcal{P}$ and $\Phi \ne \delta_1$. Then, for each $\varepsilon > 0$, there exist $\eta > 0$ and $T > 0$ such that

$$0 \le \langle\psi_1, U(t;\Phi)\rangle < \varepsilon, \quad t \ge T, \ 0 \le v' \le \eta. \tag{4.3}$$

2) Fix the parameters $\{N,v',s,m,c\}$ so that $D = (c/m) - 4Ns > 0$. Suppose further that $\Phi \in \mathcal{P}$ and $\Phi \ne \delta_0$. Then, for each $\varepsilon > 0$, there exist $\eta > 0$ and $T > 0$ such that

$$1 - \varepsilon < \langle\psi_1, U(t;\Phi)\rangle \le 1, \quad t \ge T, \ 0 \le v \le \eta. \tag{4.4}$$

For the proof of Theorem 2, we will make use of the difference analogue method used in [7; § 3]. Thus we are concerned with the diferetial equations

$$\langle \mathcal{D}_{\langle\psi_1, U\rangle} f + (c(\psi_1 - \langle\psi_1, U\rangle) - \alpha) f, U\rangle = -\alpha\langle f, \Phi\rangle, \quad f \in C^2[0,1], \tag{4.5}$$

$$\langle \mathcal{D}_y f + (c(\psi_1 - y, U\rangle) - \alpha) f, U\rangle = -\alpha\langle f, \Phi\rangle, \quad f \in C^2[0,1] \tag{4.6}$$

for $\Phi \in \mathcal{P}$, $\alpha > c$ and $y \in [0,1]$ (see [7; §3 (7)]). As is shown in

[7; Lemma 3.1], the equation (4.6) has a unique solution $U_y(\alpha,\Phi) \in \mathcal{M}$ and its moment sequence $\gamma(y;\Phi) = (\gamma_n(y;\Phi))_{n=0}^{\infty}$ is a unique bounded solution of the difference equation

$$(\mathcal{G}_y\gamma)_n + c(\gamma_{n+1} - y\gamma_n) - \alpha\gamma_n = -\alpha\langle\psi_n,\Phi\rangle, \quad n \in Z_+, \tag{4.7}$$

where $(\mathcal{G}_y\gamma)_0 = 0$ by convention. Further, due to [7; Lemma 3.2], the equation (4.5) has a solution $U = U(\alpha,\Phi) \in \mathcal{P}$ with the smallest mean $\bar{x} \in [0,1]$. Following [7; Proof of Lemma 3.2], we also let

$$E_0 = \{y \in [0,1]: \gamma_0(y;\Phi) = 1\}, \quad E_1 = \{y \in [0,1]: \gamma_1(y;\Phi) = y\}$$

and $E = E_0 \cap E_1$. Notice that the solution $U_y(\alpha,\Phi)$ of (4.6) solves the equation (4.5), if and only if $y \in E$. Further we can show that

$$E = E_1 \subset E_0. \tag{4.8}$$

Indeed, if $c = 0$, then (4.8) is clear since $E_0 = [0,1]$. Suppose next that $c > 0$ and $y_1 \in E_1$. It then follows from (4.7) with $n = 0$ that

$$(\alpha + cy_1)(\gamma_0(y_1;\Phi) - 1) = 0,$$

which proves $y_1 \in E_0$.

In the following lemmas, we use the similar notation such as $\gamma_n(y;\Phi;\xi)$ and $U(\alpha,\Phi;\xi)$ to that in Theorem 2. Further, we assume $\Phi_1, \Phi_2 \in \mathcal{P}$ and denote $a \vee b = \max\{a,b\}$.

Lemma 4.1. 1) Let

$$\xi_1 < \xi_2 \quad \text{and} \quad \langle\psi_n,\Phi_1\rangle \le \langle\psi_n,\Phi_2\rangle, \ n \in Z_+. \tag{4.9}$$

Then, for $\xi = v'$,

$$\gamma_n(y;\Phi_1;\xi_1) \le \gamma_n(y;\Phi_2;\xi_2), \quad n \in Z_+, \ y \in [0,1], \tag{4.10}$$

and for $\xi = c$,

$$\gamma_n(y;\Phi_1;\xi_1) \le \gamma_n(y;\Phi_2;\xi_2), \quad n \in Z_+ \ \text{for all}$$

$$0 \le y \le \{\gamma_1(y;\Phi_1;\xi_1)/\gamma_0(y;\Phi_1;\xi_1)\} \vee \{\gamma_1(y;\Phi_2;\xi_2)/\gamma_0(y;\Phi_2;\xi_2)\}. \tag{4.11}$$

2) Let

$$\xi_1 < \xi_2 \quad \text{and} \quad \langle\psi_n,\Phi_1\rangle \ge \langle\psi_n,\Phi_2\rangle, \ n \in Z_+. \tag{4.12}$$

Then, for $\xi = N$, s or v,

$$\gamma_n(y;\Phi_1;\xi_1) \ge \gamma_n(y;\Phi_2;\xi_2), \quad n \in Z_+, \ y \in [0,1], \tag{4.13}$$

and for $\xi = m$,

$$\gamma_n(y;\Phi_1;\xi_1) \geq \gamma_n(y;\Phi_2;\xi_2), \quad n \in Z_+ \quad \text{for all}$$

$$0 \leq y \leq \{\gamma_1(y;\Phi_1;\xi_1)/\gamma_0(y;\Phi_1;\xi_1)\} \vee \{\gamma_1(y;\Phi_2;\xi_2)/\gamma_0(y;\Phi_2;\xi_2)\}. \quad (4.14)$$

Proof. Since the proof of Part 2) is similar to the following proof of Part 1), we only prove Part 1).

Let

$$(\mathcal{L}_y(\xi)\gamma)_n = \mu_n(\xi)\gamma_{n-1} + \lambda_n(\xi)\gamma_{n+1} - \nu_n(\xi)\gamma_n, \quad n \in Z_+,$$

where $\lambda_n(\xi)$, $\mu_n(\xi)$ and $\nu_n(\xi)$ are those in (2.12) considered as functions in one of the parameters $\{N, v', v, s, m, c\}$. Let further $\gamma_n^{(i)} = \gamma_n(y;\Phi_i;\xi_i)$, $n \in Z_+$, $i = 1,2$ be the solution of the equation

$$(\mathcal{L}_y(\xi_i)\gamma)_n - \alpha\gamma_n = -\alpha\langle\psi_n,\Phi_i\rangle, \ n \in Z_+. \quad (4.15)$$

It then follows that

$$\begin{aligned}
&(\mathcal{L}_y(\xi_2)(\gamma^{(2)}-\gamma^{(1)}))_n - \alpha(\gamma^{(2)}-\gamma^{(1)})_n \\
&= -\alpha(\langle\psi_n,\Phi_2\rangle - \langle\psi_n,\Phi_1\rangle) - (\mu_n(\xi_2) - \mu_n(\xi_1))\gamma_{n-1}^{(1)} \\
&- (\lambda_n(\xi_2) - \lambda_n(\xi_1))\gamma_{n+1}^{(1)} + (\nu_n(\xi_2) - \nu_n(\xi_1))\gamma_n^{(1)}, \ n \in Z_+. \quad (4.16)
\end{aligned}$$

Assume now (4.9) and let $\xi = v'$. Then the right hand side of (4.16) is reduced to

$$-\alpha(\langle\psi_n,\Phi_2\rangle - \langle\psi_n,\Phi_1\rangle) - n(\xi_2 - \xi_1)(\gamma_{n-1}^{(1)} - \gamma_n^{(1)}),$$

which is non-positive (notice that $(\gamma_n^{(1)})_{n=0}^{\infty}$ is the moment sequence of $U_y(\alpha,\Phi_1;\xi_1)$). Hence, due to the maximum principle (see [7; Lemma A.4] e.g.), we have $(\gamma^{(2)}-\gamma^{(1)})_n \geq 0$, $n \in Z_+$. This proves (4.10).

Suppose next that $\xi = c$. Then the right hand side of (4.16) is reduced to

$$-\alpha(\langle\psi_n,\Phi_2\rangle - \langle\psi_n,\Phi_1\rangle) - (\xi_2 - \xi_1)(\gamma_{n+1}^{(1)} - y\gamma_n^{(1)}). \quad (4.17)$$

On the other hand, for a moment sequence $\gamma = (\gamma_n)_{n=0}^{\infty}$, we generally have $\gamma_n^2 \leq \gamma_{n-1}\gamma_{n+1}$, $n \in Z_+$ by Schwarz inequality, so that

$$\gamma_{n+1}/\gamma_n \geq \gamma_n/\gamma_{n-1} \geq \dots \geq \gamma_1/\gamma_0.$$

Hence the quantity (4.17) is non-positive, provided $0 \leq y \leq \gamma_1^{(1)}/\gamma_0^{(1)}$. Thus, due to the maximum principle again, we obtain (4.10) for $0 \leq y \leq$

$\gamma_1^{(1)}/\gamma_0^{(1)}$. Using the formula

$$(\mathcal{L}_y(\xi_1)(\gamma^{(2)}-\gamma^{(1)}))_n - \alpha(\gamma^{(2)}-\gamma^{(1)})_n$$
$$= -\alpha(\langle\psi_n,\Phi_2\rangle - \langle\psi_n,\Phi_1\rangle) - (\mu_n(\xi_2) - \mu_n(\xi_1))\gamma_{n-1}^{(2)}$$
$$- (\lambda_n(\xi_2) - \lambda_n(\xi_1))\gamma_{n+1}^{(2)} + (\nu_n(\xi_2) - \nu_n(\xi_1))\gamma_n^{(2)}, \ n \in Z_+$$

in place of (4.16), we also obtain (4.11) for $0 \le y \le \gamma_1^{(2)}/\gamma_0^{(2)}$. Thus the inequalities (4.11) are proved. q.e.d.

<u>Lemma 4.2</u>. 1) Suppose that (4.9) holds. Then, for ξ = v' or c,

$$\langle\psi_n,U(\alpha,\Phi_1;\xi_1\rangle \le \langle\psi_n,U(\alpha,\Phi_2;\xi_2)\rangle, \ n \in Z_+. \tag{4.18}$$

2) Suppose that (4.12) holds. Then, for ξ = N, v, s or m,

$$\langle\psi_n,U(\alpha,\Phi_1;\xi_1\rangle \ge \langle\psi_n,U(\alpha,\Phi_2;\xi_2)\rangle, \ n \in Z_+. \tag{4.19}$$

<u>Proof.</u> Since the proof of Part 2) is similar to the following proof of Part 1), we only prove Part 1).

Assume that (4.9) holds and let ξ = v'. Since the sequence $\gamma_n(y;\Phi_i;\xi_i) = \langle\psi_n,U_y(\alpha;\Phi_i;\xi_i)\rangle$, $n \in Z_+$ is the unique bounded solution of the equation (4.15), it follows from Lemma 4.1 that

$$\gamma_0(y;\Phi_1;\xi_1) \le \gamma_0(y;\Phi_2;\xi_2), \quad \gamma_1(y;\Phi_1;\xi_1) \le \gamma_1(y;\Phi_2;\xi_2), \ y \in [0,1].$$

Hence, by the same argument as in [7; Proof of Lemma 3.2], we have

$$\langle\psi_1,U(\alpha,\Phi_1;\xi_1)\rangle \le \langle\psi_1,U(\alpha,\Phi_2;\xi_2)\rangle. \tag{4.20}$$

On the other hand, by the same argument as in Proof of Lemma 4.1, the sequences $\gamma_n^{(i)} = \langle\psi_n,U(\alpha,\Phi_i;\xi_i)\rangle$, $n \in Z_+$, $i = 1,2$ satisfy

$$(\mathcal{L}_{\langle\psi_1,U(\alpha,\Phi_2;\xi_2)\rangle}(\xi_2)(\gamma^{(2)}-\gamma^{(1)}))_n - \alpha(\gamma^{(2)}-\gamma^{(1)})_n$$
$$= -\alpha(\langle\psi_n,\Phi_2\rangle-\langle\psi_n,\Phi_1\rangle) - n(\xi_2-\xi_1)(\gamma_{n-1}^{(1)}-\gamma_n^{(1)})$$
$$- (\langle\psi_1,U(\alpha,\Phi_2;\xi_2)\rangle- \langle\psi_1,U(\alpha,\Phi_1;\xi_1)\rangle)(nm\gamma_{n-1}^{(1)}-c\gamma_n^{(1)}), \quad n \in \mathbf{N} \tag{4.21}$$

and $(\gamma^{(1)}-\gamma^{(2)})_0 = 0$. Due to (4.20), the right hand side of (4.21) is non-positive. Hence we have $(\gamma^{(2)}-\gamma^{(1)})_n \ge 0$, $n \in Z_+$ by [7; Lemma A.4] (with the case $\lambda_0 = 0$). Thus we obtain (4.18).

Let next ξ = c. In this case, (4.20) also follows from (4.8) and (4.11). Further, the sequences $\gamma_n^{(i)} = \langle\psi_n,U(\alpha,\Phi_i;\xi_i)\rangle$, $n \in Z_+$, $i = 1,2$ satisfy

$$(\mathcal{L}_{\langle\psi_1, U(\alpha,\Phi_2;\xi_2)\rangle}(\xi_2)(\gamma^{(2)}-\gamma^{(1)}))_n - \alpha(\gamma^{(2)}-\gamma^{(1)})_n$$
$$= - \alpha(\langle\psi_n,\Phi_2\rangle-\langle\psi_n,\Phi_1\rangle) - (\xi_2-\xi_1)(\gamma^{(1)}_{n+1}-\gamma^{(1)}_1\gamma^{(1)}_n)$$
$$- (\langle\psi_1,U(\alpha,\Phi_2;\xi_2)\rangle- \langle\psi_1,U(\alpha,\Phi_1;\xi_1)\rangle)(nm\gamma^{(1)}_{n-1}-\xi_2\gamma^{(1)}_n),\ n \in \mathbf{N} \quad (4.22)$$

and $(\gamma^{(1)}-\gamma^{(2)})_0 = 0$. Hence, due to the assumption $\xi_2 = c_2 \le m$, [7: Lemma A.4] implies $(\gamma^{(2)}-\gamma^{(1)})_n \ge 0$, $n \in Z_+$, proving (4.18) again.

q.e.d.

Proof of Theorem 2. Since the proof of Part 2) is similar to the following proof of Part 1), we only prove Part 1).

Let $\alpha > c$, $\xi = v'$ or c. For each $\Phi \in \mathcal{P}$, we inductively define a sequence of probabilities $(U(k;\alpha,\Phi;\xi))_{k=0}^{\infty}$ by

$$U(0;\alpha,\Phi;\xi) = \Phi,$$
$$U(k+1;\alpha,\Phi;\xi) = U(\alpha,U(k;\alpha,\Phi;\xi);\xi),\quad k \in Z_+. \quad (4.23)$$

We then combine these by

$$U_\alpha(t;\Phi;\xi) = \alpha\{(k+1)h-t\}U(k;\alpha,\Phi;\xi) + \alpha\{t-kh\}U(k+1;\alpha,\Phi;\xi),$$
$$\text{for}\quad t \in [kh,(k+1)h),\quad k \in Z_+, \quad (4.24)$$

where $h = 1/\alpha$. By the exactly same way as in [9; § 6], it follows that

$$\lim_{\alpha\to\infty} U_\alpha(t;\Phi;\xi) = U(t;\Phi;\xi),\quad t \ge 0. \quad (4.25)$$

Suppose now that $\xi_1 < \xi_2$. Then, by virtue of Lemma 4.2, we obtain by induction that

$$\langle\psi_n,U(k;\alpha,\Phi;\xi_1)\rangle \le \langle\psi_n,U(k;\alpha,\Phi;\xi_2)\rangle,\quad k \in Z_+,\ \alpha > c.$$

Hence (4.24) with (4.25) proves (4.1). q.e.d.

Proof of Theorem 3. Since the proof of Part 2) is similar to the following proof of Part 1), we only prove Part 1).

Suppose that the assumptions of Theorem as well as those in Part 1) are satisfied. Let also $\xi = v'$ and $\eta > 0$. Due to Theorem 2, it then holds that

$$\langle\psi_1,U(t;\Phi;\xi)\rangle \le \langle\psi_1,U(t;\Phi;\eta)\rangle,\quad t \ge 0,\quad 0 \le \xi < \eta. \quad (4.26)$$

Further, by Theorems C and 1, we have

$$\lim_{t\to\infty} \langle\psi_1, U(t;\Phi;\eta)\rangle = \bar{x}(\eta), \tag{4.27}$$

where $\bar{x}(\eta)$ is a solution in $[0,1)$ of (2.17) with $\eta = v'$. Now, by the same argument as in [7; Proof of Theorem 5], for each $\varepsilon > 0$, we can choose an $\eta > 0$ such that $\bar{x}(\eta) < \varepsilon/2$. This with (4.26) and (4.27) ensures (4.3). q.e.d.

References

[1] Ikeda, N. and S. Watanabe, Stochastic Differential Equations and Diffusion processes. North-Holland/Kodansha, 1981.

[2] Itô, K. and H. P. McKean, Jr., Diffusion Processes and their Sample Paths. Springer, 1965.

[3] Kimura, M., Diffusion model of intergroup selection, with special reference to evolution of an altruistic character. Proc. Nat. Acad. Sci. U.S.A., 80(1983), pp.6317-6321.

[4] Kimura, M., Evolution of an altruistic trait through group selection as studied by diffusion equation model. IMA Journ. Math. Apllied to Medicine and Biology 1-1(1984), pp.1-15.

[5] Kimura, M., Diffusion model of population genetics incorporating group selection, with special reference to an altruistic trait. 15-th Conference on Stochastic Processes and their Applications, Nagoya, 1985.

[6] McKean, H. P., Jr., Elementary solutions for certain parabolic differential equations, Trans. Amer. Math. Soc. 82(1956), pp.519-548.

[7] Ogura, Y. and N. Shimakura, Stationary solutions and their stability for Kimura's diffusion model with intergroup selection. to appear in J. Math. Kyoto Univ.

[8] Shiga, T., Existence and uniqueness of solutions for a class of nonlinear diffusion equations. submitted to J. Math. Kyoto Univ.

[9] Shimakura, N., Existence and uniqueness of solutions for a diffusion model of intergroup selection. J. Math. Kyoto Univ. 25-4(1985), pp.775-788.

II. MEASURE-VALUED DIFFUSION PROCESSES RELATED TO POPULATION GENETICS

THE INFINITELY-MANY-ALLELES MODEL WITH SELECTION AS A MEASURE-VALUED DIFFUSION

S. N. Ethier
Department of Mathematics
University of Utah
Salt Lake City, UT 84112

T. G. Kurtz
Department of Mathematics
University of Wisconsin, Madison
Madison, WI 53706

1. Introduction. In [4], a diffusion model is constructed for a genetic system in which all alleles are selectively neutral and all mutants are new. The state of this model is the vector of order statistics of the gene frequencies. This reordering of the frequencies is necessary because of the assumption on mutation. Fixing the order of the alleles results in a model in which the sum of the gene frequencies is less than one for all positive time. Unfortunately, reordering makes it virtually impossible to study models with selection using this approach.

In [7] Fleming and Viot introduce measure-valued diffusion processes for the purpose of approximating genetic models involving selection, mutation, and random genetic drift. In these models the set of possible alleles or "types" is represented by a compact metric space E. Each such process takes values in $\mathcal{P}(E)$, the set of Borel probability measures on E with the topology of weak convergence, and depends on a (possibly unbounded) linear operator B on $C(E)$ (the mutation operator) and a symmetric function $\sigma \in C(E^2)$ (the selection intensity function).

In the present paper we show how the infinitely-many-alleles model of [4] can be reformulated as a measure-valued process of the type introduced by Fleming and Viot. In addition we generalize the characterization theorem of Fleming and Viot by allowing σ to be an arbitrary symmetric, bounded Borel function on E^2 and E to be a locally compact, separable metric space and by only requiring B to be the generator of a Feller semigroup on $\hat{C}(E)$, the space of continuous functions on E vanishing at infinity. Examples of models which when reformulated as measure-valued diffusions involve discontinuous σ include those in [10] and [13].

In Section 2 we introduce the appropriate martingale problem and show that it is well posed and (for compact E and continuous σ) that solutions are limits in distribution of sequences of measure-valued Wright-Fisher models. For the infinitely-many-alleles models in which we are primarily interested B is bounded, and in this case we show that solutions of the martingale problem take values in the set of purely atomic probability measures. In the selectively neutral case the vector of descending order statistics of the sizes of these atoms gives the model developed in [4]. In Section 3 we prove continuous dependence on the "parameters" B and σ as well as convergence in distribution of a sequence of diploid genetic models.

For further work on measure-valued genetic diffusions, see [2],

[3], [5] (Section 10.4), [7], [9] (Chapter 10), [11] and [12]. The survey article [8] has additional references.

A further paper is planned in which we will consider the case of bounded B in greater detail.

2. Characterization of the processes. We begin by describing a measure-valued version of the Wright-Fisher model involving selection, mutation, and random genetic drift. Let E, the space of types, be a locally compact, separable metric space, and let σ be a symmetric function in $B(E^2)$. For each positive integer $M > \|\sigma\|$, let $P_M(x,\Gamma)$ be a one-step transition function on $E\times\mathcal{B}(E)$, and define $w_M(x,y) = 1 + M^{-1}\sigma(x,y)$. ($M$ is the number of individuals or gametes in the population, $P_M(x,\Gamma)$ is the probability of a mutation from type x to a type in Γ, and $w_M(x,y)$ is the fitness of the genotype (x,y).) Using these parameters, we define a Markov chain $\{Y^M(\tau), \tau = 0,1,\ldots\}$ in the M-fold product space $E^M = E\times E\times\cdots\times E$ in which $Y_i^M(\tau)$ represents the type of the ith individual in generation τ. Each of the M individuals in generation $\tau+1$ independently selects a "parent" from generation τ. The jth individual in generation τ is selected with probability

$$(2.1)\qquad \sum_{k=1}^{M} w_M(x_j,x_k) \Big/ \sum_{\ell,m=1}^{M} w_M(x_\ell,x_m) ,$$

where $x_1,\ldots,x_M$ are the types of the M individuals in generation τ. If the parent is of type x, then the offspring's type belongs to Γ with probability $P_M(x,\Gamma)$. In particular,

$$(2.2)\qquad E[\prod_{i=1}^{n} f_i(Y_{j_i}^M(1))\,|\,Y^M(0)=(x_1,\ldots,x_M)]$$

$$= \prod_{i=1}^{n}\Big\{ \sum_{j,k=1}^{M} w_M(x_j,x_k)\int f_i(y)P_M(x_j,dy) \Big/ \sum_{\ell,m=1}^{M} w_M(x_\ell,x_m)\Big\}$$

if $j_1,\ldots,j_n \in \{1,\ldots,M\}$ are distinct and $f_1,\ldots,f_n \in B(E)$, since the components of $Y^M(1)$ are conditionally independent given $Y^M(0)$.

Define $\xi_M : E^M \to \mathcal{P}(E)$ by $\xi_M(x_1,\ldots,x_M) = M^{-1}\sum_{i=1}^M \delta_{x_i}$, and let $\{\nu_\tau^{(M)}, \tau = 0,1,\ldots\}$ be the Markov chain in $\mathcal{P}_M(E)$, the range of ξ_M, given by $\nu_\tau^{(M)} = \xi_M(Y^M(\tau))$. Under certain conditions we would like to prove the existence of a Markov process $\{\mu_t, t \geq 0\}$ with sample paths in $C_{\mathcal{P}(E)}[0,\infty)$ such that $\{\nu_{[Mt]}^{(M)}, t \geq 0\} \Rightarrow \{\mu_t, t \geq 0\}$ in $D_{\mathcal{P}(E)}[0,\infty)$.

We need to construct a generator on $B(\mathcal{P}(E))$ for the limiting process. For $\mu \in \mathcal{P}(E)$, μ^m will denote the m-fold product measure of μ in $\mathcal{P}(E^m)$, and for $f \in B(E^m)$, $\langle f,\mu^m\rangle$ will denote $\int f\, d\mu^m$.

Let B (the mutation operator) be the generator of a Feller semigroup $\{T(t)\}$ on $\hat{C}(E)$, and let σ (the selection intensity) be a symmetric function in $B(E^2)$. Let $D_m = \{ \prod_{i=1}^m f_i(x_i) : f_i \in \mathcal{D}(B),$ $i = 1,\dots,m\} \subset B(E^m)$. Define $B^{(m)}$ by setting

$$B^{(m)} f(x_1,\dots,x_m) = \sum_{i=1}^m Bf_i(x_i) \prod_{j\neq i} f_j(x_j) \tag{2.3}$$

for $f \in D_m$ and extending linearly to the span of D_m. The closure of $B^{(m)}$ generates a Feller semigroup $\{T_m(t)\}$ on $\hat{C}(E^m)$, i.e., the semigroup corresponding to m independent copies of the process corresponding to $\{T(t)\}$. Note that this semigroup is given by a transition function and can therefore be extended to all of $B(E^m)$.

For $f \in B(E^m)$ and $1 \leq i < j \leq m$, let $\Phi_{ij} f$ be the function in $B(E^{m-1})$ obtained from f by replacing x_j by x_i and renumbering the variables, and define $K_{im} : B(E^m) \to B(E^{m+2})$ for $1 \leq i \leq m$ by

$$K_{im} f(x_1,\dots,x_{m+2}) = \frac{\sigma(x_i,x_{m+1}) - \sigma(x_{m+1},x_{m+2})}{\bar{\sigma}} f(x_1,\dots,x_m) , \tag{2.4}$$

where $\bar{\sigma}$ is a positive constant satisfying $\bar{\sigma} \geq \sup \{|\sigma(x,y) - \sigma(y,z)| :$ $x,y,z \in E\}$. Define $A \subset B(\mathcal{P}(E)) \times B(\mathcal{P}(E))$ by

$$\begin{aligned} A = \{(\langle f,\mu^m\rangle, \langle B^{(m)} f,\mu^m\rangle + \sum_{i<j} (\langle \Phi_{ij} f, \mu^{m-1}\rangle - \langle f,\mu^m\rangle) \\ + \bar{\sigma} \sum_{i=1}^m \langle K_{im} f, \mu^{m+2}\rangle) : f \in \mathcal{D}(B^{(m)}),\ m = 1,2,\dots\} . \end{aligned} \tag{2.5}$$

A $\mathcal{P}(E)$-valued process $\{\mu_t, t \geq 0\}$ is a solution of the martingale problem for A if for each $(\varphi,\psi) \in A$

$$\varphi(\mu_t) - \int_0^t \psi(\mu_s)\, ds \tag{2.6}$$

is an $\{\mathcal{F}_t^\mu\}$-martingale (where $\mathcal{F}_t^\mu = \sigma(\mu_s : s \leq t)$). As a special case of (2.5), we see that for $f \in \mathcal{D}(B)$,

$$\begin{aligned} (\langle f,\mu\rangle^m, m\langle Bf,\mu\rangle\langle f,\mu\rangle^{m-1} + \frac{m(m-1)}{2}(\langle f^2,\mu\rangle - \langle f,\mu\rangle^2)\langle f,\mu\rangle^{m-2} \\ + m\bar{\sigma}\langle K_{11} f,\mu^3\rangle\langle f,\mu\rangle^{m-1}) \in A. \end{aligned} \tag{2.7}$$

The following lemma and (2.7) imply that if $\{\mu_t, t \geq 0\}$ is a solution of the $D_{\mathcal{P}(E)}[0,\infty)$ martingale problem for A, then for each $f \in \mathcal{D}(B)$,

$\{\langle f,\mu_t\rangle, t \geq 0\}$ has sample paths in $C_{\mathbb{R}}[0,\infty)$ almost surely, and hence $\{\mu_t, t \geq 0\}$ has sample paths in $C_{\mathcal{P}(E)}[0,\infty)$ almost surely.

Lemma 2.1. Suppose X is a stochastic process with sample paths in $D_{\mathbb{R}}[0,\infty)$ and U and V are measurable stochastic processes satisfying

$$(2.8) \qquad \int_0^t |U(s)|\, ds < \infty, \qquad \int_0^t |V(s)|\, ds < \infty,$$

for all $t > 0$. Suppose X, U, and V are adapted to a filtration $\{\mathcal{F}_t\}$, and for $m = 1,2,3,4$,

$$(2.9) \qquad X^m(t) - \int_0^t (m(m-1)U(s)X^{m-2}(s) + mV(s)X^{m-1}(s))\, ds$$

is an $\{\mathcal{F}_t\}$-martingale. Then almost all sample paths of X are continuous.

Proof. Without loss of generality we can consider the process stopped at the first time that $|X|$ or either of the integrals in (2.8) exceeds K. A straightforward calculation then shows that for each $t > 0$

$$(2.10) \qquad \lim E[\Sigma(X(t_{i+1}) - X(t_i))^4] = 0 ,$$

where $\{t_i\}$ is a partition of $[0,t]$ and the limit is taken as $\max (t_{i+1} - t_i) \to 0$. The continuity of X follows. □

Next observe that if $\{\mu_t, t \geq 0\}$ is a solution of the $C_{\mathcal{P}(E)}[0,\infty)$ martingale problem for A, then for $f \in B(E^m)$,

$$(2.11) \qquad \langle T_m(t_0-t)f,\mu_t^m\rangle - \int_0^t \Big[\sum_{i<j}(\langle \Phi_{ij}T_m(t_0-s)f,\mu_s^{m-1}\rangle - \langle T_m(t_0-s)f,\mu_s^m\rangle) + \bar{\sigma}\sum_{i=1}^m \langle K_{im}T_m(t_0-s)f,\mu_s^{m+2}\rangle\Big]\, ds$$

is an a.s. continuous martingale for $0 \leq t \leq t_0$. (For $f \in \mathcal{D}(B^{(m)})$, this follows by Lemma 4.3.4 of [5], and the collection of f for which the assertion holds is closed under bounded pointwise convergence.)

Lemma 2.2. Let $\Gamma \in \mathcal{B}(E)$, and suppose that $T(t)\chi_\Gamma \leq \chi_\Gamma$ for all $t \geq 0$. If $\{\mu_t, t \geq 0\}$ is a solution of the $C_{\mathcal{P}(E)}[0,\infty)$ martingale problem for A and $\mu_0(\Gamma) = 0$ a.s., then $\mu_t(\Gamma) = 0$ a.s. for all $t \geq 0$. If, in addition, for each $t_0 > 0$, there exists an $\varepsilon > 0$ such that $T(t)\chi_\Gamma \geq \varepsilon\chi_\Gamma$ for $0 \leq t \leq t_0$, then $\mu_0(\Gamma) = 0$ a.s. implies $\sup_t \mu_t(\Gamma) = 0$ a.s.

Proof. Since (2.11) is a martingale, it follows that

$$(2.12)\qquad Z(t) = \langle T(t_0-t)\chi_\Gamma, \mu_t\rangle \exp\left\{-\int_0^t \bar{\sigma}\, \frac{\langle K_{11}T(t_0-s)\chi_\Gamma, \mu_s^3\rangle}{\langle T(t_0-s)\chi_\Gamma, \mu_s\rangle}\, ds\right\},$$

is a nonnegative martingale (see for example Corollary 2.3.3 of [5]). (If the denominator in the integrand is zero, take the ratio to be zero.) Since $Z(0) = 0$ a.s., $Z(t) = 0$ for all t a.s. (see Proposition 2.2.15 of [5]), and the lemma follows. □

Theorem 2.3. a) The $C_{\mathcal{P}(E)}[0,\infty)$ martingale problem for A is well posed.

b) Suppose σ is continuous and E is compact. For $M > \|\sigma\|$, let the Markov chain $\{\nu_\tau^{(M)}, \tau = 0,1,\ldots\}$ in $\mathcal{P}_M(E)$ be as above, and define Q_M and B_M on $B(E)$ by

$$(2.13)\qquad Q_M f(x) = \int f(y)P_M(x,dy), \qquad B_M = M(Q_M - I)\ .$$

Suppose that

$$(2.14)\qquad B \subset \underset{M\to\infty}{\text{ex-lim}}\, B_M\ .$$

(For information on the extended limit, see Chapter 1 of [5].) Let $\{\mu_t, t \ge 0\}$ be a solution of the $C_{\mathcal{P}(E)}[0,\infty)$ martingale problem for A, and suppose that $\nu_0^{(M)} \Rightarrow \mu_0$ in $\mathcal{P}(E)$. Then $\{\nu_{[Mt]}^{(M)}, t \ge 0\} \Rightarrow \{\mu_t, t \ge 0\}$ in $D_{\mathcal{P}(E)}[0,\infty)$.

Proof. a) Existence of solutions for continuous σ and compact E will be a consequence of the relative compactness proved for the approximating sequence in part (b), and existence for bounded measurable σ and locally compact E follows as in the proof of Theorem 3.1(a). Uniqueness follows by a duality argument. (See Proposition 4.4.7 of [5].) To identify the correct duality relationship, define $F:\mathcal{P}(E)\times \bigcup_{m=1}^\infty B(E^m) \to \mathbb{R}$ by $F(\mu,f) = \langle f,\mu^m\rangle$ for $f \in B(E^m)$, and write

$$(2.15)\qquad AF(\mu,f) = \langle B^{(m)}f,\mu^m\rangle + \sum_{i<j}(\langle \Phi_{ij}f,\mu^{m-1}\rangle - \langle f,\mu^m\rangle) + \bar{\sigma}\sum_{i=1}^m \langle K_{im}f,\mu^{m+2}\rangle$$

$$= \langle B^{(m)}f,\mu^m\rangle + \sum_{i<j}(\langle \Phi_{ij}f,\mu^{m-1}\rangle - \langle f,\mu^m\rangle) + \bar{\sigma}\sum_{i=1}^{m}(\langle K_{im}f,\mu^{m+2}\rangle - \langle f,\mu^m\rangle) + \bar{\sigma}m\langle f,\mu^m\rangle$$

$$= CF(\mu,f) + \bar{\sigma}mF(\mu,f) \ ,$$

where A operates on $F(\mu,f)$ as a function of μ, and C, which is defined by the last equality, operates on $F(\mu,f)$ as a function of f. C is the generator of the dual process which will be a process with state space $\bigcup_{m=1}^{\infty} B(E^m)$. Unfortunately, if B is unbounded, (2.15) only makes sense if $f \in \mathcal{D}(B^{(m)})$ or $\mu \in \mathcal{D}(B^*)$, where B^* is the usual functional analytic dual of B defined on the space of finite signed measures by the requirement that $\langle f,B^*\mu\rangle = \langle Bf,\mu\rangle$ for all $f \in \mathcal{D}(B)$. Consequently, Theorem 4.4.11 of [5] does not apply directly to give the desired duality relationship, and we must proceed in a slightly different manner.

Let $M = \{M(t), t \geq 0\}$ be a jump Markov process in $\mathbb{N}$ with transition intensities $q_{m,m+2} = \bar{\sigma}m$, $q_{m,m-1} = m(m-1)/2$, and $q_{i,j} = 0$ for all other $i \neq j$, let $\{\tau_k\}$ be the sequence of jump times of M (take $\tau_0 = 0$), and let $\{\Gamma_k\}$ be a sequence of random operators which are conditionally independent given M and satisfy

$$\text{(2.16)} \qquad P\{\Gamma_k = \Phi_{ij}|M\} = \frac{2}{m(m-1)}\chi_{\{M(\tau_k-) = m,\ M(\tau_k) = m-1\}}$$

for $1 \leq i < j \leq m < \infty$, and

$$\text{(2.17)} \qquad P\{\Gamma_k = K_{im}|M\} = \frac{1}{m}\chi_{\{M(\tau_k-) = m,\ M(\tau_k) = m+2\}}$$

for $1 \leq i \leq m < \infty$. Then the dual process is given by

$$\text{(2.18)} \qquad Y(t) = T_{M(\tau_k)}(t-\tau_k)\Gamma_k T_{M(\tau_{k-1})}(\tau_k-\tau_{k-1})\Gamma_{k-1}\cdots\Gamma_1 T_{M(0)}(\tau_1)Y(0) \ , \quad \tau_k \leq t < \tau_{k+1} \ , \ k = 0,1,\ldots,$$

where $Y(0) \in B(E^{M(0)})$.

Uniqueness follows from the duality identity

$$\text{(2.19)} \qquad E[\langle f,\mu_t^m\rangle] = E[\langle Y(t),\mu_0^{M(t)}\rangle \exp\{\bar{\sigma}\int_0^t M(u)\,du\}] \ ,$$

(where $Y(0) = f$ and $M(0) = m$) by Proposition 4.4.7 of [5]. To establish (2.19), write the difference of the two sides as the telescoping sum of terms of the form

$$(2.20)\qquad E[\langle Y(s+h),\mu_{t-s-h}^{M(s+h)}\rangle \exp\{\bar\sigma\int_0^{s+h} M(u)\,du\}] - E[\langle Y(s),\mu_{t-s}^{M(s)}\rangle \exp\{\bar\sigma\int_0^{s} M(u)\,du\}]$$

and show that each such term is $o(h)$. Using the definition of Y and elementary properties of M, we can decompose the first term in (2.20) in terms of the values of $M(s+h) - M(s)$ to obtain

$$(2.21)\qquad E[E[\langle Y(s+h),\mu_{t-s-h}^{M(s+h)}\rangle \exp\{\bar\sigma\int_0^{s+h} M(u)\,du\} \mid \mathcal{F}_s^Y]]$$
$$= E[\langle T_{M(s)}(h)Y(s),\mu_{t-s-h}^{M(s)}\rangle \exp\{\bar\sigma\int_0^{s} M(u)\,du - M(s)(M(s)-1)h/2\}]$$
$$+ E[\sum_{i<j}\int_0^h \langle T_{M(s)-1}(h-r)\Phi_{ij}T_{M(s)}(r)Y(s),\mu_{t-s-h}^{M(s)-1}\rangle$$
$$\times\exp\{\bar\sigma\int_0^{s} M(u)\,du - M(s)(M(s)-1)h/2 + (M(s)-1)(h-r)\}\,dr]$$
$$+ E[\sum_{i=1}^{M(s)}\bar\sigma\int_0^h \langle T_{M(s)+2}(h-r)K_{iM(s)}T_{M(s)}(r)Y(s),\mu_{t-s-h}^{M(s)+2}\rangle$$
$$\times\exp\{\bar\sigma\int_0^{s} M(u)\,du - M(s)(M(s)-1)h/2 - (2M(s)+1)(h-r)\}\,dr]$$
$$+ o(h).$$

Using the fact that (2.11) is a martingale, the second term in (2.20) equals

$$(2.22)\qquad E[\langle T_{M(s)}(h)Y(s),\mu_{t-s-h}^{M(s)}\rangle \exp\{\bar\sigma\int_0^{s} M(u)\,du\}]$$
$$+ E\Big[\int_0^h\Big\{\sum_{i<j}(\langle \Phi_{ij}T_{M(s)}(r)Y(s),\mu_{t-s-r}^{M(s)-1}\rangle - \langle T_{M(s)}(r)Y(s),\mu_{t-s-r}^{M(s)}\rangle)$$
$$+ \bar\sigma\sum_{i=1}^{M(s)}\langle K_{iM(s)}T_{M(s)}(r)Y(s),\mu_{t-s-r}^{M(s)+2}\rangle\Big\}\,dr\,\exp\{\bar\sigma\int_0^{s} M(u)\,du\}\Big].$$

Formally it is now easy to see that the difference between (2.21) and (2.22) is $o(h)$. The proof again requires the use of the fact that (2.11) is a martingale, since we are not assuming $Y(s)$ takes values in $\hat{C}(E^{M(s)})$ and hence $T_{M(s)}(r)Y(s)$ need not be a continuous function of r.

b) Let $f_i \in \mathcal{D}(B)$, $i = 1,\dots,m$, and define $f \in D_m$ by $f(x_1,\dots,x_m) = \prod_{i=1}^m f_i(x_i)$. Since $B \subset \text{ex-lim } B_M$, there exist $f_i^M \in B(E)$ such that $\lim_{M\to\infty} f_i^M = f_i$ and $\lim_{M\to\infty} B_M f_i^M = Bf_i$ (where the convergence is in the sup norm). Let $f^M(x_1,\dots,x_m) = \prod_{i=1}^m f_i^M(x_i)$, and set $\varphi_M(\mu) = \langle f^M,\mu^m\rangle$ and $\varphi(\mu) = \langle f,\mu^m\rangle$. Then $\lim_{M\to\infty}\sup_{\mu\in\mathcal{P}_M(E)}|\varphi_M(\mu) - \varphi(\mu)| = 0$, and arguing as in the proof of Theorem 10.4.1 of [5]

$$\lim_{M\to\infty} \sup_{\mu\in\mathcal{P}_M(E)} |ME[\varphi_M(\nu_1^{(M)}) - \varphi_M(\mu)\,|\,\nu_0^{(M)} = \mu] - A\varphi(\mu)| = 0 . \tag{2.23}$$

Using Corollary 4.8.17 of [5], (2.23) and the uniqueness proved in part (a) imply that if $\nu_0^{(M)} \Rightarrow \mu_0$, the sequence of processes $\{\nu_{[M\cdot]}^{(M)}\}$ is relatively compact in $D_{\mathcal{P}(E)}[0,\infty)$ and converges to the unique solution of the martingale problem for A with initial distribution that of μ_0. □

Let $\mathcal{P}_a(E)$ denote the collection of purely atomic measures in $\mathcal{P}(E)$, and let $\bar{\nabla}_\infty = \{(x_1,x_2,\ldots): x_1 \ge x_2 \ge \ldots \ge 0,\ \Sigma\, x_i \le 1\}$. Define $\gamma: \mathcal{P}(E) \to \bar{\nabla}_\infty$ by letting $\gamma(\mu)$ be the vector of descending order statistics of the sizes of the atoms of μ.

__Theorem 2.4__. a) Let B be a bounded linear operator on $B(E)$ of the form

$$Bf(x) = \theta(x)\int (f(y) - f(x))P(x,dy) , \tag{2.24}$$

where $\theta \in B(E)$ is nonnegative and $P(x,\Gamma)$ is a one-step transition function on $E\times\mathcal{B}(E)$, and let σ be a symmetric function in $B(E^2)$. Define A as in (2.5) taking $\mathcal{D}(B)$ to be any sub-algebra of $\bar{C}(E)$ that separates points, and suppose that $\{\mu_t, t \ge 0\}$ is a solution of the $C_{\mathcal{P}(E)}[0,\infty)$ martingale problem for A. Then

$$P\{\mu_t \in \mathcal{P}_a(E) \text{ for all } t > 0\} = 1. \tag{2.25}$$

b) Assume in addition that θ is a constant, that $\sigma \equiv 0$, and that for each $x \in E$, $P(x,\cdot)$ has no atoms. Let $X(t) = \gamma(\mu_t)$ for $t \ge 0$. Then X is a solution of the $C_{\bar{\nabla}_\infty}[0,\infty)$ martingale problem for the infinite-dimensional differential operator

$$G = \frac{1}{2}\sum_{i,j=1}^{\infty} x_i(\delta_{ij}-x_j)\frac{\partial^2}{\partial x_i \partial x_j} - \theta\sum_{i=1}^{\infty} x_i\frac{\partial}{\partial x_i} , \tag{2.26}$$

with $\mathcal{D}(G)$ taken to be the algebra generated by $\{1,\varphi_2,\varphi_3,\ldots\}$, where $\varphi_m(x) = \Sigma_{i=1}^{\infty} x_i^m$, that is, X is the infinitely-many-neutral-alleles diffusion of [4] (with $\theta/2$ in [4] replaced by θ).

__Remark 2.5__. a) We are not assuming that B generates a Feller semigroup, so the existence assertion in Theorem 2.3 does not apply here.

In the case $\sigma \equiv 0$, existence can easily be obtained by directly constructing the semigroup corresponding to A. This involves verifying the range condition in the Hille-Yosida Theorem and showing that the process corresponding to the semigroup has a version with continuous sample paths. Existence for $\sigma \not\equiv 0$ then follows by the absolute continuity discussed in the proof of part (b).

b) Under the conditions of part (b), (2.25) is just the assertion that $P\{\sum X_i(t) = 1 \text{ for all } t > 0\} = 1$, which is Theorem 2.6 of [4].

c) The assertion in (2.25) could be proved by a slight modification of the proof of Theorem 10.4.5 of [5]. (The definition of φ_γ in that proof is incorrect for $\gamma < 1$. In that case φ_γ should simply be defined as the limit of $\varphi_{n,\gamma}$.)

<u>Proof</u>. a) We reduce part (a) to the assertion of part (b). The distribution of the process (restricted to the time interval $[0,T]$) with bounded measurable σ is absolutely continuous with respect to the distribution of the process with $\sigma \equiv 0$. (See [1].) The Radon-Nikodym derivative is given by

$$(2.27)\quad L_T = \exp\Big\{\tfrac{1}{2}\Big[\langle\sigma,\mu_T\rangle - \langle\sigma,\mu_0\rangle - \int_0^T\Big[\langle B^{(2)}\sigma,\mu_s^2\rangle + \langle\Phi_{12}\sigma,\mu_s\rangle - \langle\sigma,\mu_s^2\rangle + \bar{\sigma}\langle K_{12}\sigma,\mu_s^4\rangle\Big]ds\Big]\Big\}.$$

Consequently, we may as well assume $\sigma \equiv 0$.

Next, let $\tilde{E} = E\times[0,1]$, $\bar{\theta} = \sup_x \theta(x)$, and define

$$(2.28)\quad \tilde{B}f(x,u) = \bar{\theta}\Big[\frac{\theta(x)}{\bar{\theta}}\int_0^1\int (f(y,v) - f(x,u))P(x,dy)dv + \frac{\bar{\theta}-\theta(x)}{\bar{\theta}}\int_0^1 (f(x,v) - f(x,u))\,dv\Big].$$

Then $\tilde{B}$ satisfies the conditions of part (b). Let $\tilde{A}$ be defined by (2.5) with B replaced by $\tilde{B}$ and $\sigma \equiv 0$. If $\{\tilde{\mu}_t, t \geq 0\}$ is a solution of the $C_{\mathcal{P}(\tilde{E})}[0,\infty)$ martingale problem for $\tilde{A}$ and $\mu_t(\Gamma) = \tilde{\mu}_t(\Gamma\times[0,1])$ for all $t \geq 0$, then $\{\mu_t, t \geq 0\}$ is a solution of the martingale problem for A. Clearly, if $P\{\tilde{\mu}_t \in \mathcal{P}_a(E\times[0,1])$ for all $t > 0\} = 1$, then (2.22) holds. Hence it is enough to prove part (b).

b) Let $\{\mu_t, t \geq 0\}$ be a solution of the $C_{\mathcal{P}(E)}[0,\infty)$ martingale problem for A. Let $\{E_i^n\}$, $n = 1,2,\ldots$, be a sequence of partitions of E into Borel sets satisfying $\max_i \operatorname{diam}(E_i^n) \to 0$. Let $X^n(t) \in \bar{\nabla}_\infty$ be the vector of descending order statistics of $\{\mu_t(E_1^n), \mu_t(E_2^n), \ldots\}$. Then $X = \lim_{n\to\infty} X_n$. Let $\varphi_m^n(\mu) = \Sigma_i \mu(E_i^n)^m$. Then

$$(2.29) \qquad A\varphi_m^n(\mu) = \sum_{i=1}^{\infty}\Big[\, m\theta(\langle P(\cdot,E_i^n),\mu\rangle - \mu(E_i^n))\mu(E_i^n)^{m-1} + \frac{m(m-1)}{2}(\mu(E_i^n) - \mu(E_i^n)^2)\mu(E_i^n)^{m-2}\Big] ,$$

and hence

$$(2.30) \qquad \varphi_m(X^n(t)) - \int_0^t A\varphi_m^n(\mu_s)\, ds$$

is an $\{\mathcal{F}_t^\mu\}$-martingale. Since $P(x,\cdot)$ has no atoms, as $n \to \infty$ (2.30) converges to

$$(2.31) \qquad \varphi_m(X(t)) - \int_0^t G\varphi_m(X(s))\, ds ,$$

which is therefore an $\{\mathcal{F}_t^X\}$-martingale. (Note that the sequence given in (2.30) is bounded.) Similar calculations work for the other elements in $\mathcal{D}(G)$, and it follows that X is a solution of the $C_{\overline{\nabla}_\infty}[0,\infty)$ martingale problem for G. □

3. <u>Convergence theorems</u>. We now consider in what sense the processes introduced in Section 2 depend continuously on the parameters B and σ.

<u>Theorem 3.1</u>. a) Let B be the generator of a Feller semigroup on $\hat{C}(E)$, and let $\sigma_1, \sigma_2, \ldots$ be a sequence of symmetric functions in $B(E^2)$ which converges boundedly and pointwise to $\sigma \in B(E^2)$. Let A_n be given by (2.5) with σ replaced by σ_n, and let $\{\mu_t^n, t \geq 0\}$ be a solution of the $C_{\mathcal{P}(E)}[0,\infty)$ martingale problem for A_n. If $\{\mu_t, t \geq 0\}$ is a solution of the $C_{\mathcal{P}(E)}[0,\infty)$ martingale problem for A and $\mu_0^n = \mu_0$ for $n = 1,2,\ldots$, then $\{\mu_t^n, t \geq 0\} \Rightarrow \{\mu_t, t \geq 0\}$.

b) For $n = 1,2, \ldots$, let E_n and E be locally compact, separable metric spaces; let $\eta_n : E_n \to E$ be continuous and define $\pi_n : \overline{C}(E) \to \overline{C}(E_n)$ by $\pi_n f = f \circ \eta_n$ and $\hat{\eta}_n : \mathcal{P}(E_n) \to \mathcal{P}(E)$ by $\hat{\eta}_n \mu = \mu\eta_n^{-1}$; let B_n and B generate Feller semigroups on $\hat{C}(E_n)$ and $\hat{C}(E)$; let σ_n and σ be symmetric functions in $B(E_n^2)$ and $\overline{C}(E^2)$; using E_n, B_n, σ_n and E, B, σ

define A_n and A as in (2.5); let $\{\mu_t^n, t \geq 0\}$ and $\{\mu_t, t \geq 0\}$ be solutions of the $C_{\mathcal{P}(E_n)}[0,\infty)$ martingale problem for A_n and the $C_{\mathcal{P}(E)}[0,\infty)$ martingale problem for A. If

$$(3.1) \qquad B \subset \operatorname*{ex-lim}_{n\to\infty} B_n \quad (\text{with respect to } \{\pi_n\}),$$

if

$$(3.2) \qquad \lim_{n\to\infty} \sup_{x,y\in E_n} |\sigma_n(x,y) - \sigma(\eta_n(x),\eta_n(y))| = 0 ,$$

and if $\hat{\eta}_n \mu_0^n \Rightarrow \mu_0$ in $\mathcal{P}(E)$, then $\{\hat{\eta}_n \mu_t^n, t \geq 0\} \Rightarrow \{\mu_t, t \geq 0\}$ in $C_{\mathcal{P}(E)}[0,\infty)$.

Remark 3.2. A simple example of a setting in which part (b) applies is to take $E_n = \{k/n : 0 \leq k \leq n\}$ and $E = [0,1]$, and to let η_n be the natural embedding.

Proof. a) Let $E^\Delta = E\cup\{\Delta\}$ be the one-point compactification of E. Relative compactness in $C_{\mathcal{P}(E^\Delta)}[0,\infty)$ for the sequence follows from the fact that $\{A_n F\}$ is bounded for functions in $\{F : F(\mu) = \langle f, \mu^m\rangle,\ f \in \bigcup_{m=1}^\infty \mathcal{D}(B^{(m)})\}$, and that the linear span of this collection of functions is dense in $C(\mathcal{P}(E^\Delta))$. (See Theorems 3.9.1 and 3.9.4 of [5].) Note that convergence in distribution in $C_{\mathcal{P}(E^\Delta)}[0,\infty)$ will imply convergence in distribution in $C_{\mathcal{P}(E)}[0,\infty)$, since by Lemma 2.2 all processes involved have sample paths in $C_{\mathcal{P}(E)}[0,\infty)$. (See Corollary 3.3.2 of [5].) It remains to show convergence of the finite-dimensional distributions.

Convergence of the finite-dimensional distributions can be obtained using the duality relationship (2.19). First note that the dual process Y_n for A_n, $n = 1,2,\ldots$, and the dual Y for A can all be constructed on the same probability space in such a way that $\lim_{n\to\infty} Y_n(t) = Y(t)$. (Let $\bar{\sigma}$ be sufficiently large so that we can take $\bar{\sigma}_n = \bar{\sigma}$, and replace σ by σ_n in the definition of the dual, keeping M the same.) Then

$$(3.3) \qquad \begin{aligned} \lim_{n\to\infty} E[\langle f, \mu_t^{nm}\rangle] &= \lim_{n\to\infty} E[\langle Y_n(t), \mu_0^{M(t)}\rangle \exp\{\bar{\sigma}\int_0^t M(u)\,du\}] \\ &= E[\langle Y(t), \mu_0^{M(t)}\rangle \exp\{\bar{\sigma}\int_0^t M(u)\,du\}] \\ &= E[\langle f, \mu_t^m\rangle] , \end{aligned}$$

where $f = Y(0) = Y_n(0)$ and $m = M(0)$. Convergence of the one-dimensional distributions follows. For the two-dimensional convergence, let $f \in \overline{C}(E^m)$ and $g \in \overline{C}(E^\ell)$. Then

$$(3.4)\qquad \lim_{n\to\infty} E[\langle f,\mu_{t_2}^{nm}\rangle\langle g,\mu_{t_1}^{n\ell}\rangle]$$

$$= \lim_{n\to\infty} E\Big[\langle Y_n(t_2-t_1),\mu_{t_1}^{nM(t_2-t_1)}\rangle\langle g,\mu_{t_1}^{n\ell}\rangle \exp\{\overline{\sigma}\int_0^{t_2-t_1} M(u)\,du\}\Big]$$

$$= \lim_{n\to\infty} E\Big[\langle \tilde{Y}_n(t_1),\mu_0^{\tilde{M}(t_1)}\rangle \exp\Big\{\overline{\sigma}\Big[\int_0^{t_1}\tilde{M}(u)\,du + \int_0^{t_2-t_1} M(u)\,du\Big]\Big\}\Big]$$

$$= E\Big[\langle \tilde{Y}(t_1),\mu_0^{\tilde{M}(t_1)}\rangle \exp\Big\{\overline{\sigma}\Big[\int_0^{t_1}\tilde{M}(u)\,du + \int_0^{t_2-t_1} M(u)\,du\Big]\Big\}\Big]$$

$$= E[\langle f,\mu_{t_2}\rangle\langle g,\mu_{t_1}\rangle]\ ,$$

where $\tilde{Y}_n$ is a version of the dual with $\tilde{Y}_n(0) = Y_n(t_2-t_1)\times g$ (which makes $\tilde{M}(0) = M(t_2-t_1) + \ell$) and is conditionally independent of Y_n given $Y_n(t_2-t_1)$. The higher-dimensional distributions are handled in a similar way.

b) If E were compact, then the result would follow easily from convergence of the generators and uniqueness for the martingale problem. The convergence in (3.1) implies

$$(3.5)\qquad \lim_{n\to\infty}\ \sup_{x\in E_n^m} |T_m^n(t)(f\circ\eta_n)(x) - T_m(t)f(\eta_n(x))| = 0,\quad f \in \hat{C}(E_n^m),$$

where $\{T_m^n(t)\}$ is the semigroup generated by $B_n^{(m)}$. The proof is now essentially the same as that of part (a), although somewhat more care must be taken in showing that the duals converge. □

Although we artificially imposed a diploid selection scheme on our formulation of the Wright-Fisher model, the latter is really a haploid model. Here we describe a true diploid model and obtain the corresponding limit theorem. When E is finite, the model reduces to the monoecious multinomial-sampling model in [6].

Let E be a compact metric space. Then E^2 is the set of ordered pairs (x,y) of elements of E. Let $E^{(2)}$ be the set of unordered pairs $\{x,y\}$ of elements of E. (Note that if $x,y \in E$, then $(x,y) \neq (y,x)$ unless $x = y$, but $\{x,y\} = \{y,x\}$ always.) $E^{(2)}$ is the set of genotypes. If r is a metric for E, then

$$(3.6)\qquad r^{(2)}(\{x,y\},\{z,w\}) = (r(x,z) + r(y,w))\wedge(r(x,w) + r(y,z))$$

defines a metric for $E^{(2)}$, and the function $\rho: E^2 \to E^{(2)}$ given by $\rho(x,y) = \{x,y\}$ is continuous.

Define $\beta: E^2 \to E^2$ by $\beta(x,y) = (y,x)$. Given $\mu \in \mathcal{P}(E^{(2)})$ we define its <u>symmetrization</u> $\hat{\mu} \in \mathcal{P}(E^2)$ by

$$(3.7) \qquad \hat{\mu}(\Gamma) = \mu(\rho(\Gamma \cap \beta(\Gamma))) + \tfrac{1}{2}\mu(\rho(\Gamma \cap \beta(\Gamma)^c)) .$$

For example, if $\mu = \delta_{\{x,y\}}$, then $\hat{\mu} = \frac{1}{2}(\delta_{(x,y)} + \delta_{(y,x)})$. We say that $\mu \in \mathcal{P}(E^{(2)})$ is in <u>Hardy-Weinberg form</u> if $\hat{\mu}$ is a product measure, hence if $\hat{\mu} = (\hat{\mu}\pi^{-1})^2$, where $\pi: E^2 \to E$ is given by $\pi(x,y) = x$.

We now describe our model. Let $\sigma \in \overline{C}(E^2)$ be symmetric. For each positive integer $N > \|\sigma\|/2$, let $P_N(x,\Gamma)$ be a one-step transition function on $E \times \mathcal{B}(E)$, and define $w_N(x,y) = 1 + (2N)^{-1}\sigma(x,y)$. Given $\mu \in \mathcal{P}(E^{(2)})$, define μ^* and μ^{**} in $\mathcal{P}(E^{(2)})$ by

$$(3.8) \qquad d\hat{\mu}^* = w_N \, d(\hat{\mu}\pi^{-1})^2 / \langle w_N, (\hat{\mu}\pi^{-1})^2 \rangle$$

and

$$(3.9) \qquad \hat{\mu}^{**}(d\xi, d\eta) = \int_{E^2} \tfrac{1}{2}[P_N(x,d\xi)\times P_N(y,d\eta) + P_N(y,d\xi)\times P_N(x,d\eta)]\,\hat{\mu}^*(dx,dy).$$

Note that μ^{**} is in Hardy-Weinberg form if μ^* is, and μ^* is in Hardy-Weinberg form if there exists $v_N \in B(E)$ such that $w_N(x,y) \equiv v_N(x)v_N(y)$, but not in general. See [6] for further discussion.

We let $\{\nu_\tau^{(N)}, \tau = 0,1,\dots\}$ be the Markov chain in

$$(3.10) \qquad \mathcal{P}_N(E^{(2)}) = \{\mu \in \mathcal{P}(E^{(2)}) : \mu = N^{-1}\sum_{i=1}^N \delta_{\{x_i,y_i\}}\}$$

such that, given $\nu_\tau^{(N)} = \mu \in \mathcal{P}_N(E^{(2)})$, the conditional distribution of $\nu_{\tau+1}^{(N)}$ is that of $\mu' = N^{-1}\sum_{i=1}^N \delta_{\{x_i',y_i'\}}$, where $\{x_1',y_1'\},\dots,\{x_N',y_N'\}$ are i.i.d. μ^{**}.

Define $\varsigma: \mathcal{P}(E^{(2)}) \to \mathcal{P}(E)$ by $\varsigma\mu = \hat{\mu}\pi^{-1}$. If μ is the distribution of genotypes, then $\varsigma\mu$ is the distribution of alleles. We remark that if μ^{**} is in Hardy-Weinberg form for each $\mu \in \mathcal{P}(E^{(2)})$, then $\{\varsigma\nu_\tau^{(N)}, \tau = 0,1,\dots\}$ is the Wright-Fisher model (with $M = 2N$), but this is not true in general.

<u>Theorem 3.3</u>. For positive integers $N > \|\sigma\|/2$, let $\{\nu_\tau^{(N)}, \tau = 1,2,\dots\}$ in $\mathcal{P}_N(E^{(2)})$ be as above. Define Q_N on $B(E)$ as in (2.13), let $B_N = 2N(Q_N - I)$, and suppose that (2.14) holds. If $\{\mu_t, t \geq 0\}$ is a solution

of the $C_{\mathcal{P}(E)}[0,\infty)$ martingale problem for A, and if $\xi\nu_0^{(N)} \Rightarrow \mu_0$ in $\mathcal{P}(E)$, then $\{\xi\nu_{[2Nt]}^{(N)}, t \geq 0\} \Rightarrow \{\mu_t, t \geq 0\}$ in $D_{\mathcal{P}(E)}[0,\infty)$.

Proof. With φ and φ_N as in the proof of Theorem 2.3, it is easy to show that

$$(3.11) \qquad \lim_{N\to\infty} \sup_{\mu\in\mathcal{P}_N(E^{(2)})} |2NE[\varphi_N(\xi\nu_1^{(N)}) - \varphi_N(\xi\mu) | \nu_0^{(N)} = \mu] - A\varphi(\xi\mu)| = 0 .$$

As in the proof of Theorem 2.3, this implies convergence in distribution in $D_{\mathcal{P}(E)}[0,\infty)$. □

References

[1] Dawson, D. A. (1978). Geostochastic calculus. Canad. J. Statist. 6, 143-168.

[2] Dawson, D. A. and Hochberg, K. J. (1982). Wandering random measures in the Fleming-Viot model. Ann. Probab. 10, 554-580.

[3] Ethier, S. N. and Griffiths, R. C. (1987). The infinitely-many-sites model as a measure-valued diffusion. Ann. Probab. 15, to appear.

[4] Ethier, S. N. and Kurtz, T. G. (1981). The infinitely-many-neutral-alleles diffusion model. Adv. Appl. Probab. 13, 429-452.

[5] Ethier, S. N. and Kurtz, T. G. (1986). Markov Processes: Characterization and Convergence. Wiley, New York.

[6] Ethier, S. N. and Nagylaki, T. (1980). Diffusion approximations of Markov chains with two time scales and applications to population genetics. Adv. Appl. Probab. 12, 14-49.

[7] Fleming, W. H. and Viot, M. (1979). Some measure-valued Markov processes in population genetics theory. Indiana Univ. Math. J. 28, 817-843.

[8] Hochberg, K. J. (1986). Stochastic population theory: Mathematical evolution of a genetical model. In New Directions in Applied and Computational Mathematics. Springer-Verlag, to appear.

[9] Kurtz, T. G. (1981). Approximation of Population Processes. CBMS-NSF Regional Conference Series in Applied Mathematics 36. SIAM, Philadelphia.

[10] Li, W. H. (1978). Maintenance of genetic variability under the joint effects of mutation, selection, and random drift. Genetics 90, 349-382.

[11] Shiga, T., Shimizu, A., and Tanaka, H. (1986). Some measure-valued diffusion processes associated with genetical diffusion models, preprint.

[12] Shimizu, A. (1985). Diffusion approximation of an infinite allele model incorporating gene conversion. In Population Genetics and Molecular Evolution. Ohta, T. and Aoki, K. eds. Springer-Verlag, Berlin, pp. 243-255.

[13] Watterson, G. A. (1977). Heterosis or neutrality? Genetics 85, 789-814.

MULTI-ALLELIC GILLESPIE-SATO DIFFUSION MODELS AND THEIR EXTENSION TO INFINITE ALLELIC ONES

Tokuzo Shiga
Tokyo Institute of Technology

Summary

We first consider a multi-allelic Markov chain model for which one-step transition consists of three stages — independent reproduction, mutation and random sampling. Taking account of difference among alleles in means and variances of offspring numbers we discuss a diffusion approximation of the Markov chain model both in a finite-allelic case and in a countably infinite-allelic case. This diffusion approximation was derived by Gillespie heuristically in a di-allelic case, and by Sato in a multi-allelic case, neglecting any mutation factor. Our result extends Sato's one.

We next consider a continuum limit of the alleles space in the diffusion model. The limiting process is then a measure-valued diffusion process. Particularly if the alleles space is one-dimensional and the mutation operator is the Laplacian, we can derive an infinite dimensional stochastic differential equation of which solution defines a probability-density-valued diffusion process.

1. Introduction

In population genetics theory discrete time stochastic models are first considered to describe evolution of gene frequencies. However in order to analyze the discrete time models diffusion approximations are often used. Such resultant diffusion processes are also an interesting mathematical object since the corresponding diffusion operators are completely degenerate on the boundary of their state space. A typical example is a diffusion approximation of the Wright-Fisher model, which is a diffusion process on a (d-1)-dimensional closed simplex K_{d-1}

$$(1.1)\qquad K_{d-1} = \{x = (x_1,\cdots,x_{d-1}) \in R^{d-1} : x_1 \geq 0,\cdots,x_{d-1} \geq 0, \sum_{p=1}^{d-1} x_p \leq 1\},$$

of which infinitesimal generator is

$$(1.2)_a\qquad L = \frac{\sigma^2}{2}\sum_{p=1}^{d-1}\sum_{q=1}^{d-1} x_p(\delta_{pq} - x_q)\frac{\partial^2}{\partial x_p \partial x_q} + \sum_{p=1}^{d-1} b_p(x)\frac{\partial}{\partial x_p}$$

$$(1.2)_b \qquad b_p(x) = \sum_{q=1}^{d} x_q\lambda_{qp} + x_p(\gamma_p - \sum_{q=1}^{d} \gamma_q x_q)$$

with $x_d = 1 - \sum_{p=1}^{d-1} x_p$, $\sigma^2 \geq 0$, $\lambda_{pq} \geq 0$ for $p \neq q$, $\lambda_{pp} = -\sum_{\substack{q=1\\q\neq p}}^{d} \lambda_{pq}$,

γ_p real, and δ_{pq} the Kronecker symbol. In this model d possible alleles $A_1,\cdots,A_d$ are considered at one locus. λ_{pq} stands for mutation rate from A_p to A_q and γ_p is selection rate of A_p. The domain $\mathcal{D}(L)$ of L is $C^2(K_{d-1})$, the set of all C^2-functions defined on K_{d-1}.

There have been many works concerning diffusion approximations of several kinds of discrete time stochastic models by the diffusion process associated with L of (1.2). (e.q. See [6], [10].)

In the present report we are concerned with diffusion processes on K_{d-1} associated with L of the following (1.3) and their generalization to (both countably and continuously) infinite-allelic cases,

$$(1.3)_a \qquad L = \frac{1}{2}\sum_{p=1}^{d-1}\sum_{q=1}^{d-1}(\delta_{pq}\beta_p x_p + x_p x_q(\sum_{r=1}^{d}\beta_r x_r - \beta_p - \beta_q))\frac{\partial^2}{\partial x_p \partial x_q} + \sum_{p=1}^{d-1} b_p(x)\frac{\partial}{\partial x_p}$$

$$(1.3)_b \qquad b_p(x) = \sum_{q=1}^{d} x_q\lambda_{qp} + x_p(\gamma_p - \sum_{q=1}^{d} \gamma_q x_q)$$

with $x_d = 1 - \sum_{p=1}^{d-1} x_p$, $\beta_p \geq 0$, λ_{pq} and γ_p the same as in (1.2). Notice that (1.3) is reduced to (1.2) if β_p is independent of $1 \leq p \leq d$.

We will first discuss a diffusion approximation of a Markov chain model by the diffusion process associated with L of (1.3). This diffusion approximation was derived by Gillespie [5] (heuristically) in a di-allelic case and by Sato [11] in a multi-allelic case, neglecting any mutation factor. Incorporating mutation into the Markov chain model considered by Gillespie and Sato, we will in the section 2 generalize Sato's diffusion approximation in [11] in a multi-allelic case (possibly in an infinite-allelic case). Even in the presence of mutation Sato's argument is still valid for the proof of tightness. Accordingly our main task is to prove the well-posedness of the diffusion process associated with L of (1.3). The well-posedness problem will be solved in the section 3 in an infinite-allelic setting, which extends the result by Ethier [3]. In the final section some measure-valued diffusion models and their stochastic differential equations are derived by taking a continuum limit of the spaces of alleles.

2. Diffusion approximation of Gillespie-Sato model incorporating mutation

Following Sato [11] we consider a Markov chain model of a haploid population of a fixed size N with non-overlapping generations with the possible d-alleles $A_1, \cdots, A_d$ in one locus. In the model selection is incorporated in the form of difference not only of the means but also of the variances of the offspring numbers of the alleles, but mutation is neglected. In this report, assuming that mutation (possibly immigration) is also incorporated, we will discuss convergence of the Markov chain to a diffusion process associated with L of (1.3).

Let $X_p^{(N)}(n)$ be the number of individuals of allele A_p among N individuals in the n-th generation. We assume that transition from the n-th generation to the (n+1)-th consists of three stages. The first stage is reproduction, where each individual gives birth to a random number of offspring independently. Offspring of an individual of allele A_p are of allele A_p and the probability distribution of their number may depend on p. The second stage is mutation, where each individual changes its type of alleles independently. Composition of these two stages yields a branching process with multi-types. The final stage is sampling of N individuals from the offspring individuals.

Let Z_+^d be the set of d-dimensional cubic lattice points with non-negative components and $J^{(N)}$ be the set of $i = (i_1, \cdots, i_d) \in Z_+^d$ such that $|i| \equiv i_1 + \cdots + i_d = N$. For any large N (say, $N \geq N_0$), let $X^{(N)}(n) = (X_1^{(N)}(n), \cdots, X_d^{(N)}(n))$, $n = 0, 1, \cdots$, be a Markov chain on $J^{(N)}$ with stationary probability $P_{ik}^{(N)}$ defined as follows. We are given three objects $f_p^{(N)}$, λ_{pq} and $Q_{jk}^{(N)}$ such that for each $p, j \in Z_+^d$ and $N \geq N_0$

(i) $f_p^{(N)}(s)$ is a generating function of a probability distribution on Z_+^1,

(ii) $\lambda_{pq}^{(N)}$ is a probability vector on $\{1, 2, \cdots, d\}$, and

(iii) $Q_{jk}^{(N)}$ is a probability distribution $J^{(N)}$.

(i), (ii) and (iii) correspond to offspring, mutation and sampling, respectively. For each $N \geq N_0$ and $i \in J^{(N)}$, let $c_{ij}^{(N)}$ is a probability distribution on Z_d^+ with generating function

$$\sum_{j \in Z_+^d} c_{ij}^{(N)} s_1^{j_1} \cdots s_d^{j_d} = \prod_{p=1}^{d} g_p^{(N)}(\underline{s})^{i_p} \tag{2.1}$$

with

$$g_p^{(N)}(\underline{s}) = f_p^{(N)}\Big(\sum_{q=1}^{d} \lambda_{pq}^{(N)} s_q\Big). \tag{2.2}$$

$P_{ik}^{(N)}$ is defined by

$$(2.3)\qquad P_{ik}^{(N)} = \sum_{j\in Z_+^d} c_{ij}^{(N)} Q_{jk}^{(N)}.$$

Noting that $X_1^{(N)}(n)+\cdots+X_d^{(N)}(n) = N$, we normalize and interpolate by

$$(2.4)\qquad Y^{(N)}(t) = (X_1^{(N)}(n)/N,\cdots,X_{d-1}^{(N)}(n)/N) \qquad \text{for } t = n/N$$

$$(2.5)\qquad Y^{(N)}(t) = (n+1-Nt)Y^{(N)}(n/N) + (Nt-n)Y^{(N)}((n+1)/N)$$

$$\text{for } n/N \le t \le (n+1)/N.$$

Then $Y^{(N)}(t)$ is a K_{d-1}-valued continuous stochastic process. Let $\Omega = C([0,\infty),K_{d-1})$, the space of continuous paths $\omega : [0,\infty) \to K_{d-1}$ endowed with the topology of uniform convergence on compact time intervals, let $X_t(\omega) = \omega(t)$ be the coordinate function at $t \ge 0$, and let $F(F_t)$ be the σ-field generated by $\{X_t(\omega) : t \ge 0\}$ $(\{X_s(\omega) : 0 \le s \le t\})$. We denote by $P^{(N)}$ the probability measure on (Ω,F) induced by the process $Y^{(N)}(t)$, $t \ge 0$. Then it will be shown that $P^{(N)}$ converges as $N \to \infty$ to a diffusion measure associated with L of the same type as (1.3).

Let $M_p^{(N)}$ and $V_p^{(N)}$ be the mean and the variance of the offspring distribution generated by $f_p^{(N)}$, and for the sampling distribution $Q_{jk}^{(N)}$, set

$$(2.6)\qquad m_p^{(N)}(j) = \sum_{k\in J^{(N)}} k_p Q_{jk}^{(N)}.$$

Our basic assumption is

Assumption A

$$(2.7)\qquad M_p^{(N)} = \alpha(1+N^{-1}\gamma_p) + O(N^{-2})$$

$$(2.8)\qquad V_p^{(N)} = \alpha^2\beta_p + O(N^{-1})$$

$$(2.9)\qquad \lambda_{pq}^{(N)} = \delta_{pq} + N^{-1}\lambda_{pq} + O(N^{-2})$$

as $N \to \infty$ with $\alpha > 0$, $\beta_p \ge 0$, γ_p real, δ_{pq} the Kronecker symbol, $\lambda_{pq} \ge 0$ for $p \ne q$, $\lambda_{pp} = -\sum_{p\ne q} \lambda_{pq}$, and

$$(2.10)\qquad m_p^{(N)}(j) = Nj_p/|j| \qquad \text{for } j \in Z_+^d \setminus \{0\}.$$

Note that $\alpha\beta_p + \alpha - 1 \ge 0$ holds automatically. We further impose the following technical conditions.

Assumption B.

(2.11) $\quad \alpha\beta_p + \alpha - 1 > 0.$

There is an $\varepsilon > 0$ such that, for every N and p, $f_p^{(N)}(s)$ has convergence radius $> 1 + \varepsilon$, and moreover

(2.12) $\quad (f_p^{(N)})''(1-s) = (f_p^{(N)})''(1) + O(s)$

uniformly in N as $s \to 0$.

Assumption C. Let

(2.13) $\quad \mu_{pq}^{(N)}(j) = \sum_{k \in J^{(N)}} (k_p - m_p^{(N)}(j))(k_q - m_q^{(N)}(j)) Q_{jk}^{(N)}$

(2.14) $\quad \mu_{pppp}^{(N)}(j) = \sum_{k \in J^{(N)}} (k_p - m_p^{(N)}(j))^4 Q_{jk}^{(N)}.$

For each $j \in Z_+^d \setminus \{0\}$ and $1 \leq p \leq d$

(2.15) $\quad \sup_{i \in J^{(N)}} N^{-3} \sum_{j \neq 0} c_{ij}^{(N)} \mu_{pppp}^{(N)}(j) \to 0$

and for some $\sigma^2 \geq 0$

(2.16) $\quad \sup_{i \in J^{(N)}} |N^{-1} \sum_{j \neq 0} c_{ij}^{(N)} \mu_{pq}^{(N)}(j) - \sigma^2 (N^{-1} i_p)(\delta_{pq} - N^{-1} i_q)| \to 0$

as $N \to \infty$.

In order to describe the limit measure of $P^{(N)}$ let us introduce the following differential operator on K_{d-1}, which is the same as (1.3) up to parameters.

(2.17)$_a$ $\quad L = \frac{1}{2} \sum_{p=1}^{d-1} \sum_{q=1}^{d-1} a_{pq}(x) \frac{\partial^2}{\partial x_p \partial x_q} + \sum_{p=1}^{d-1} b_p(x) \frac{\partial}{\partial x_p}$

with

(2.17)$_b$ $\quad a_{pq}(x) = \sigma^2 x_p(\delta_{pq} - x_q) + x_p x_q (\sum_{r=1}^{d} \beta_r x_r - \beta_p - \beta_q) + \delta_{pq}\beta_p x_p$

(2.17)$_c$ $\quad b_p(x) = \sum_{q=1}^{d} x_q \lambda_{qp} + x_p \sum_{q=1}^{d} (\gamma_q - \beta_q)(\delta_{pq} - x_q).$

Recall that $\mathcal{D}(L)$ is the set of all C^2-functions defined on K_{d-1}. For each $f \in \mathcal{D}(L)$, let

(2.18) $$M_f(t) = f(x(t)) - \int_0^t Lf(x(s))ds.$$

Given $x \in K_{d-1}$, a probability measure P on $(\Omega, \mathcal{F})$ is called a solution of the (K_{d-1}, L, x)-martingale problem if $P(x(0) = x) = 1$ and $(M_f(t), \mathcal{F}_t, P)$ is a martingale for each $f \in \mathcal{D}(L)$. If P_x is the unique solution of the (K_{d-1}, L, x)-martingale problem for each $x \in K_{d-1}$ then $(x(t), P_x)_{x \in K_{d-1}}$ defines a diffusion process on K_{d-1}, which is called the (K_{d-1}, L)-diffusion. Then we can extend Sato's result in [11] to the case incorporating mutation as follows.

<u>Theorem 2.1.</u> Suppose that $Y^{(N)}(0) = x^{(N)}$ are non-random and $x^{(N)} \to x$ as $N \to \infty$. Then, under Assumptions A, B and C, $P^{(N)}$ converges weakly to a probability measure P_x as $N \to \infty$. Furthermore, $(x(t), P_x)$ is the (K_{d-1}, L)-diffusion with L of (2.17).

<u>Remark.</u> A typical sampling satisfying Assumption C is given by multinomial distribution on $J^{(N)}$, i.e., for each $j \in Z_+^d \setminus \{0\}$

(2.19) $$Q_{jk}^{(N)} = N! \prod_{p=1}^{d} (k_p!)^{-1} (j_p / |j|)^{k_p}.$$

Moreover, sampling by multivariate hypergeometric distribution, that by multivariate Pólya-Eggenberger distribution and nearly non-random sampling also satisfy Assumption C, (see [11]).

The proof of Theorem 2.1 follows by modifying Sato's argument in [11] paying our attentions to the mutation factor. Then a key point is to prove the uniqueness of solutions for the (K_{d-1}, L, x)-martingale problem. As is easily seen, the (K_{d-1}, L)-diffusion process is well-posed up to the hitting time of the boundary. In the absence of mutation (and immigration) the diffusion process starting at any boundary point never enters the interior of the closed domain K_{d-1}, which enable us to prove the well-posedness extremely easily. However addition of the mutation factor makes the situation more complicated. For L of (2.17) the uniqueness problem was solved by Okada [8] for $d = 3$, and was partially solved by Shiga [12] for $d \geq 4$, but this problem has been remained unsolved in a case involving mutation and immigration for general d. In the next section we will solve it in a quite general setting which covers not only multi-allelic cases but also infinite-allelic cases.

3. Infinite-allelic Gillespie-Sato diffusion model

Let S be the set of alleles. Assuming that S is a countable (finite or infinite) set, we denote elements of S by $p, q, r, \cdots$. Let K_S be the space of gene frequencies, endowed with the weak topology as the set of probability vectors on S,

$$(3.1) \qquad K_S = \{x = (x_p)_{p\in S} : x_p \geq 0 \quad \text{and} \quad \sum_{p\in S} x_p = 1\}.$$

Let us introduce a generalized form of L of (2.17)

$$(3.2)_a \qquad L = \frac{1}{2} \sum_{p\in S} \sum_{q\in S} a_{pq}(x) \frac{\partial^2}{\partial x_p \partial x_q} + \sum_{p\in S} b_p(x) \frac{\partial}{\partial x_p}$$

with

$$(3.2)_b \qquad a_{pq}(x) = x_p x_q \Big(\sum_{r\in S} \beta_r x_r - \beta_p - \beta_q\Big) + \delta_{pq}\beta_p x_p$$

and $b_p(x)$, $p \in S$ are continuous functions defined on K_S such that

$$(3.3) \qquad b_p(x) \geq 0 \quad \text{if} \quad x \in K_S \quad \text{and} \quad x_p = 0$$

$$(3.4) \qquad \sum_{p\in S} b_p(x) = 0 \qquad \text{(uniformly convergent in } x \in K_S)$$

where β_p, $p \in S$ are non-negative constants satisfying $\sup_p \beta_p < +\infty$. The domain $\mathcal{D}(L)$ of L is chosen so that each element is a C^2-function defined on an open set R^S containing K_S, and depends only on finitely many components. We note that the conditions (3.3) and (3.4) are necessary for the L-diffusion to be confined into K_S.

Assumption D. There is an $S \times S$-matrix Q_{pq} satisfying that $Q_{pq} \geq 0$, $\sup_{p\in S} \sum_{q\in S} Q_{pq} < \infty$

$$(3.5) \qquad |b_p(x) - b_p(x')| \leq \sum_{q\in S} Q_{pq}|x_q - x'_q|$$

for every $x \in K_S$, $x' \in K_S$ and $p \in S$.
Then we have the following.

Theorem 3.1. Let L be the diffusion operator of (3.2). Suppose that (3.3), (3.4) and the Assumption D are fulfilled. Then, for every $x \in K_S$, the (K_S, L, x)-martingale problem has a unique solution.

For the proof of Theorem 3.1 we consider a stochastic differential equation (SDE),

$$(3.6) \qquad dx_p(t) = \sum_{q\in S} \alpha_{pq}(x(t))dB_q(t) + b_p(x(t))dt \qquad (p \in S)$$

where $B_p(t)$, $p \in S$, are independent one dimensional Brownian motions, and $\alpha_{pq}(x)$, $p \in S$, $q \in S$, is an $S \times S$-matrix satisfying

$$(3.7) \qquad \sum_{r\in S} \alpha_{pr}(x)\alpha_{qr}(x) = a_{pq}(x).$$

It is well-known that to show the existence and uniqueness of solutions of the (K_S, L, x)-martingale problem is equivalent to show that the SDE has a unique K_S-valued solution satisfying $x(0) = x$. Here notice that $\alpha_{pq}(x)$ can be chosen as follows:

$$(3.8) \qquad \alpha_{pq}(x) = (\delta_{pq} - x_p)\sqrt{\beta_q x_q}.$$

We actually consider a simpler SDE (3.9) rather than (3.6), of which solution takes values in Y,

$$(3.9) \qquad dy_p(t) = \sqrt{\beta_p y_p(t)}\, d\tilde{B}_p(t) + \tilde{b}_p(y(t))dt \qquad (p \in S)$$

$$(3.10) \qquad Y = \{y = (y_p)_{p\in S} : y_p \geq 0 \quad \text{and} \quad 0 < \sum_{p\in S} y_p < +\infty\},$$

where $\tilde{B}_p(t)$, $p \in S$, are independent one-dimensional Brownian motions, and

$$(3.11) \qquad \tilde{b}_p(y) = b_p(\Pi y) + c\Pi_p y + \Pi_p y(\beta_p - \sum_{q\in S} \beta_q \Pi_q y)$$

with $\Pi_p y = y_p / \sum_q y_q$, $\Pi y = (\Pi_p y)$ and c is a fixed constant satisfying $c > \frac{1}{2} \sup_p \beta_p$. The SDE (3.9) is easily solved by using a one-dimensional technique of Yamada-Watanabe [15]. The SDE (3.9) is closely related to the SDE (3.6) through normalization and time change as follows: Let $y(t)$ be a Y-valued solution of the SDE (3.9), and set

$$r(t) = \sum_{p\in S} y_p(t) \quad \text{and} \quad A(t) = \int_0^t r(s)^{-1} ds.$$

Then $A(t)$ is strictly increasing and $\lim_{t\to\infty} A(t) = \infty$ a.s.. Denoting by $A^{-1}(t)$ the inverse function of $A(t)$ we define a new process $x(t)$ by

$$x(t) = y(A^{-1}(t)) / r(A^{-1}(t)).$$

Then we can show that $x(t)$ satisfies the SDE (3.6) for some independent one-dimensional Brownian motions $B_p(t)$, $p \in S$. Conversely, if one starts from a K_S-valued solution $x(t)$ of the SDE (3.6) he can trace the same procedure as the above toward the opposite direction by introducing a new total mass process. Thus the well-posedness problem of K_S-valued solutions of the SDE (3.6) is reduced to that of Y-valued solutions of the SDE (3.9). See [13] for the detail.

Finally it would be worthy of remark that the Y-valued diffusion associated with (3.9) is like a continuous state branching process, which should be obtained as a diffusion approximation of the Markov chain model without the sampling stage of the previous section.

4. Some measure-valued diffusions and their SDE

We will next discuss some measure-valued diffusion processes obtained as a continuum limit of the space of alleles in an infinite-allelic Gillespie-Sato diffusion model. Let $S = Z^n$ and consider the following SDE, which is an infinite-allelic version of (2.7) with nearest interacting mutation:

$$(4.1)\qquad dx_p(t) = \sqrt{\beta_p x_p(t)}\, dB_p(t) - \sum_{q\in Z^d} x_p(t)\sqrt{\beta_q x_q(t)}\, dB_q(t)$$

$$+ \frac{m}{2n}\sum_{q\in Z^n,\, |q-p|=1} (x_q(t) - x_p(t))dt$$

$$+ x_p(t)\sum_{q\in Z^n} (\lambda_q - \beta_q)(\delta_{pq} - x_q(t))dt,$$

where $\{\beta_p\}_{p\in Z^n}$ is a non-negative bounded sequence, $\{\gamma_p\}_{p\in Z^n}$ is a real sequence satisfying $\sum_p |\gamma_p - \beta_p| < +\infty$, $m > 0$ and $B_p(t)$, $p\in Z^n$, are independent one-dimensional Brownian motions.

In order to formulate a continuum limit of the SDE (4.1) we start with two bounded continuous functions $\beta(u)$ and $\gamma(u)$ defined on R^n such that $\gamma(u) - \beta(u) \equiv c(u)$ is Lebesgue integrable and further that $\sum_p |c(p/N)| < +\infty$ for every $N \geq 1$. For each $N \geq 1$, set

$$(4.2)\qquad \beta_p^{(N)} = \beta(p/N),\quad m^{(N)} = N^2 \quad\text{and}\quad \gamma_p^{(N)} - \beta_p^{(N)} = c(p/N).$$

For any continuous probability density $X(u)$ on R^n, set

$$(4.3)\qquad x_p^{(N)} = \int_{V_p^{(N)}} X(u)du$$

where $V_p^{(N)}$ is the cube centered at p/N with the edge-length $1/N$. Then by virtue of Theorem 3.1 there is a unique solution $x_p^{(N)}(t)$, $p\in Z^n$, of the SDE (4.1) starting at $x_p^{(N)}$, $p\in Z^n$, with β_p, c_p and m replaced by $\beta_p^{(N)}$, $c_p^{(N)}$ and N^2 respectively. For the solution $x_p^{(N)}(t)$, $p \in Z^n$, one can define a probability-density-valued process $X_t^{(N)}(u)$, $u \in R^n$ by a suitable interpolation so that

$$(4.4) \qquad X_t^{(N)}(u) = N^n x_p^{(N)}(t) \qquad \text{for } u = p/N \qquad (p \in Z^n).$$

Clearly $X_t^{(N)}(u)$ satisfies the following stochastic differential equation (SDE),

$$(4.5) \qquad X_t^{(N)}(p/N) = X_0^{(N)}(p/N) + \int_0^t \sqrt{\beta(p/N)X_s^{(N)}(p/N)}\, dB_s^{(N)}(p/N)$$

$$- \int_0^t X_s^{(N)}(p/N)\,(N^{-n}\sum_q \sqrt{\beta(q/N)X_s^{(N)}(q/N)}\, dB_s^{(N)}(q/N))ds$$

$$+ \int_0^t \frac{1}{2}\Delta_N X_s^{(N)}(p/N)ds$$

$$+ \int_0^t X_s^{(N)}(p/N)\,(c(p/N) - N^{-n}\sum_q c(q/N)X_s^{(N)}(q/N))ds$$

where $\Delta_N X(p/N) = (N^2/d)\sum_{q:|q-p|=1}(X(q/N) - X(p/N))$, and $B_t^{(N)}(p/N) = N^{n/2}B_p(t)$.

To formulate a continuum limit of the SDE (4.5) let us introduce an infinite dimensional standard Brownian motion. Let $\mathcal{S}(R^n)$ be the space of rapidly decreasing C^∞-functions on R^n, equipped with the Schwartz topology, and let $\mathcal{S}'(R^n)$ be its topological dual, namely $\mathcal{S}'(R^n)$ is the space of tempered distributions. An $\mathcal{S}'(R^n)$-valued continuous process B_t is called an $\mathcal{S}'(R^n)$-valued standard Brownian motion if, for each $\phi \in \mathcal{S}(R^n)$, $\langle B_t, \phi \rangle$ is a one-dimensional Gaussian process with

$$(4.6) \qquad E\langle B_t,\phi\rangle = 0 \quad \text{and} \quad E(\langle B_t,\phi\rangle\langle B_t\ \psi\rangle) = (\phi,\psi)\min\{t,s\}$$

where $(\phi,\psi) = \int_{R^n}\phi(u)\psi(u)du$.

Suppose one can show that $X_t^{(N)}(u)$ converges as $N \to \infty$ to a probability-density-valued process $X_t(u)$. Then it should satisfy the following stochastic differential equation (SDE):

$$(4.7) \qquad X_t(u) = X_0(u) + \int_0^t \sqrt{\beta(u)X_s(u)}\, dB_s(u)$$

$$- \int_0^t \int_{R^n} X_s(u)\sqrt{\beta(v)X_s(v)}\, dB_s(v)dv$$

$$+ \int_0^t \frac{1}{2} \Delta X_s(u) ds$$

$$+ \int_0^t X_s(u)(c(u) - \int_{R^n} c(v) X_s(v) dv) ds$$

where Δ stands for the Laplace operator on R^n.

Let $P(R^n)$ be the totality of probability measures equipped with the topology of weak convergence. Regarding $X_t^{(N)}$ as a $P(R^n)$-valued continuous process we denote by $P^{(N)}$ the probability distribution on the path space $C([0,\infty), P(R^n))$ induced by $X_t^{(N)}$, $t \geq 0$. Then it can be shown that $P^{(N)}$, $N \geq 1$, is tight, and any limit point of $P^{(N)}$, $N \geq 1$, is a solution of the $(P(R^n), L)$-martingale problem with

$$\text{(4.8)} \qquad LF(\mu) = \frac{1}{2} \int_{R^n} \mu(du) \beta(u) \frac{\delta^2 F}{\delta\mu(u)^2}$$

$$- \frac{1}{2} \int_{R^n \times R^n} \mu(du)\mu(dv)(<\mu,\beta> - \beta(u) - \beta(v)) \frac{\delta^2 F}{\delta\mu(u)\delta\mu(v)}$$

$$+ \int_{R^n} \mu(du) \frac{1}{2} \Delta(\frac{\delta F}{\delta\mu})(u)$$

$$+ \int_{R^n} \mu(du)(c(u) - <\mu,c>) \frac{\delta F}{\delta\mu(u)} \qquad (\mu \in P(R^n))$$

where $<\mu,\phi>$ denotes the integral of ϕ by μ, the domain $\mathcal{D}(L)$ of L consists of such $F(\mu) = f(<\mu,\phi_1>, \cdots, <\mu,\phi_k>)$ with $\phi_1, \cdots, \phi_k \in C_b^2(R^n)$ and $f \in C_b^2(R^k)$, and

$$\frac{\delta F}{\delta\mu(u)} = \lim_{\varepsilon \downarrow 0} \frac{F(\mu + \varepsilon\delta_u) - F(\mu)}{\varepsilon} \qquad \text{(if exists)}$$

with δ_u the Dirac measure at $u \in R^n$. In particular, if $\beta(u)$ and $c(u)$ are constant, then L of (4.8) is nothing but the generator of Fleming-Viot model with $\Delta/2$ as its mutation operator, which defines a $P(R^n)$-valued diffusion process (X_t, P_μ) uniquely. It is known that, for each $t > 0$, the random measure X_t is singular w.r.t. the Lebesgue measure P_μ-a.e. if $n \geq 3$, and furthermore, it is plausible that the same conclusion may hold even for $n = 2$, but if $n = 1$, then, for each $t > 0$, X_t would have an L^2_{loc}-density w.r.t. the Lebesgue measure P_μ-a.e. since the corresponding measure-valued branching process has these properties ([1], [2], [9]).

We would here like to assert that the SDE (4.7) not only makes sense but also is well-posed as an $S'(R^1)$-valued SDE as far as $n = 1$ is concerned. Consequently the solution defines a diffusion process taking values in a nice state space E,

$$(4.9) \qquad E = \{X(u)\,;\,[0,\infty) \to R_+ \text{ continuous}, \int_{R^1} X(u)du = 1, \text{ and}$$

$$\sup_u e^{-\lambda|u|}|X(u)| < +\infty \text{ for every } \lambda > 0\}.$$

Let $n = 1$. Supposing that $\beta(u)$ and $c(u)$ in (4.8) are constant, we denote by (X_t, P_μ) the $P(R^1)$-valued diffusion process associated with L of (4.8). Then we have the following.

Theorem 4.1. Let an arbitrary $\mu \in P(R^1)$ be fixed. Then
(i) X_t has a density $X_t(u)$ w.r.t. the Lebesgue measure for all $t > 0$ and $t \to X_t(\cdot)$ is an E-valued continuous function, P_μ-almost surely.
(ii) X_t satisfies the following SDE:

$$X_t(u) = X_{t_0}(u) + \int_{t_0}^t \sqrt{X_s(u)}\, dB_s(u) - \int_{t_0}^t \int_{R_1} X_s(u)\sqrt{X_s(v)}\, dB_s(v)dv$$

$$+ \int_{t_0}^t \frac{1}{2}\Delta X_s(u)ds \quad \text{for all } 0 < t_0 < t, \ P_\mu\text{-almost surely.}$$

Finally it would be an important problem to find a "true state space" of the Fleming-Viot process for $n \geq 2$. Then, as is seen in the above, one cannot expect that the SDE (4.7) makes sense. But if we take account of an integral operator such as a generator of a jump-type Markov process in place of $\Delta/2$ in (4.8), it is possible to characterize the state space of the associated Fleming-Viot process as a set of discrete probability measures by making use of another kind of stochastic equations [14].

References

[1] D. Dawson and K. Hochberg, The carrying dimension of a stochastic measure diffusion, Ann. Prob. 7, 693-703 (1979).

[2] D. Dawson, Measure-valued processes; construction, qualitative behavior and stochastic geometry, Technical report series of the Laboratory for Research in Statistics and Probability No.53, Carleton Univ. (1985).

[3] S. N. Ethier, A class of infinite dimensional diffusions occurring in population genetics, Indiana Univ. Math. J. 30, 925-935 (1981).

[4] W. H. Fleming and M. Viot, Some measure-valued Markov processes in population genetics theory, Indiana Univ. Math. J. 28 817-843 (1979).

[5] J. H. Gillespie, Natural selection for within-generation variance in offspring number, Genetics 76, 601-606 (1974).

[6] S. Karlin and J. McGregor, On some stochastic models in genetics, "Stochastic Models in Medicine and Biology" ed. by J. Gurland, Univ. of Wisconsin Press, Madison, 245-279 (1964).

[7] N. Konno and T. Shiga, Some measure-valued diffusion processes and their stochastic differential equations, (in preparation).

[8] N. Okada, On the uniqueness problem of two dimensional diffusion processes occurring in population genetics, Z. Wahr. verw. Geb. 56, 63-74 (1981).

[9] Roelly-Coppoleta, Un critère de convergence pour les lois de processus a valeurs measures, application aux processus de branchments, (preprint).

[10] K. Sato, Diffusion processes and a class of Markov chains related to population genetics, Osaka J. Math. 13, 631-659 (1976).

[11] K. Sato, Convergence to a diffusion of a multi-allelic model in population genetics, Adv. Appl. Prob. 10, 538-562 (1978).

[12] T. Shiga, Diffusion processes in population genetics, J. Math. Kyoto Univ. 21, 133-151 (1981).

[13] T. Shiga, A certain class of infinite dimensional diffusion processes arising in population genetics, (to appear in J. Math. Soc. Japan).

[14] T. Shiga, A. Shimizu and H. Tanaka, A stochastic equation for some measure-valued diffusion, (in preparation).

[15] T. Yamada and S. Watanabe, On the uniqueness of solutions of stochastic differential equations, J. Math. Kyoto Univ. 11, 155-167 (1971).

STATIONARY DISTRIBUTION OF A DIFFUSION PROCESS TAKING VALUES IN PROBABILITY DISTRIBUTIONS ON THE PARTITIONS

Akinobu Shimizu
Department of Mathematics
Nagoya Institute of Technology
Nagoya 466, Japan

Summary

The diffusion process, which will be discussed in this paper, is closely related to a genetical model which has been investigated by T. Ohta. We will discuss an n locus haploid model in which mutation, gene conversion and random drift are taken into consideration. Since we are concerned only with the average identity probability at different loci on one chromosome, random partitions of the number n determined by chromosomes with n loci should be investigated. The diffusion process describes the time evolution of distributions of the random partitions.

The average probability of types of chromosomes at equilibrium, that is, the mean vector of the stationary distribution can be obtained exactly. It is written in a form similar to the Ewens sampling formula. This result will be applied to calculation of the average identity probability at different loci on one chromosome.

1. Construction of a sequence of Markov chains

First, we will explain partitions of a natural number n. The set of natural numbers is denoted by $\underline{N}$. Define a partition of n to be a sequence

$$X = (x_1, \ x_2, \ \ldots., \ x_k) \in \underline{N}^k$$

such that $\sum_i x_i = n$ and $x_1 \geq x_2 \geq x_3 \geq \cdots \geq x_k \geq 1$.

The terms x_i are called the parts of X and we say X has k parts. If the partition X has α_i parts equal to i, then we write

$$X = \langle 1^{\alpha_1}, 2^{\alpha_2}, \dots, n^{\alpha_n} \rangle, \ \alpha_i \geq 0, \ \sum_i i\,\alpha_i = n.$$

For instance,

$$(3, 2, 1, 1) = \langle 1^2, 2^1, 3^1, 4^0, 5^0, 6^0, 7^0 \rangle.$$

The set of partitions of n with k parts is denoted by S_k^n. S_n^n has a single element (1, 1, 1,...., 1), and S_1^n consists of an element (n). Obviously, $S^n = \sum_k S_k^n$.

Next, we explain the meaning of a partition

$$X = (x_1, x_2, \dots, x_k) = \langle 1^{\alpha_1}, 2^{\alpha_2}, \dots, n^{\alpha_n} \rangle$$

in the application to population genetics. We consider n locus model, so we find n genes on a chromosome. A partition X describes a state of a chromosome. X means that there exist k kinds of alleles which occupy x_1 loci, x_2 loci,...., x_k loci. In other words, X describes that there exist α_i kinds of alleles occupying i loci for each i. Since we are concerned with the average identity probability of genes at different loci on one chromosome, it is sufficient to consider a Markov chain taking values in probability distributions on S^n.

Mutation. The concept, mutation, which will be discussed in this paper, follows the infinite allele model proposed by Kimura and Crow [4]. Assume that every mutant is new, and that the decreasing rate of gene frequencies is equal to v(1/N) per generation. Here, N stands for the number of population, and 1/N equals the time of one generation in diffusion approximation. Let us consider a partition

$$X = \langle 1^{\alpha_1}, 2^{\alpha_2}, \dots, i^{\alpha_i}, \dots, n^{\alpha_n} \rangle$$

such that $\alpha_i > 0$ for some $i > 2$. If a gene of the alleles occupying i loci is changed by mutation, the partition X is replaced by

$$X' = \langle 1^{\alpha_1+1}, 2^{\alpha_2}, \dots, (i-1)^{\alpha_{i-1}+1}, i^{\alpha_i-1}, \dots, n^{\alpha_n} \rangle$$

with the rate $i\alpha_i v(1/N)$ per generation. Suppose that $\alpha_i > 0$ for $i = 2$. A partition

$$X = \langle 1^{\alpha_1}, 2^{\alpha_2}, \ldots, n^{\alpha_n} \rangle$$

is changed to

$$X' = \langle 1^{\alpha_1+2}, 2^{\alpha_2-1}, \ldots, n^{\alpha_n} \rangle$$

with the rate $2\alpha_2 v(1/N)$. A partition X is not changed when a gene of the alleles occupying a single locus is changed by mutation.

If X can be changed to X' by mutation, we call X' to be a consequent of X by mutation. If $X \in S_k^n$ ($k < n$) and X' is a consequent of X by mutation, then $X' \in S_{k+1}^n$.

<u>Gene conversion.</u> The concept, gene conversion, which was introduced by T.Ohta [6], can be formulated as follows: If a gene conversion occurs between a gene of the alleles occupying i_1 loci and a gene of the alleles occupying i_2 loci, a partition

$$X = \langle 1^{\alpha_1}, 2^{\alpha_2}, \ldots, i_1^{\alpha_{i_1}}, \ldots, i_2^{\alpha_{i_2}}, \ldots, n^{\alpha_n} \rangle,$$

$$\alpha_{i_1}, \alpha_{i_2} > 0, \quad i_1 + 2 < i_2,$$

is changed to

$$X' = \langle 1^{\alpha_1}, 2^{\alpha_2}, \ldots,$$
$$(i_1-1)^{\alpha_{i_1-1}+1}, i_1^{\alpha_{i_1}-1}, \ldots, i_2^{\alpha_{i_2}-1}, (i_2+1)^{\alpha_{i_2+1}+1}, \ldots, n^{\alpha_n} \rangle$$

or

$$X'' = \langle 1^{\alpha_1}, 2^{\alpha_2}, \ldots, i_1^{\alpha_{i_1}-1}, (i_1+1)^{\alpha_{i_1+1}+1}, \ldots,$$
$$(i_2-1)^{\alpha_{i_2-1}+1}, i_2^{\alpha_{i_2}-1}, \ldots, n^{\alpha_n} \rangle.$$

Each rate of the both changes equals $i_1\alpha_{i_1} \cdot i_2\alpha_{i_2} \cdot \lambda\ (1/N)$ per generation. A partition

$$X = \langle 1^{\alpha_1}, 2^{\alpha_2}, \ldots, i_1^{\alpha_{i_1}}, \ldots, i_2^{\alpha_{i_2}}, \ldots, n^{\alpha_n} \rangle,$$

$$\alpha_{i_1}, \alpha_{i_2} > 0, \ i_1 + 2 = i_2,$$

is changed to

$$X' = \langle 1^{\alpha_1}, 2^{\alpha_2}, \ldots, (i_1-1)^{\alpha_{i_1-1}+1}, i_1^{\alpha_{i_1}-1}, \ldots,$$
$$i_2^{\alpha_{i_2}-1}, (i_2+1)^{\alpha_{i_2+1}+1}, \ldots, n^{\alpha_n} \rangle$$

or

$$X'' = \langle 1^{\alpha_1}, 2^{\alpha_2}, \ldots, i_1^{\alpha_{i_1}-1}, (i_1+1)^{\alpha_{i_1+1}+2}, i_2^{\alpha_{i_2}-1}, \ldots, n^{\alpha_n} \rangle.$$

Each rate is equal to $i_1\alpha_{i_1} \cdot i_2\alpha_{i_2} \cdot \lambda\ (1/N)$.

A partition

$$X = \langle 1^{\alpha_1}, 2^{\alpha_2}, \ldots, i_1^{\alpha_{i_1}}, i_2^{\alpha_{i_2}}, \ldots, n^{\alpha_n} \rangle,$$

$\alpha_{i_1}, \alpha_{i_2} > 0$, $i_1 + 1 = i_2$, moves to

$$X' = \langle 1^{\alpha_1}, 2^{\alpha_2}, \ldots, (i_1-1)^{\alpha_{i_1-1}+1}, i_1^{\alpha_{i_1}-1},$$
$$i_2^{\alpha_{i_2}-1}, (i_2+1)^{\alpha_{i_2+1}+1}, \ldots, n^{\alpha_n} \rangle$$

with the rate $i_1\alpha_{i_1} \cdot i_2\alpha_{i_2} \cdot \lambda \cdot (1/N)$. If a gene conversion occurs between two genes of different kinds of the alleles occupying i loci, a partition

$$X = \langle 1^{\alpha_1}, 2^{\alpha_2}, \ldots, i^{\alpha_i}, \ldots, n^{\alpha_n} \rangle, \ \alpha_i \geq 2,$$

is changed to

$$X' = \langle 1^{\alpha_1}, \ldots, (i-1)^{\alpha_{i-1}+1}, i^{\alpha_i-2}, (i+1)^{\alpha_{i+1}+1}, \ldots, n^{\alpha_n} \rangle$$

with the rate $i\alpha_i \cdot i(\alpha_i - 1) \cdot \lambda \cdot (1/N)$.

In the above explanation, the symbol X', which is written four times, should be slightly changed according to each case when i_1 or i = 1. It is obvious that we do not need to write anything on the alleles occupying (i - 1) loci when i = 1.

If X can be changed to X' by gene conversion, X' is called a consequent of X by gene conversion. If $X \in S_k^n$ $(k > 1)$ and X' is a consequent of X by gene conversion, then $X' \in S_k^n$ or $X' \in S_{k-1}^n$.

We can see easily the following facts:

(I) The statements (a) and (a') are equivalent;

(a) $X \in S_k^n$, $1 \leq k < n$, and $X' \in S_{k+1}^n$ is a consequent of X by mutation, (a') $X' \in S^n_{k+1}$, $1 \leq k < n$, and $X \in S^n_k$ is a consequent of X' by gene conversion.

(II) The statements (b) and (b') are equivalent;

(b) $X \in S^n_k$, $1 < k < n$, and $X' \in S^n_k$ is a consequent of X by gene conversion,

(b') $X' \in S^n_k$, $1 < k < n$, and $X \in S^n_k$ is a consequent of X' by gene conversion.

(III) The statements (c) and (d) hold;

(c) If distinct partitions X' and X'' are consequents of X by mutation, then X' (X'') is a consequent of X'' (X') by gene conversion respectively.

(d) If $X \in S^n_k$, $1 \leq k < n$, is changed to X' by mutation, and if X' is changed to $X'' \in S^n_k$ by gene conversion, then X'' (X) is a consequent of X (X'') by gene conversion respectively.

The facts (I) (II) (III) tell us that there exist triangles of the following three types (A),(B) and (C):

(A) $X \in S^n_k$, X',X''(distinct) $\in S^n_{k+1}$, $1 < k < n$. X' and X'' are consequents of X by mutation (i.e. X' and X'' can be changed to X by gene conversion). X' and X'' can be changed to each other by gene conversion.

(B) X, $X' \in S^n_k$ ($1 < k < n$) are distinct, and $X'' \in S^n_{k+1}$. X and X' can be changed to X'' by mutation (i.e. X'' can be changed to X and X' by gene conversion). X and X' can be changed to each other by gene conversion.

(C) X, X', $X'' \in S^n_k$, $1 < k < n$. Any two partitions of X, X' and X'' can be changed to each other by gene conversion.

We can see that , for each $X \in S^n_k$ ($1 < k < n -1$), there exist at least one triangles including x as a vertex in some manner among the three types (A),(B) and (C).

Let $q_{X_1 X_2} \cdot (1/N)$ be the rate of mutation or gene conversion from X_1 to X_2 per generation. If X_2 is not a consequent from X_1 in any sense, then $q_{X_1 X_2} = 0$. The next lemma will play a basic role to calculate the mean vector of the stationary distribution of the diffusion process which is the limiting process of the sequence of Markov chains being constructed in this section.

Lemma 1.1. For any distinct elements X_1, X_2 and X_3 of S^n, the equality

$$q_{X_1X_2} \cdot q_{X_2X_3} \cdot q_{X_3X_1} = q_{X_1X_3} \cdot q_{X_3X_2} \cdot q_{X_2X_1}$$

holds.

Proof. Though we should consider several cases, here we discuss only a case for simplicity. Put

$$X_1 = \langle 1^{\alpha_1}, \ldots, i^{\alpha_i}, \ldots, j^{\alpha_j}, \ldots, n^{\alpha_n} \rangle,$$

$$X_2 = \langle 1^{\alpha_1+1}, \ldots, (i-1)^{\alpha_{i-1}+1}, i^{\alpha_i-1}, \ldots, j^{\alpha_j}, \ldots, n^{\alpha_n} \rangle,$$

$$X_3 = \langle 1^{\alpha_1+1}, \ldots, i^{\alpha_i}, \ldots, (j-1)^{\alpha_{j-1}+1}, j^{\alpha_j-1}, \ldots, n^{\alpha_n} \rangle.$$

Here, we assume that α_i, α_j are strictly positive, and that $2 < i < j-1$. X_1 can be changed to X_2 and X_3 by mutation (i.e. X_1 is a consequent of X_2 and X_3 by gene conversion), besides X_2 and X_3 can be changed to each other by gene conversion. We have

$$q_{X_1X_2} = i \cdot \alpha_i \cdot v, \qquad q_{X_2X_1} = (\alpha_1+1)(i-1)(\alpha_{i-1}+1)\lambda,$$

$$q_{X_2X_3} = (i-1)(\alpha_{i-1}+1)\, j\alpha_j\, \lambda, \qquad q_{X_3X_2} = i\alpha_i(j-1)(\alpha_{j-1}+1)\,\lambda,$$

$$q_{X_3X_1} = (\alpha_1+1)(j-1)(\alpha_{j-1}+1)\lambda, \qquad q_{X_1X_3} = j\alpha_j v.$$

Obviously, the equality holds. In other cases, the equality can be verified analogously.

Define $q_{XX} = -\sum_{Y \neq X} q_{XY}$. Let $p(n)$ be the total number of partitions of n, whose generating function is given by

$$\sum_{n \geq 0} p(n)\, u^n = \prod_{k \geq 1} (1 - u^k)^{-1}.$$

Note that the matrix $\{ q_{XY} \}_{X,Y \in S^n}$ generates a continuous time Markov chain with $p(n)$ states, which has a unique stationary distribution.

Sequence of Markov chains. Let $M(S^n)$ be the set of probability distributions $p = (p_X)_{X \in S^n}$, where $p_X \geqq 0$ and $\sum_X p_X = 1$. p_X means the frequency of chromosomes of type X. By a usual method, we construct a sequence of Markov chains incorporating mutation, gene conversion and random drift. Let N be a positive integer, which means the total number of population. The frequency of chromosomes of type X is assumed to change to $\gamma_X^N(p)$, $X \in S^n$, from $p_N = (p_X)_{X \in S^n}$ by mutation and gene conversion. $\gamma_X(p)$ is given by

$$\gamma_X^N(p) = p_X + (1/N) \sum_Y p_Y q_{YX} ,$$

where 1/N is the time interval in the continuous path space which means one generation.

Let Z_+ be the set of non-negative integers. Put $K_N = \{ A/N \in M(S^N) : A$ is a mapping of S^N into $Z_+ \}$. Define Ω_N to be the space of functions ω defined on Z_+ which take values in K_N. It is endowed with the topology of pointwise convergence on Z_+, and let $\underline{M}^{(N)}$ be the class of Borel sets in Ω_N. Define the coordinate map $Y(m)$ of Ω_N to K_N by $Y(m)(\omega) = \omega(m)$, and let $\underline{M}_m^{(N)}$ be the σ-algebra of subsets of Ω_N generated by $Y(k)$, $k = 0,1,\ldots,m$.

A sequence of Markov chains $(Q_p^N , Y(m))$, $p \in M(S^n)$, $m \in Z_+$, with the discrete time parameter m is defined as follows. Let Q_p^N be the unique probability measure on $(\Omega_N, \underline{M}^{(N)})$ for each N such that $Q_p^N (Y(0) = p) = 1$, and

$$Q_p^N (Y(m+1) = A/N \mid \underline{M}_m^N) = N! \prod_X (A_x!)^{-1} \{ \gamma_x^N(Y(m)) \}^{A_X},$$

where $A = (A_X)_{X \in S^n}$, $A_X \in Z_+$, $\sum_X A_X = N$.

2. Diffusion Approximation to the Markov chains

Let Ω be the space $C([0,\infty), M(S^n))$ with the topology of uniform convergence on compact sets, and $\underline{M}$ denotes the class of Borel sets in Ω. Define the coordinate map $p(t)$ of Ω to $M(S^n)$ by $p(t)(\omega) = \omega(t)$, $\omega \in \Omega$, for each $t \geq 0$. Let $\underline{M}_t$ be the σ-algebra of subsets of Ω generated by $p(s)$, $0 \leq s \leq t$, for each t. Define the map η_N of Ω_N to Ω by

$$p(t)\cdot \eta_N = Y([Nt]) + (Nt - [Nt])\{ Y([Nt] +1) - Y([Nt]) \},$$

for $t \geq 0$, where $[Nt]$ denotes the integral part of Nt. Let $P_p^{(N)}$ be the probability measure on $(\Omega, \underline{M})$ defined by

$$P_p^{(N)} = Q_p^{(N)} \cdot \eta_N^{-1}, \quad p \in K_N ,$$

where K_N is contained in $M(S^n)$.

Define the degenerate differential operator

$$(2.1) \quad L = (1/2) \sum_{X,Y \in S^n} (p_X \delta_{XY} - p_X p_Y) \partial^2 / \partial p_X \partial p_Y + \sum_{X \in S^n} b_X(p) \partial / \partial p_X ,$$

where $b_X(p)$ is given by

$$(2.2) \quad b_X(p) = \sum_Y p_Y q_{YX} .$$

The operator L operates on smooth functions defined on $M(S^n)$. A solution to the martingale problem for L starting $p \in M(S^n)$ is a probability measure P_p on $(\Omega, \underline{M})$ for which $P_p(p(0) = p) = 1$ and

$$\{ f(p(t)) - \int_0^t (Lf)(p(s))ds, \underline{M}_t , t \geq 0 \}$$

is a P_p- martingale for every $f \in C^2(M(S^n))$. The uniqueness of solutions to this martingale problem has been established by Ethier [2]. The Sato's result [9] combined with the uniqueness tells us the following fact: Let $p \in M(S^n)$. If $p_N \in K_N$ for $N = 1,2,...$ and $\{ p_N\}$ converges to p, then the sequence of probability measures $P_{p_N}^{(N)}$

converges to the solution P_p to the martingale problem as N tends to the infinity.

Hence, we say that the sequence of Markov chains constructed in the section 1 can be approximated by the diffusion process with the generator L given by (2.1) and (2.2). Note that the operator L has the same form as the generator of the diffusion describing a p(n)-allele model incorporating mutation and random drift with single locus, but we should give a remark that the matrix $\{ q_{XY}\}$ depends on the combinatorial structure of the partitions.

3. Stationary distribution of the diffusion process

The diffusion process with the generator L given by (2.1) and (2.2) is easily shown to be ergodic, since the matrix $\{q_{XY}\}$ generates an ergodic Markov chain. Hence, the diffusion has a unique stationary distribution $\mu(dp)$ on $M(S^n)$. In this section, we will discuss only the mean vector of the stationary distribution μ. Noting that the coefficients $b_X(p)$ given by (2.2) are expressed by linear combinations of p_X, $X \in S^n$, we can obtain the next lemma.

Lemma 3.1. The mean vector $\bar{p} = \{ \bar{p}_X \}_{X \in S^n}$ of the stationary distribution $\mu(dp)$ satisfies the system of linear equations (3.1) and (3.2):

$$(3.1) \qquad b_X(\bar{p}) = \sum_Y \bar{p}_Y \, q_{YX} = 0,$$

$$(3.2) \qquad \sum_X \bar{p}_X = 1.$$

The system of linear equations (3.1) and (3.2) has a unique solution.

Proof. Let P_p be the solution to the martingale problem stated in the section 2, and let $p(t) = (p_X(t))_{X \in S^n}$ be the coordinate map. The fact that P_p is the solution to the martingale problem implies the equality

$$E_\mu[p_X(t)] - E_\mu[p_X(0)] = \int_0^t E_\mu[(Lp_X)(p(s))] \, ds.$$

The left-hand side is equal to zero because μ is the stationary distribution. On the other hand, $Lp_X = b_X(p)$, hence the right-hand side equals

$$\int_0^t \langle b_X(p), \mu \rangle ds = t \langle b_X(p), \mu \rangle = t\, b_X(\bar{p}).$$ Thus, (3.1) holds.

(3.2) holds obviously. The uniqueness of solutions to (3.1) and (3.2) follows from the facts that the Markov chain generated by the matrix $\{q_{XY}\}$ has a unique stationary distribution , and that a solution to (3.1) and (3.2) is a stationary distribution of the Markov chain.

A finite sequence $\{X_1, X_2, \ldots, X_J\}$ of partitions is called (X_1, X_J)-chain if X_{j+1} is a consequent of X_j by mutation or gene conversion for each $j = 1,2,\ldots,J-1$. Lemma 1.1 shows that the value

$$(q_{X_1X_2}/ q_{X_2X_1})(q_{X_2X_3}/ q_{X_3X_2}).....(q_{X_{J-1}X_J}/ q_{X_JX_{J-1}})$$

does not depend on the choice of (X_1, X_J)- chains.

Let X be any partition of n, and let $(X_1, X_2, \ldots, X_J)$ be a $((n), X)$-chain. Put

$$(3.3) \qquad p_X' = \prod_{j=1}^{J-1} (q_{X_jX_{j+1}} / q_{X_{j+1}X_j}), \text{ and } p'_{(n)} = 1,$$

then, we can see easily that $(p'_X)_{X \in S^n}$ satisfies (3). Therefore,

$$\bar{p}_X = p'_X / \sum_Y p'_Y, \; X \in S^n,$$

satisfies (3.1) and (3.2).

Let $X = \langle 1^{\alpha_1}, 2^{\alpha_2}, \ldots, n^{\alpha_n} \rangle$, and put $\alpha(X) = \sum_i \alpha_i$. Let the set $\{\alpha_{i_1}, \alpha_{i_2}, \ldots, \alpha_{i_d}\}$ be the collection of α_i such that $\alpha_i > 0$. We can suppose that $i_1 < i_2 < \ldots < i_d$. Consider a $((n), X)$-chain of the following type : First, mutation occurs successively $\{\alpha(X)-1\}$ times. That is,

$X_1 = (n)$, $X_2 = (n-1, 1), \ldots, X_{\alpha(X)} = (n - \alpha(X) + 1,1,1,\ldots,1)$.

After that, gene conversion occurs successively $\{n - \alpha(X) - (i_d - 1)\}$ times, such that the number of genes of each allele, except the one that exists initially, is increasing monotonously, and the chain includes the partitions

$$(n - [\alpha(X)-1]-[i_d-1], i_d, 1, 1, \dots, 1),$$
$$(n - [\alpha(X)-1]-2[i_d-1], i_d, i_d, 1, 1, \dots, 1),$$
$$\dots\dots$$
$$(n - [\alpha(X)-1]-(\alpha_{i_d}-1)[i_d-1], i_d, \dots, i_d, 1, \dots, 1),$$
$$(n-[\alpha(X)-1]-(\alpha_{i_d}-1)[i_d-1]-\alpha_{i_{d-1}}[i_{d-1}-1], i_d, \dots, i_d, i_{d-1}, \dots, i_{d-1}, 1, \dots, 1),$$
$$\dots\dots\dots .$$

<u>Lemma 3.2.</u> Let $\{ X_1, X_2, \dots, X_J\}$ be a $((n), X)$-chain of the type stated above. Then, the equalities

$$\prod_{j=1}^{J-1} q_{X_j X_{j+1}} = \{ n! / i_d! (i_d-1)! \} \prod_{i=1}^{n} \{ (i-1)! \}^{\alpha_i} \{ (\alpha(X)-1)! / \alpha_1! \} v^{\alpha(X)-1} \lambda^{n-\alpha(X)-i_d+1},$$

and

$$\prod_{j=1}^{J-1} q_{X_{j+1} X_j} = \{ (n-1)!/ i_d!(i_d-1)! \} \prod_{i=2}^{n} \alpha_i! \prod_{i=1}^{n} (i!)^{\alpha_i} (\alpha(X)-1)! \lambda^{n-i_d},$$

hold.

Lemma 3.2 is shown by a simple combinatorial calculation. By Lemma 3.2, we can see that $\bar{p}'_X$ given by (3.3) is written as follows,

$$\bar{p}'_X = \{ n / \prod_{i=1}^{n} \alpha_i! i^{\alpha_i}\} (v / \lambda)^{\alpha(X)-1}.$$

By making use of the well-known equality (See [8], p.70),

$$\sum_{X \in S^n} n! \prod_{i=1}^{n} \{ t^{\alpha_i} / \alpha_i! i^{\alpha_i}\} = t(t+1)(t+2)\dots\dots(t+n-1),$$

we see

$$\sum_{X} \bar{p}'_X = \{ 1/ (n-1)! \} \{ (v/\lambda)+1 \}\{ (v/\lambda)+2 \}\dots\dots\{ (v/\lambda)+n-1\}.$$

Hence, we obtain the next theorem.

<u>Theorem 3.1.</u> The mean vector $p = \{\bar{p}_X\}$, $X \in S^n$, of the stationary distribution of the diffusion process with the generator L given by (3.1) and (3.2) can be written in the form:

$$\bar{p}_X = \{ n! / \theta(\theta+1)(\theta+2)\dots\dots(\theta+n-1) \} \prod_{j=1}^{n} \{ \theta^{\alpha_j} / j^{\alpha_j} \alpha_j! \},$$

where $\theta = v / \lambda$.

This result will be applied in the section 5, and it will be useful in the discussion in [7].

4. Infinite allele model with single locus and the Ewens sampling formula

Recall the infinite allele model proposed by Kimura and Crow [4], and the Ewens sampling formula ([1], [3], [5], [11]).

Let Δ be the set of sequences ($x_1, x_2, \dots, x_j, \dots$) such that

$x_j \geqq x_{j+1} \geqq 0$ for each j, and $\sum_j x_j = 1$. The Poisson-Dirichlet distribution was first defined as a probability measure on the space Δ in the following way (Kingman [5]): Suppose that $x_1, x_2, \dots, x_m$ are random variables with the Dirichlet distribution having probability density function

$$\text{const. } x_1^{\alpha_1 - 1} x_2^{\alpha_2 - 1} \dots x_m^{\alpha_m - 1} dx_1 dx_2 \dots dx_{m-1}.$$

Assume that $\alpha_1 = \alpha_2 = \dots = \alpha_m = \theta/m$, and let $x_{(1)} \geqq x_{(2)} \geqq \dots \geqq x_{(m)}$ be the descending order statistics of these variables. The Poisson-Dirichlet distribution, which is denoted by $\mu_{PD}(dx)$, can be defined as the limiting distribution, as m tends to infinity, of the random variable

$$(x_{(1)}, x_{(2)}, \dots, x_{(m)}, 0, 0, \dots)$$

taking values in Δ.

Let a point $\bar{x} = (x_1, x_2, \dots, x_j, \dots) \in \Delta$ be fixed, and let $Z_1, Z_2, \dots, Z_n$ be independent identically distributed random variables such that $P[Z_j = k] = x_k$, $k=1,2,\dots$. Denote by $\alpha_i(Z) = \alpha_i(Z_1, Z_2, \dots, Z_n)$ the cardinality of the set { k : exactly i random variables of $Z_1, Z_2, \dots, Z_n$ are equal to k }. The random partition $\langle 1^{\alpha_1(Z)}, 2^{\alpha_2(Z)}, \dots, n^{\alpha_n(Z)} \rangle$ induces a probability distribution on S^n, which is denoted by $p_{\bar{x}}(X)$, $X \in S^n$. The next statement is known as the Ewens sampling formula [2].

$$(4.1) \quad \int p_{\bar{x}} (\langle 1^{\alpha_1}, 2^{\alpha_2}, \dots, n^{\alpha_n} \rangle) \mu_{PD}(d\bar{x}) =$$

$$= \{ n! / \theta(\theta+1) \ldots (\theta+n-1) \} \prod_{j=1}^{n} (\theta^{\alpha_j} / j^{\alpha_j} \alpha_j!).$$

In the references in population genetics, the parameter θ which appears in this formula is considered to be equal to 4Nv. Here, N stands for the effective population size, and v denotes the rate of mutation. It seems well-known that there exists some difference in parameters between mathematical references and genetical ones. From the mathematical point of view, the limiting diffusion processes are obtained by making the population size N tend to the infinity. So, in our formulation, the parameter θ in (4.1) is considered to be equal to 2v, where v(1/N) (or v(1/2N) in diploid model) means the mutation rate in Markov chains.

The Poisson-Dirichlet distribution is the stationary distribution of the diffusion process describing the infinite allele model with single locus in some sense. It seems clearer if a measure valued diffusion process of Fleming-Viot type is considered describing the infinite allele model. By the argument similar to [10], the measure valued diffusion process is shown to be ergodic. The stationary distribution of this process should be called Dirichlet random measure, which can be regarded as the limiting distribution of the sequence of finite dimensional Dirichlet distributions. Note that we do not need the order statistics in the above discussion of this paragraph. The Ewens sampling formula can be proved , replacing the Poisson-Dirichlet distribution by the Dirichlet random measure. More general arguments on measure valued diffusion processes and the Poisson random measure will appear in [11].

5. Average identity probability of genes at different loci on one chromosome

Let F_n be a function defined on the set of partitions S^n. $\mu(dp)$ denotes the stationary distribution of the diffusion as before. Consider the infinite allele model with mutation rate (v/λ)(1/2N) (or $(v/\lambda)(1/4N)$ in case of diploid model). The Poisson-Dirichlet distribution is considered to be defined for this mutation rate in the following. Theorem 1 and the argument of the previous section give that

(5.1) $\bar{p}_X = \int p_{\bar{x}}(X)\, \mu_{PD}(d\bar{x}).$

Let $X = \langle 1^{\alpha_1}, 2^{\alpha_2}, \ldots, n^{\alpha_n} \rangle$ be fixed. The probability that arbitrarily chosen j objects from n ones belong to the same kind is determined by the partition X. So, the probability is a function defined on S^n, and it will be denoted by $F_{n,j}$. We obtain the next theorem.

Theorem 5.1. The equality

$$(5.2) \quad \sum_{X \varepsilon S^n} \bar{p}_X F_{n,j}(X) = \lambda^{j-1}(j-1)! \,/\, \{v+\lambda\}\{v+2\lambda\}\ldots\{v+(j-1)\lambda\}.$$

holds.

Proof. First, we note the next fact:

$$\sum_{X \varepsilon S^n} p_{\bar{X}}(X) F_{n,j}(X) = P[\text{ arbitrarily chosen } j \text{ random variables } Z_{i_1}, Z_{i_2}, \ldots, Z_{i_j} \text{ from } Z_1, Z_2, \ldots, Z_n \text{ take the same values}]$$

$$= P[\, Z_1 = Z_2 = \ldots = Z_j \,]$$

$$= \sum_{X \varepsilon S^j} p_{\bar{X}}(X) F_{j,j}(X).$$

$$= p_{\bar{X}}(\,(j)\,).$$

By (5.1) and Theorem 3.1, we can see that the equality (5.2) holds.

Remark. Put $j = 2$ in Theorem 5.1. Then, the left-hand side is the average identity probability of genes at different loci on one chromosome discussed by Ohta, and the right-hand side is equal to $\lambda \,/\, (\lambda + v)$. This agrees with the corresponding part of the Ohta's results [6].

References

[1] Donnelly, P. (1985) Partition structures, Polya urns, the Ewens sampling formula and the ages of alleles. (preprint).

[2] Ethier, S.N. (1976) A class of degenerate diffusion processes occuring in population genetics. Comm.Pur Appl.Math., 29, 483-

493.

[3] Ewens, W. (1972) The sampling theory of selectively neutral alleles. Theor. Pop. Biol. 3, 87-112.

[4] Kimura, M. and Crow, J.F. (1964) The number of alleles that can be maintained in a finite population. Genetics 49, 725-736.

[5] Kingman J.F.C.(1978) Random partitions in population genetics. Proc.Roy.Soc.A.361, 1-20.

[6] Ohta, T. (1983) On the evolution of multigene families. Theor.Pop.Biol. 23, 216-240.

[7] Ohta, T. (1985) Actual number of alleles contained in a multigene family. Genet. Res. (to appear).

[8] Riordan, J. (1958) An introduction to Combinatorial Analysis. Wily Publications in Statistics, John Wily & Sons,Inc.,London.

[9] Sato, K. (1976) Diffusion processes and a class of Markov chains related to population genetics. Osaka J. Math. 13, 631-659.

[10] Shimizu, A. (1985) Diffusion approximation of an infinite allele model incorporating gene conversion. Population Genetics and Molecular Evolution, eds. T.Ohta, & K.Aoki, 243-255. Japan Sci. Soc. Press, Tokyo/Springer-Verlag,Berlin.

[11] Shiga, T. Shimizu, A. and Tanaka, H. (1985) Some measure-valued diffusion processes associated with genetical diffusion models. (preprint).

[12] Watterson, G.A. (1976) Stationary distribution of the infinitely-many neutral alleles diffusion model. J.Appl.Prob.13,639-651.

III. NEUROPHYSIOLOGY

Weak Convergence of Stochastic Neuronal Models

G. Kallianpur

University of North Carolina
Chapel Hill, North Carolina

Robert L. Wolpert

Duke University
Durham, North Carolina

1. Introduction to Stochastic Models for Neuronal Activity

The electrical behavior of neuronal membranes and the role of ion currents have been studied and understood since the landmark 1952 papers of Hodgkin and Huxley. The existence of ionic gates exhibiting stochastic behavior was confirmed over ten years ago with the development of the experimental patch-clamp technique, and the nature and structure of those ionic gates was illuminated dramatically in 1984 with the publication by Noda *et al.* [1984] of the complete amino acid chain comprising the sodium gating channel for the electric organ of *electrophorus electricus*. Despite all this experimental progress, and despite the wide interest in gaining a better understanding of the behavior of individual neurons and of systems of neurons, there has been little success in the efforts to develop stochastic mathematical models capable of reflecting and helping to predict neuronal activity. It is a goal of our research to develop such models in order to illuminate the connection between the microkinetic behavior of thousands of gating molecules scattered over the surface membrane of a single isolated neuron subject to a stream of excitatory and inhibitory impulses, and the macrokinetic behavior of that same neuron in generating and propagating action potentials and spike trains. We do not address the interesting questions of how networks of interconnected neurons behave.

One reason for the lack of modeling progress is the long list of major obstacles to be overcome. The easy models for mathematicians to construct and manipulate are deterministic, finite-dimensional, and linear. Models designed to reflect the interesting behavior of neurons must be stochastic, infinite-dimensional, and highly nonlinear.

The aspect of neuronal behavior most readily measured and most often modeled is the evolution of electrical voltage potential, the potential difference measured across the molecular membrane as a function of location and of time. This voltage potential difference arises in part from the selective permeability of the molecular membrane to the different ionic species (especially sodium Na^+, potassium K^+, calcium Ca^{++}, and chloride Cl^-) present within the cell and in the surrounding medium. This suggests that it may also be of interest to model the time evolution of the local permeabilities of

---

Research supported by Air Force Office of Scientific Research contract #F49620 85 C 0144.

the cell membrane to these ionic species.

Stochastic (or *random*) disturbances to a quiescent neuron arise from a number of different sources, each with a different characteristic scale of space and time.

On the slowest scale, action potentials from its neighbors periodically cause a given neuron to be flooded with a stream of vesicles of various chemicals called *neurotransmitters*. These floods arrive unpredictably and chaotically (although we naturally hope that our own neurons exhibit some pattern in their firing!), and can be modeled stochastically.

On a faster time scale, vesicles of neurotransmitters released by nearby neurons come haphazardly in both space and time. These vesicles vary in size and composition, and arrive at sites varying in their sensitivity to different neurotransmitters. Each such vesicle causes a jump in the membrane voltage potential at the site where it arrives, either up or down an amount depending upon the composition of the vesicle and the state of the neuron. Perhaps the arrivals are not truly random, but they are chaotic and (for us) unpredictable and are thus likely candidates for stochastic modeling.

On an even faster time scale, individual ionic channels selectively gate the passage of different ionic species by opening and closing thousands of times each second, with the rates of both opening and closing depending upon the voltage potential. Each time a gate opens a tiny current flows in a direction and at a rate depending upon both the membrane voltage potential and the concentration difference of each ionic species across the cell wall; these tiny pulses of current make their contributions to the membrane voltage potential in an apparently random manner, giving rise to a third source of random impulses affecting the state of the neuron.

Finally, the arrival and departure of individual ions cause extremely rapid current impulses which could be modeled using stochastic methods.

It is the second of these four sources of randomness which has received the most attention--- the haphazard arrival of individual vesicles of neurotransmitters. Motivated by our interest in the Hodgkin-Huxley equations, we are interested both in the randomness associated with vesicle arrivals and also in the third source of randomness listed above, the random opening and closing of ionic gating channels. If we scale time in such a way that individual ion channels seem to open and close in a noisy, random sequence, the passage of individual ions will seem to proceed at such a furious rate that random fluctuations are not apparent. Only the smooth mean behavior predicted by the law of large numbers would be observable. On such a time scale action potentials will occur so infrequently that we can safely focus on the behavior of the neuron in the absence of arriving action potentials, and vesicles will rarely seem to arrive.

For some modeling purposes it is not necessary to distinguish different points on the surface of the neuron; it is sufficient to model the entire neuronal membrane as a single point, and represent the (surface average of the) voltage potential as a single stochastic function of time. Even if the average ionic permeabilities must also be modeled, a finite-dimensional random function suffices. When it is necessary to distinguish the voltage potential at different locations, particularly in the course of modeling the generation and propagation of action potentials, we must regard the membrane voltage potential as a random function of both *time* and *location*, or else as a random function of time whose value at each particular instant of time must specify the value of the membrane potential at *infinitely* many points on the neuronal surface.

Several authors including Wan and Tuckwell [1979], Walsh [1981], and others have studied the membrane potential as a stochastic process indexed not by the usual one-dimensional time, but by a two-dimensional product of space and time, for the special case in which the part of the neuronal membrane of interest is a long, almost infinitely-thin cylinder which can be approximated mathematically as a line segment. The notion of an "equivalent cylinder" introduced by Rall [1978] suggests that it may be possible to model entire dendritic trees, rather than only individual dendritic fibers, using such methods. (Philologists will recognize *dendritic* as the Greek word for "treelike", so that the *dendritic tree* must be a "treelike tree"; perhaps we should christen it a "dendron" instead. By *dendritic fiber* we mean what is usually called a "process" in the biological literature. Obviously it would cause hopeless confusion for us to use that term in the present context.)

We take the other approach suggested above, and model the membrane potential as a stochastic process indexed by one-dimensional time but taking values in an infinite-dimensional space specifying the voltage potential at every point of the membrane at each instant of time. The choice of an appropriate infinite-dimensional space is not an easy one; as we shall see in examples, when the membrane is two (or more) dimensional the membrane voltage potential cannot be expected to be a smooth enough function of location for it to be chosen from a space of continuous functions, or even from a space of locally integrable functions. The natural setting for many of the problems we consider will be a space of *distributions,* also called "generalized functions" in the literature.

It has been argued by Kubo [1986] that most physical systems respond to any disturbance which pushes them away from their equilibrium condition by returning to equilibrium at rates proportional to their distances from equilibrium. This behavior, in which the rate of return is proportional to the distance from equilibrium, is termed *linear dynamics.* Unfortunately, linear dynamics cannot hope to explain the really interesting phenomena of neurophysiology such as the generation of action potentials. The neuron seems to respond to small disturbances by returning to equilibrium at a rate nearly proportional to the distance from equilibrium, but for disturbances which move the potential sufficiently far from equilibrium, the system responds with a jump even *farther* from equilibrium. This initiates a propagating action potential, a phenomenon inconsistent with linear dynamics. Thus neuronal models must be nonlinear.

In this paper we will introduce and illustrate several methods for coping with the stochastic, infinite-dimensional, nonlinear problems arising in the modeling of neuronal behavior. We do this in several steps, in order to isolate the difficulties.

In Section 2, we introduce and solve finite-dimensional non-linear stochastic integral equations suitable for modeling certain neurophysiological phenomena if it is unnecessary to distinguish the membrane potential at different points on the neuronal membrane (*i.e.* if a one-point model for the neuron is adequate). A rich collection of models is based on the idea that neuronal electrical behavior is rather simple as long as the membrane voltage potential remains below some "threshold". When the voltage potential does reach such a threshold, a propagating action potential may be generated---from that point on, the behavior is more complex. Although a restriction to finite-dimensional (*i.e.*

one-point) neurons precludes the study of propagating action potentials with such models, they are adequate for the study of the probability distribution of the time necessary to reach the threshold, even in the presence of certain nonlinearities such as those introduced by the so-called "reversal potentials."

In Section 3 we introduce and solve infinite-dimensional stochastic integral equations, suitable for the study of spatially-extended neurons, but restrict our attention to models exhibiting linear dynamics. This restriction allows us to use the mathematical tools of harmonic analysis and partial differential equations in order to obtain closed-form results in some simple cases, and explicit estimates on the smoothness and growth of membrane potentials in many other cases.

Finally in Section 4 we introduce and solve non-linear, infinite-dimensional stochastic integral equations. We use a method introduced by Krylov and Rozovskii [1979] and based on the *Galerkin* method of solving infinite-dimensional deterministic evolution equations by using finite-dimensional approximations. This allows us to apply the notation and infinite-dimensional structure introduced in Section 3 and to extend the existence and uniqueness proofs given in Section 2 to solve nonlinear infinite-dimensional problems.

The mathematical technique central to all sections of this work is that of weak convergence of probability measures. We use this technique as a tool for proving the existence of a unique "weak" (or probability-measure) solution to complicated stochastic integral equations, by solving a sequence of simpler equations and then showing that the solutions must converge to a solution to the original problem. We also prove results about weak convergence which have direct application to neuronal modeling. For example, in Section 2 we show that the probability distribution measures for a sequence of solutions to stochastic integral equations driven by (generalized) Poisson impulse processes converge weakly to the probability distribution measure for the solution to a Gaussian-driven stochastic integral equation which is, in some sense, the limit of the sequence of equations. It is a corollary of this result that the probability distributions of threshold hitting-times for the Poisson-driven processes converge weakly to those of the Gaussian-driven equation; in particular, the moments will converge. This is of interest because of the enormous amount of effort that has been devoted to studying the hitting-time distributions for Gaussian-driven processes, while most authors regard the generalized-Poisson process as a better stochastic model for the incident stream of random disturbances to the quiescent neuron. Our weak convergence result suggests that the hitting-time probability distributions for the Gaussian processes will be good approximations for those of the Poisson-driven processes, provided that the Poisson impulses are (on average) small enough and frequent enough.

We would like to express our thanks to Charles Smith, John Walsh, Gilbert Bauman, Augustus Grant, and others for interesting and useful conversations, and to Kathy Kuyper, Peggy Ravitch, and Lorraine Evans for typing the manuscript.

2. Stochastic Models for One-point neurons, with reversal potential.

Existence and Uniqueness.

Let U be a measurable space and (a,b,f) a triplet of measurable functions a: $\mathbf{R}_+ \times \mathbf{R} \to \mathbf{R}$, b: $\mathbf{R}_+ \times \mathbf{R} \to \mathbf{R}_+$, and f: $\mathbf{R}_+ \times \mathbf{R} \times U \to \mathbf{R}$. Say that (a,b,f) and the positive Borel measure μ on U satisfy Condition (A) if there exist a number $p>2$, a locally-integrable $\mathbf{R}_+$-valued Borel function $\dot{\theta}_1$, and a locally bounded function $\dot{\theta}_2$ on $\mathbf{R}_+$ such that, for every $t \geq 0$ and every pair x,y of real numbers,

$$|a_t(x) - a_t(y)|^2 + |b_t(x) - b_t(y)|^2 + \int_U |f_t(x,u) - f_t(y,u)|^2 \mu(du) \leq \dot{\theta}_1(t)|x-y|^2 \qquad (A_1)$$

$$|a_t(x)|^q \leq \dot{\theta}_2(t)(1+|x|^q), \qquad q = 1,2 \qquad (A_2)$$

$$|b_t(x)|^2 \leq \dot{\theta}_2(t)(1+|x|^2),$$

$$\int_U |f_t(x,u)|^q \mu(du) \leq \dot{\theta}_2(t)(1+|x|^q), \qquad q = 2,p.$$

Define $\theta_i(t) := \int_0^t \dot{\theta}_i(s)ds$ for $i = 1,2$, and (without loss of generality) take $\dot{\theta}_2$ to be increasing.

Let $W = (W_t)$ be a standard Wiener process on $\mathbf{R}_+$, N a Poisson random measure on $U \times \mathbf{R}_+$ with intensity measure $\mathbf{E}\, N(dudt) = \mu(du)dt$, and ξ_0 any square-integrable random variable such that W, N, and ξ_0 are mutually independent. The following result is well known (Ikeda and Watanabe, [1981, p.230]).

Theorem 2.1. There exists a unique right-continuous strong solution $\xi = (\xi_t)$ to the stochastic integral equation (SIE)

$$\xi_t = \xi_0 + \int_0^t a_s(\xi_s)ds + \int_0^t b_s(\xi_s)dW_s + \int_0^{t+}\int_U f_s(\xi_{s-},u)\tilde{N}(du,ds). \qquad (2.1)$$

Here $\tilde{N}(du\, ds)$ denotes the fully compensated Poisson measure $N(du\, ds) - \mu(du)ds$. Both stochastic integrals are martingale integrals.

For later use we need the following bounds on the moments of the solution ξ_t:

Theorem 2.2. Let θ_3 be an upper bound for the second moment of ξ_0, *i.e.*

$$\mathbf{E}|\xi_0|^2 \leq \theta_3.$$

Then

$$\mathbf{E} \sup_{0 \leq t \leq T} |\xi_t|^2 \leq 3\theta_3 + 12[\theta_3 + (T+2)\theta_2(T)]\, e^{6(T+4)\theta_1(T)}. \qquad (2.2)$$

If $p \geq 2$,

$$\mathbf{E}|\xi_t|^p \leq [1 + \mathbf{E}|\xi_0|^p]\, e^{p^2 2^p \theta_2(t)} - 1. \qquad (2.3)$$

The proof of (2.2) is straightforward. To show (2.3) one uses the Itô formula (Ikeda and Watanabe [1981, p.66]) and the elementary inequality $x^{\alpha}(1 + x^{\beta-\alpha}) \leq (1 + \alpha/\beta)(1 + x^{\beta})$, valid for $0 \leq \alpha \leq \beta$ and

$x>0$.

□

Consider a sequence of SIEs of the type (2.1) with coefficient functions $(a^k, b^k, f^k)_{k<\infty}$ and measures $(\mu^k)_{k<\infty}$ satisfying (A) where, however, it is assumed that the constants appearing in the bounds do not depend on k.

We are concerned with the convergence in distribution of the solution processes $\{\xi^k\}_{k<\infty}$ (equivalently, of the weak convergence of the sequence $\{P^k\}_{k<\infty}$ of induced probability measures) with specified initial probability distribution measures μ_0^k.

In order to investigate this convergence, it will be convenient to first truncate the coefficients as follows.

For each $n\geq 1$ define the continuous function $C_n(x)$ by

$$C_n(x) := \begin{cases} 1 & 0\leq|x|<n \\ n+1-|x| & n\leq|x|<n+1 \\ 0 & n+1\leq|x|<\infty \end{cases}$$

and define

$$a_t^{k,(n)}(x) := C_n(x)a_t^k(x)$$

$$b_t^{k,(n)}(x) := C_n(x)b_t^k(x)$$

$$f_t^{k,(n)}(x,u) := C_n(x)f_t^k(x,u).$$

Let a^k, b^k, f^k, μ_0^k, μ^k satisfy the condition

(B): There exist locally-bounded functions a: $\mathbf{R}_+\times\mathbf{R}\to\mathbf{R}$, b: $\mathbf{R}_+\times\mathbf{R}\to\mathbf{R}_+$, and c: $\mathbf{R}_+\times\mathbf{R}\to\mathbf{R}_+$, a number $p>2$, and a probability measure μ_0 on $(\mathbf{R}, \mathbf{B})$ such that for each $t\geq 0$ and $x\in\mathbf{R}$,

$$\lim_{k\to\infty} a_t^k(x) = a_t(x) \tag{B$_1$}$$

$$\lim_{k\to\infty} b_t^k(x) = b_t(x) \tag{B$_2$}$$

$$\lim_{k\to\infty}\int_U |f_t^k(x,u)|^2\mu^k(du) = c_t^2(x) \tag{B$_3$}$$

$$\mu_0^k \text{ converges weakly to } \mu_0. \tag{B$_4$}$$

For each $R\geq 0$, each $t>0$,

$$\lim_{k\to\infty}\sup_{|x|\leq R}\int_0^t\int_U |f_s^k(x,u)|^p\mu^k(du)ds = 0. \tag{B$_5$}$$

$$\int_{\mathbf{R}} |x|^q\mu_0^k(dx) \leq \theta_3 \quad \text{for } q = 2, p. \tag{B$_6$}$$

From (B$_5$),

$$\sup_{k<\infty}\sup_{|x|\leq R}\int_0^t\int_U |f_s^k(x,u)|^p\mu^k(du)ds < \infty;$$

note that the supremum over $|x|\le R$ is finite for each fixed k by condition (A_2).

Fix $n\ge 1$. Then the cut-off coefficients $(a^{k,(n)}, b^{k,(n)}, f^{k,(n)})$, μ^k also satisfy (B), with limits $a_t^{(n)}(x) := C_n(x)a_t(x)$, $b_t^{(n)}(x) := C_n(x)b_t(x)$, and $c_t^{(n)}(x) := C_n(x)c_t(x)$. Indeed condition (B_5) may be strengthened to the uniform bound:

$$\sup_{k<\infty}\sup_{|x|<\infty}\int_0^t\int_U |f_s^{k,(n)}(x,u)|^p\mu^k(du\,ds) \le \theta_2(t)[(n+1)^p + 1].$$

Of course this bound may depend on n, but not on k.

Let (W^k, N^k, ξ_0^k) be a sequence of triplets, each consisting of a standard Wiener process W^k, a Poisson measure N^k with intensity measure $\mu^k(du)ds$, and an initial value of ξ_0^k with distribution μ_0^k. We take W^k, N^k, and ξ_0^k to be mutually independent.

Since (a^k, b^k, f^k) satisfied (A) for each k, so does the cutoff $(a^{k,(n)}, b^{k,(n)}, f^{k,(n)})$; in fact, it is easy to check that $(a^{k,(n)}, b^{k,(n)}, f^{k,(n)})$, μ^k satisfy (uniformly in k):

$$|a_t^{k,(n)}(x)-a_t^{k,(n)}(y)|^2 + |b_t^{k,(n)}(x)-b_t^{k,(n)}(y)|^2 + \int_U|f_t^{k,(n)}(x,u)-f_t^{k,(n)}(y,u)|^2\mu(du) \qquad (A^+_1)$$

$$\le \dot\theta_1^{(n)}(t)|x-y|^2$$

$$|a_t^{k,(n)}(x)|^q \le \dot\theta_2(t)(1+|x|^q)1_{[|x|<n+1]} \qquad (A^+_2)$$

$$\le \dot\theta_2^{(n)}(t)\,, \quad q=1, 2$$

$$|b_t^{k,(n)}(x)|^2 \le \dot\theta_2(t)(1+|x|^2)1_{[|x|<n+1]}$$

$$\le \dot\theta_2^{(n)}(t)$$

$$\int_U|f_t^{k,(n)}(x,u)|^q\mu^k(du) \le \dot\theta_2(t)(1+|x|^q)1_{[|x|<n+1]}$$

$$\le \dot\theta_2^{(n)}(t)\,, \quad q=2, p,$$

where we set

$$\dot\theta_1^{(n)}(t) := 2\dot\theta_1(t) + 6(n+1)^2\dot\theta_2(t) \quad \text{and}$$

$$\dot\theta_2^{(n)}(t) := \dot\theta_2(t)(1+(n+1)^p).$$

Let ξ_t^k be the strong solution (from Theorem 2.1) to the stochastic integral equation

$$\xi_t = \xi_0^k + \int_0^t a_s^k(\xi_s)ds + \int_0^t b_s^k(\xi_s)dW_s^k + \int_0^t\int_U f_s^k(\xi_{s-},u)\tilde N^k(du\,ds) \qquad (2.4)$$

and $\xi_t^{k,(n)}$ the strong solution to the cut-off equation

$$\xi_t = \xi_0^k + \int_0^t a_s^{k,(n)}(\xi_s)ds + \int_0^t b_s^{k,(n)}(\xi_s)dW_s^k + \int_0^t\int_U f_s^{k,(n)}(\xi_{s-},u)\tilde N^k(du\,ds). \qquad (2.5)$$

Denote by $D := D(\mathbf{R}_+:\mathbf{R})$ the Skorokhod space of real-valued right-continuous functions with left-hand limits on $\mathbf{R}_+$, and by $\{P^k\}_{k<\infty}$ and $\{P^{k,(n)}\}_{k<\infty}$ the probability measures on D induced by $\{\xi^k\}_{k<\infty}$

and $\{\xi^{k,(n)}\}_{k<\infty}$, respectively (*i.e.*, $P^k := \mathbf{P}(\xi^k)^{-1}$, *etc.*, where $\mathbf{P}$ is the basic probability measure on the probability space on which all the $\{\xi^k\}_{k<\infty}$ are defined). We wish to show that $\{P^k\}_{k<\infty}$ converges weakly to a measure P, and to identify P. We will do this in three steps:

1) Prove that $\{P^{k,(n)}\}_{n<\infty}$ converges to P^k as $n\to\infty$, uniformly in k.
2) Prove that $\{P^{k,(n)}\}_{k<\infty}$ converges to $P^{(n)}$ as $k\to\infty$.
3) Prove that $\{P^{(n)}\}_{n<\infty}$ converges to some limit P as $n\to\infty$.

If $\delta(.,.)$ denotes a metric giving the weak topology on the space of probability measures on D and $\varepsilon>0$, then we can

1) Find n^* such that $\delta(P^{k,(n)}, P^k) < \varepsilon/3$ for all k if $n\geq n^*$.
2) Find k^* such $\delta(P^{k,(n)}, P^{(n)}) < \varepsilon/3$ for all $k\geq k^*$.
3) Find $n\geq n^*$ such that $\delta(P^{(n)}, P) < \varepsilon/3$.

It follows that

$$\delta(P^k, P) \leq \delta(P^k, P^{k,(n)}) + \delta(P^{k,(n)}, P^{(n)}) + \delta(P^{(n)}, P) \leq \varepsilon/3 + \varepsilon/3 + \varepsilon/3 = \varepsilon$$

for all $k\geq k^*$. This will prove that $\{P^k\}_{k<\infty}$ converges weakly to P and, incidentally, that $\{P^{(n)}\}_{n<\infty}$ has only one limit point and hence that $\{P^{(n)}\}_{n<\infty}$ converges weakly to P.

2.1. Uniform weak convergence of $\{P^{k,(n)}\}_{n<\infty}$ for fixed k.

The first step in our program is to prove that the sequence $\{P^{k,(n)}\}_{n<\infty}$ converges weakly to P^k *uniformly in* k as n tends to infinity. Of course, we will have to say precisely what we mean by uniform weak convergence: we introduce an appropriate metric for this notion in Lemma 2.2.

By Theorem 2.2 we have the bound

$$\mathbf{E}|\xi_t^{k,(n)}|^p \leq (1 + \mathbf{E}|\xi_0^k|^p)e^{\beta(t)},$$

with $\beta(t) = p^2\, 2^p\, \theta_2(t)$; under the uniform (in k) bound (B_6) on the initial value, *i.e.*,

$$\mathbf{E}|\xi_0^k|^q = \int |x|^q \mu_0(dx) \leq \theta_3, \quad q=2, p,$$

hence

$$\mathbf{E}|\xi_t^{k,(n)}|^q \leq \gamma_t := (1+\theta_3)\, e^{\beta(t)} \tag{2.6}$$

uniformly in k for $q = 2, p$, and it follows that the event

$$B_t^{k,(n)} := \{|\xi_t^{k,(n)}| > n+1\}$$

has probability

$$\begin{aligned} \mathbf{P}[B_t^{k,(n)}] &\leq \mathbf{E}[|\xi_t^{k,(n)}|^2/(n+1)^2] \\ &\leq \gamma_t/(n+1)^2 \\ &\leq \gamma_T/n^2 \end{aligned} \tag{2.7}$$

for $0\leq t\leq T$, $n\geq 1$.

We estimate the L^2 distance from ξ_t^k to $\xi_t^{k,(n)}$ as follows:

$$|\xi_t^k - \xi_t^{k,(n)}|^2 \le 3t\int_0^t |a_s^k(\xi_s^k) - a_s^{k,(n)}\xi_s^{k,(n)})|^2 ds \tag{2.8}$$

$$+ 3|\int_0^t (b_s^k(\xi_s^k) - b_s^{k,(n)}(\xi_s^{k,(n)}))dW_s|^2$$

$$+ 3|\int_0^{t+}\int_U (f_s^k(\xi_{s-}^k,u) - f_s^{k,(n)}(\xi_{s-}^{k,(n)},u))\tilde{N}(du\, ds)|^2.$$

By Doob's martingale maximal inequality and some routine (but tedious) calculations, it can be shown that the function $g^{k,(n)}(T) := \mathbf{E}\sup_{0\le t\le T}|\xi_t^k - \xi_t^{k,(n)}|^2$ satisfies

$$g^{k,(n)}(T) \le 3(T+8)\theta_2(T)\gamma_T/n^2 + (\gamma_T/n^2)^{1-2/p}T(1+\theta_3)^{2/p}e^{(p2^{p+1}\theta_2(T))} + 3(T+4)\int_0^t g^{k,(n)}(s)d\theta_1(s).$$

If we denote by $\alpha_n(T)$ the sum of the first two terms above, Gronwall's inequality yields

$$g^{k,(n)}(T) \le \alpha_n(T)e^{3(T+4)\theta_1(T)}$$

Since both α_n and θ_1 are independent of k, and since $\alpha_n(T) = O(n^{-2(p-2)/p})$ as $n\to\infty$, we have shown that $g^{k,(n)}(T) \to 0$ uniformly in k as $n \to \infty$ for each fixed $T > 0$ and so have proved

Lemma 2.1. Let (a^k, b^k, f^k), μ^k satisfy condition (A), all with the same functions $\dot{\theta}_1$ and $\dot{\theta}_2$. For each $k<\infty$ let (W^k, N^k, ξ_0^k) be a triplet of a mutually independent Wiener process, Poisson measure (with intensity measure $\mu^k(du)dt$), and random variable ξ_0^k satisfying $\mathbf{E}|\xi_0^k|^q \le \theta_3$ for $q = 2,p$, uniformly in k. Then the strong solutions $\{\xi^k\}_{k<\infty}$ and $\{\xi^{k,(n)}\}_{k<\infty}$ to equation (2.1) with coefficients (a^k, b^k, f^k) and $(a^{k,(n)}, b^{k,(n)}, f^{k,(n)})$ respectively satisfy

$$\lim_{n\to\infty}\sup_k \mathbf{E}\sup_{0\le t\le T}|\xi_t^k - \xi_t^{k,(n)}|^2 = 0$$

for each $T\ge 0$.

□

Let ρ denote any metric which determines the usual Prokhorov topology on D and satisfies the inequality

$$\rho(x,y) \le \sup_{0\le t\le T}|x_t - y_t| + e^{-T} \tag{2.9}$$

for all $T\ge 0$ (see Kallianpur and Wolpert [1984]). Let $\mathbf{D}$ denote the Borel sets in (D,ρ) and $\mathbf{M}$ the space of probability measures on $\mathbf{D}$.

Lemma 2.2. The space $\mathbf{M}$ is a complete separable metric space in the metric

$$\delta(P,Q) := \inf\{\varepsilon>0: P(A) \le Q(A^\varepsilon) + \varepsilon,\ Q(A) \le P(A^\varepsilon)) + \varepsilon \text{ for all } A\in\mathbf{D}\}. \tag{2.10}$$

Here A^ε denotes $\{x\in\mathbf{D}: \rho(x,y) <\varepsilon \text{ for some } y\in A\}$ for $\varepsilon>0$ and $A\in\mathbf{D}$. Obviously A^ε is open and hence measurable. This follows directly from the results in Appendix III of Billingsley [1968].

□

Theorem 2.3. Let (P^k) and $(P^{k,(n)})$ denote the measures induced on **D** by $\{\xi^k\}_{k<\infty}$ and $\{\xi^{k,(n)}\}_{k<\infty}$, respectively. Then $\delta(P^k, P^{k,(n)})$ converges to zero uniformly in k as n tends to infinity.

Proof. Fix $\varepsilon > 0$ and find $T > 0$ so that $e^{-T} < \varepsilon/2$. Using Lemma 2.1, find n^* so that

$$\mathbf{E} \sup_{0\le t\le T} |\xi_t^k - \xi_t^{k,(n)}|^2 < \varepsilon^3/4 \tag{2.11}$$

for every k and every $n \ge n^*$. Fix any $n \ge n^*$, and denote by Q the measure on $\mathbf{D}\times\mathbf{D}$ induced by $(\xi^k, \xi^{k,(n)})$; the first and second marginals of Q are P^k and $P^{k,(n)}$, respectively. Set

$$\Delta_\varepsilon := \{(x,y)\colon \sup_{0\le t\le T} |x_t - y_t| < \varepsilon/2\}$$

By (2.11),

$$\begin{aligned} Q(\Delta_\varepsilon^c) &\le 4 \int_{\Delta_\varepsilon^c} \sup_{0\le t\le T} |x_t - y_t|^2/\varepsilon^2 \, dQ \\ &\le 4\varepsilon^{-2} \int_{D\times D} \sup_{0\le t\le T} |x_t - y_t|^2 \, dQ \\ &\le 4\varepsilon^{-2}\, \mathbf{E} \sup_{0\le t\le T} |\xi_t^k - \xi_t^{k,(n)}|^2 \\ &\le \varepsilon. \end{aligned}$$

Using the above inequality it is easy to show that for any $A \in \mathbf{D}$,

$$\begin{aligned} P^k(A) &= Q(A\times D) \\ &\le P^{k,(n)}(A^\varepsilon) + \varepsilon. \end{aligned}$$

Similarly $P^{k,(n)}(A) \le P^k(A^\varepsilon) + \varepsilon$, so $\delta(P^k, P^{k,(n)}) < \varepsilon$. We have used the fact that $(x,y) \in (A\times D)\cap\Delta_\varepsilon$ implies $x \in A$ and $\sup_{0\le t\le T} |x_t - y_t| < \varepsilon/2$, hence by (2.9) $\rho(x,y) < \varepsilon/2 + e^{-T} < \varepsilon$ and $y \in A^\varepsilon$.

□

2.2. Weak Convergence of $\{P^{k,(n)}\}_{k<\infty}$ for Fixed n.

In this section we first prove tightness and then convergence (as $k \to \infty$) to $P^{(n)}$ of $\{P^{k,(n)}\}_{k<\infty}$.

For convenience we collect here the conditions (introduced above) we will require of the coefficient functions $(a^{k,(n)}, b^{k,(n)}, f^{k,(n)})$ and measure $\mu^{k,(n)}$, $\mu_0^{k,(n)}$:

(A^+) There exist a number $p > 2$, a locally integrable function $\dot\theta_1$, and an increasing function $\dot\theta_2$ such that $(a^{k,(n)}, b^{k,(n)}, f^{k,(n)})$ and $\mu^{k,(n)}$ satisfy (uniformly in k):

$$|a_t^{k,(n)}(x) - a_t^{k,(n)}(y)|^2 + |b_t^{k,(n)}(x) - b_t^{k,(n)}(y)|^2 + \int_U |f_t^{k,(n)}(x,u) - f_t^{k,(n)}(y,u)|^2 \, \mu^{k,(n)}(du) \tag{A^+_1}$$

$$\leq \dot{\theta}_1(t)|x-y|^2$$

$$|a_t^{k,(n)}(x)|^q \leq \dot{\theta}_2(t), \qquad q = 1, 2 \tag{A^+_2}$$

$$|b_t^{k,(n)}(x)|^2 \leq \dot{\theta}_2(t)$$

$$\int_U |f_t^{k,(n)}(x,u)|^q \, \mu^{k,(n)}(du) \leq \dot{\theta}_2(t), \qquad q = 2, p.$$

(B) There exist a real number $\theta_3 > 0$, locally bounded functions $a_t(x)$, $b_t(x)$, and $c_t(x)$, and a probability measure μ_0 such that for each $R>0$, $t>0$, and $x \in \mathbf{R}$,

$$\lim_{k\to\infty} a_t^{k,(n)}(x) = a_t(x) \tag{B_1}$$

$$\lim_{k\to\infty} b_t^{k,(n)}(x) = b_t(x) \tag{B_2}$$

$$\lim_{k\to\infty} \int_U (f_t^{k,(n)}(x,u))^2 \, \mu^k(du) = c_t^2(x) \tag{B_3}$$

$$w\text{-}\lim_{k\to\infty} \mu_0^k = \mu_0 \tag{B_4}$$

$$\lim_{k\to\infty} \sup_{|x|\leq R} \int |f_t^{k,(n)}(x,u)|^p \, \mu^k(du) = 0 \qquad \text{for each } R<\infty \tag{B_5}$$

$$\int |x|^q \mu_0^k(dx) \leq \theta_3\,, \quad q = 2, p, \quad k<\infty. \tag{B_6}$$

We leave the (n)-dependence of a_t, b_t, and c_t implicit.

To establish tightness under conditions (A^+) and (B), we proceed as follows: Write

$$Y_t^{k,(n)} := \int_0^t \int_U f_s^k(\xi_{s-}^{k,(n)}, u) \tilde{N}^{k,(n)}(duds).$$

Then the quadratic variation process is given by

$$\langle Y^{k,(n)} \rangle_t = \int_0^t \int_U |f_s^k(\xi_{s-}^{k,(n)}, u)|^2 \, \mu^k(du)ds.$$

Lenglart's inequality (Liptser and Shiryaev [1984]) yields the following, for any positive quantities a and b:

$$\mathbf{P}\Big[\sup_{0\leq t\leq T} |Y_t^{k,(n)}| \geq a\Big] \leq \frac{b}{a^2} + \mathbf{P}\Big[\langle Y^{k,(n)}\rangle_T \geq b\Big] \tag{2.12}$$

$$\leq \frac{b}{a^2} + \frac{\mathbf{E}\langle Y^{k,(n)}\rangle_T}{b}$$

$$\leq \frac{b}{a^2} + \frac{T\dot{\theta}_2(T)}{b}.$$

For any stopping time $\tau_k \leq T$ and $\delta>0$,

$$\mathbf{P}\Big[\sup_{0\leq s\leq\delta} |Y_{\tau_k+s}^{k,(n)} - Y_{\tau_k}^{k,(n)}| \geq a\Big] \leq \frac{b}{a^2} + \mathbf{P}\Big[\langle Y^{k,(n)}\rangle_{\tau_k+\delta} - \langle Y^{k,(n)}\rangle_{\tau_k} \geq b\Big] \tag{2.13}$$

$$\le \frac{b}{a^2} + \mathbf{P}\left[\int_{\tau_k}^{\tau_k+\delta}\int_U |f_s^k(\xi_{s-}^{k,(n)}, u)|^2\mu^k(du) \ge b\right]$$

$$\le \frac{b}{a^2} + \frac{\dot\theta_2(T)\delta}{b}.$$

From (2.12) and using the bounds on $a_s^{k,(n)}$ and $\mathbf{E}|\xi_0^k|$, we have

$$\mathbf{P}\left[\sup_{0\le t\le T}|\xi_t^{k,(n)}|\ge a\right] \le \frac{3(\theta_3 + T\dot\theta_2(T))}{a} + \frac{9b}{a^2} + \frac{T\dot\theta_2(T)}{b}.$$

From the arbitrariness of b it follows that

$$\lim_{a\to\infty}\sup_{k<\infty}\mathbf{P}\left[\sup_{0\le t\le T}|\xi_t^{k,(n)}|\ge a\right] = 0. \tag{2.14}$$

Next,

$$\sup_{0\le s\le\delta}|\xi_{\tau_k+s}^{k,(n)} - \xi_{\tau_k}^{k,(n)}| \le \int_{\tau_k}^{\tau_k+\delta}|a^{k,(n)}(s,\xi_s^{k,(n)})|\,ds + \sup_{0\le s\le\delta}|Y_{\tau_k+s}^{k,(n)} - Y_{\tau_k}^{k,(n)}|$$

so that using (2.13),

$$\mathbf{P}\left[\sup_{0\le s\le\delta}|\xi_{\tau_k+s}^{k,(n)} - \xi_{\tau_k}^{k,(n)}|\ge a\right] \le \frac{2\dot\theta_2(T)\delta}{a} + \frac{4b}{a^2} + \frac{\dot\theta_2(T)\delta}{b}. \tag{2.15}$$

Now let $\varepsilon>0$ be arbitrary and choose $b<\frac{a^2\varepsilon}{8}$, $\delta<\frac{a^2\varepsilon^2}{4}\dot\theta_2(T)(5 + a\varepsilon)$. Then from (2.15),

$$\sup_{k\le\infty}\mathbf{P}\left[\sup_{0\le s\le\delta}|\xi_{\tau_k+s}^{k,(n)} - \xi_{\tau_k}^{k,(n)}|\ge a\right] < \varepsilon. \tag{2.16}$$

Formula (2.14) and inequality (2.16) imply tightness of the sequence $\{P^{k,(n)}\}_{k<\infty}$, as is shown by Liptser and Shiryaev [1984, Lemma 2.3]. It remains to show that the sequence has only one possible limit point and to identify that limit point.

We now complete the second step in our program by proving (as Theorem 2.4) that under specified conditions the sequence $\{P^{k,(n)}\}_{k<\infty}$ of measures converges weakly as k tends to infinity to a limiting measure of $P^{(n)}$. We do this in the usual way, *i.e.*, having proved that $\{P^{k,(n)}\}_{k<\infty}$ is tight for each fixed n we merely identify the only possible limit point $P^{(n)}$.

Let $(\xi_t^{(n)})$ be a diffusion process with initial distribution μ_0, drift $a_t^{(n)}$, and diffusion rate $\sigma_t^{(n)} = ((b_t^{(n)})^2 + (c_t^{(n)})^2)^{1/2}$, *i.e.*, a solution to the stochastic integral equation

$$\xi_t = \xi_0 + \int_0^t a_s^{(n)}(\xi_s)ds + \int_0^t \sigma_s^{(n)}(\xi_s)dW_s \tag{2.17}$$

for some independent pair (ξ_0, W) consisting of a random variable ξ_0 with distribution μ_0 and a standard Wiener process W. Let $P^{(n)}$ be the measure induced on $(D, \mathbf{D})$ by $(\xi_t^{(n)})$; we will show in Theorem 2.4 that $P^{k,(n)}$ converges weakly to $P^{(n)}$.

The processes $\xi^{k,(n)}$ and $\xi^{(n)}$ are Markov and from Gikhman and Skorokhod [1972, Theorem 2, p. 291] we can identify (restrictions of) their generators as $L^{k,(n)}$ and $L^{(n)}$, given by

$$L_t^{k,(n)}\phi(x) := a_t^{k,(n)}(x)\phi'(x) + \tfrac{1}{2}(b_t^{k,(n)}(x))^2\phi''(x) \qquad (2.18a)$$
$$+ \int_U [\phi(x + f_t^{k,(n)}(x,u)) - \phi(x) - f_t^{k,(n)}(x,u)\phi'(x)]\mu^k(du)$$

$$L_t^{(n)}\phi(x) := a_t^{(n)}(x)\phi'(x) + \tfrac{1}{2}(\sigma_t^{(n)}(x))^2\phi''(x) \qquad (2.18b)$$

for sufficiently smooth (*e.g.*, C_b^2) functions ϕ.

For each $t\geq 0$ let $\mathbf{D}_t \subset \mathbf{D}$ be the sigma-algebra generated by sets of the form $\{x: x_s < a\}$ for $a \in \mathbf{R}$, $s\leq t$. For each $\phi \in C_b^2$ and $x = (x_s) \in D$, define processes

$$M_t^{\phi,k,(n)}(x) := \phi(x_t) - \phi(x_0) - \int_0^t L_s^{k,(n)}\phi(x_s)ds \quad \text{for } k < \infty,$$

$$M_t^{\phi,(n)}(x) := \phi(x_t) - \phi(x_0) - \int_0^t L_s^{(n)}\phi(x_s)ds.$$

Then, $M_t^{\phi,k,(n)} := M_t^{\phi,k,(n)}(\xi_t^{k,(n)})$ is a square-integrable martingale on $(D, \mathbf{D}, (\mathbf{D}_t), P^{k,(n)})$ for each $k<\infty$ and $\phi \in C_b^2$. Similarly $M_t^{\phi,(n)} := M_t^{\phi,(n)}(\xi_t^{(n)})$ is an L^2 martingale on $(D, \mathbf{D}, (\mathbf{D}_t), P^{(n)})$.

Our method for proving that $\{P^{k,(n)}\}_{k<\infty}$ converges weakly to $P^{(n)}$ is to show that any limit point P^* of $\{P^{k,(n)}\}_{k<\infty}$ has the property that $(M_t^{\phi,(n)})_{t\geq 0}$ is a $(D, \mathbf{D}, (\mathbf{D}_t), P^*)$-martingale for every $\phi \in C_c^\infty$. Since at most one measure can have that property, we conclude that $P^* = P^{(n)}$ is the weak limit of $\{P^{k,(n)}\}_{k<\infty}$. The rather lengthy argument which establishes this will only be summarized here.

We mention only the key steps in the proof.

(i) $M_s^{\phi,k,(n)}(x) \to M_s^{\phi,(n)}(x)$ as $k \to \infty$ uniformly in $x \in K$ for each compact set K of $C := C(\mathbf{R}_+) \subset D$ and $s\leq t$;

(ii) If P^* is any limit point of $\{P^{k,(n)}\}_{k<\infty}$, then $P^*(C) = 1$;

(iii) For any $\phi \in C_b^3$, $\{M_t^{\phi,(n)}\}_{t\geq 0}$ is a $\{D, \mathbf{D}, \{\mathbf{D}_t\}, P^*\}$ martingale.

To conclude the proof, note that $\{M_t^{\phi,(n)}\}_{t\geq 0}$ is a martingale on $\{D, \mathbf{D}, (\mathbf{D}_t), P^{(n)}\}$ for every compactly supported C^∞ function ϕ. By (iii) this property is also shared by P^*. A theorem of Stroock and Varadhan [1979, p. 152] asserts that at most one measure enjoys this property, so that $P^* = P^{(n)}$.

Thus the sequence $\{P^{k,(n)}\}_{k<\infty}$ converges weakly to its unique limit point, $P^{(n)}$.

We have just proven

Theorem 2.4. Let the sequences (a^k, b^k, f^k) of coefficient functions and μ^k, μ_0^k of measures satisfy conditions (A^+) and (B). Let (W^k, N^k, ξ_0^k) be an independent standard Wiener process, Poisson measure with intensity measure $\mu^k(du)dt$, and random variable with distribution measure μ_0^k. For fixed $n\geq 1$ let $(a^{k,(n)}, b^{k,(n)}, f^{k,(n)})$ be the cutoff coefficients constructed above, $(\xi_t^{k,(n)})_{t\geq 0}$ and $(\xi_t^{(n)})_{t\geq 0}$ the processes constructed in Theorem 2.1 as solutions to the stochastic integral equations (2.1) and (2.17), respectively, with these cutoff coefficients. Let $P^{k,(n)}$ and $P^{(n)}$ be the probability measures induced on $(D, \mathbf{D})$ by $\xi^{k,(n)}$ and $\xi^{(n)}$. Then $\{P^{k,(n)}\}_{k<\infty}$ converges to $P^{(n)}$ as k tends to infinity, for each fixed n.

□

We need to state one more result to complete the third step of our program, *i.e.* prove that $\{P^{(n)}\}_{n<\infty}$ converges to some P, to gather all the ingredients for the derivation of our principal theorem.

Theorem 2.5. Let the coefficient functions $a_t(x)$, $\sigma_t(x)$ satisfy the conditions (for each $t\geq 0$, $x,y \in \mathbf{R}$)

$$|a_t(x) - a_t(y)|^2 + |\sigma_t(x) - \sigma_t(y)|^2 \leq \dot{\theta}_1(t)|x - y|^2 \tag{2.19}$$

$$|a_t(x)|^2 \leq \dot{\theta}_2(t)(1 + |x|^2)$$

$$|\sigma(x)|^2 \leq \dot{\theta}_2(t)(1 + |x|^2)$$

for some locally-integrable $\dot{\theta}_1$ and increasing $\dot{\theta}_2$. For each $n\geq 1$ let $a_t^{(n)}(x)$, $\sigma_t^{(n)}(x)$ satisfy

$$a_t^{(n)}(x) = a_t(x), \qquad \sigma_t^{(n)}(x) = \sigma_t(x) \qquad \text{if } |x|<n \tag{2.20}$$

$$a_s^{(n)}(x) \leq 2\dot{\theta}_2(t)(n+1)^2, \qquad |\sigma_s^{(n)}(x)| \leq 2\dot{\theta}_2(t)(n+1)^2 \qquad \text{if } s\leq t.$$

Then for any square-integrable random variable ξ_0 and independent standard Wiener process W there are unique processes $\xi^{(n)}$ and ξ satisfying the stochastic integral equations

$$\xi_t^{(n)} = \xi_0 + \int_0^t a_s^{(n)}(\xi_s^{(n)})\, ds + \int_0^t \sigma_s^{(n)}(\xi_s^{(n)})\, dW_s \tag{2.21}$$

$$\xi_t = \xi_0 + \int_0^t a_s(\xi_s)\, ds + \int_0^t \sigma_s(\xi_s)\, dW_s.$$

Furthermore, the measures $P^{(n)}$ induced on $(D, \mathbf{D})$ by $(\xi_t^{(n)})_{t\geq 0}$ converge weakly to the measure P induced by $(\xi_t)_{t\geq 0}$.

Proof. The existence and uniqueness follow from Theorem 2.1, the convergence from theorems 6.3.4 and 11.1.4 of Stroock and Varadhan [1979, pp. 152 and 264].

□

In our applications the coefficient functions a_t, b_t, $a_t^{(n)}$, *etc.*, and function $\dot{\theta}_1$, $\dot{\theta}_2$, *etc.*, will be those introduced in conditions (A^+) and (B).

We are now in a position to state our main results.

Theorem 2.6. Let the sequences $(a^k, b^k, f^k)_{k<\infty}$ of coefficient functions and $(\mu^k)_{k<\infty}$, $(\mu_0^k)_{k<\infty}$ of measures satisfy (A) and (B), and let P^k be the measure induced on $(D, \mathbf{D})$ by the unique solution $(\xi_t^k)_{t\geq 0}$ to the stochastic integral equation (2.1). Then P^k converges weakly as k tends to infinity to the measure P induced on $(D, \mathbf{D})$ by the solution $(\xi_t)_{t\geq 0}$ to the stochastic integral equation

$$\xi_t = \xi_0 + \int_0^t a_s(\xi_s)ds + \int_0^t (b_s^2(\xi_s) + c_s^2(\xi_s))^{1/2} dW_s,$$

where ξ_0 is a random variable with distribution measure μ_0 which is independent of the standard

Wiener process W.

Proof. Fix $\varepsilon>0$, and let δ be the metric on the space of probability measures on D given in Lemma 2.2. Use Theorem 2.3 to find $n_1 \geq 1$ so that the measures $\{P^{k,(n)}\}$ constructed above satisfy $\delta(P^k, P^{k,(n)}) < \varepsilon/3$ for all k if $n \geq n_1$. Set $\sigma_t(x) := (b_t^2(x) + c_t^2(x))^{1/2}$ and note that the coefficient functions (a_t, σ_t) satisfy (2.19), while $(a_t^{(n)}, \sigma_t^{(n)})$ satisfy (2.20); here $\sigma_t^{(n)} := ((b_t^{(n)}(x))^2 + (c_t^{(n)}(x))^2)^{1/2}$. Thus Theorem 2.5 applies and allows us to find $n_2 \geq n_1$ so that $\delta(P^{(n)}, P) < \varepsilon/3$ for $n \geq n_2$. Now fix such an n and apply Theorem 2.4 to find k^* such that $\delta(P^k, P^{k,(n)}) < \varepsilon/3$ for $k \geq k^*$; then for any such k,

$$\delta(P^k, P) \leq \delta(P^k, P^{k,(n)}) + \delta(P^{k,(n)}, P^{(n)}) + \delta(P^{(n)}, P) < \varepsilon.$$

□

Remark. It is only for notational convenience that we have confined ourselves to real-valued processes. A version of Theorem 2.6 appropriate for $\mathbf{R}^d$-valued processes can be given which may prove to be useful in subjecting Hodgkin and Huxley's work to a stochastic analysis.

2.3. Diffusion approximations.

Let us associate with each neuron a firing threshold c and a resting potential x_0, both assumed to be constants (for simplicity) with $c>x_0$. Vesicles reaching the cell membrane contribute positive ("excitatory") or negative ("inhibitory") charge increments of various magnitudes to the voltage potential; if (as in Ricciardi and Sacerdote [1979]) there are p possible magnitudes a_e^j ($j = 1, \cdots, p$) of excitatory increments and q possible magnitudes a_i^l ($l = 1, \cdots, q$) of inhibitory increments arriving in independent Poisson processes N_e^j and N_i^l with rates f_e^j and f_i^l respectively, then it is reasonable to suppose that the voltage potential V_t at time t should obey the stochastic differential equation (SDE)

$$dV_t = -\beta V_t\, dt + \sum_{j=1}^{p} a_e^j dN_e^j(t) - \sum_{l=1}^{q} a_i^l dN_i^l(t)$$

or its equivalent stochastic integral equation (SIE)

$$V(t) = x_0 - \int_0^t \beta V_s\, ds \;+ \sum_{j=1}^{p} a_e^j N_e^j(t) - \sum_{l=1}^{q} a_i^l N_i^l(t). \tag{2.22}$$

Here $\beta > 0$ denotes the rate at which the potential decays (due to some sort of leakage across the cell membrane, perhaps). This is a simple example of the class of models we have considered; it is of the form (2.1):

$$\xi_t = \xi_0 + \int_0^t a_s(\xi_s)ds + \int_0^t b_s(\xi_s)dW_s + \int_0^t\int_U f_s(\xi_{s-},u)\tilde{N}(duds) \tag{2.23}$$

with $\xi_0 = x_0$, $a_s(x) = -\beta x + \lambda$, $b_s(x) = 0$, $U = \mathbf{R}$, and $f_s(x,u) = u$. Here $\lambda := \sum_j a_e^j f_e^j - \sum_l a_i^l f_i^l$ and $\tilde{N}$ is the fully compensated Poisson measure with intensity $\mu(du)ds$, where μ is the finite sum of a point mass of magnitude f_e^j (resp., f_i^l) at each point $u = a_e^j$ (resp., $u = -a_i^l$). The condition (A) is easy to verify. A sequence of such coefficient functions $a_s^k(x) = -\beta^k(x) + \lambda^k$, $b^k = 0$, $f_s^k(x, u) = u$, and intensity measures μ^k will satisfy (B), if there exists some $\beta > 0$, $\lambda \in \mathbf{R}$, and $\sigma > 0$ for which

$$\beta^k \to \beta \tag{2.24}$$

$$\lambda^k := \sum_j a_e^{j,k} f_e^{j,k} - \sum_l a_i^{l,k} f_i^{l,k} \to \lambda$$

$$\sum_j (a_e^{j,k})^2 f_e^{j,k} + \sum_l (a_i^{l,k})^2 f_i^{l,k} \to \sigma^2$$

$$\sup_{j,l}\{a_e^{j,k},\, a_i^{l,k}\} \to 0.$$

In this case the solutions V^k to (2.22) (*i.e.*, the solutions ξ^k to (2.23)) converge in distribution to the process ξ satisfying

$$d\xi_t = (-\beta\xi_t + \lambda)dt + \sigma dW_t. \tag{2.25}$$

The solution $\xi_t = \zeta_t + \lambda/\beta$ of (2.25) differs only by the constant λ/β from the well-known Ornstein-Uhlenbeck (OU) process ζ_t, a Gaussian Markov process satisfying the Langevin equation $d\zeta_t = -\beta\zeta_t\, dt + \sigma\, dW_t$. A somewhat more general treatment of the diffusion approximation (2.25) is available in Kallianpur [1982].

2.4. Reversal potentials.

As indicated in the Introduction, one of our concerns in this article is to derive (under appropriate conditions) diffusion approximations for the discontinuous "point" neuron model which take into account the phenomenon of reversal potentials. Let us first briefly describe the discontinuous model introduced by Stein [1965] and developed by Cope and Tuckwell [1979] and Wan and Tuckwell [1979].

These authors introduce a "reversal potential" V_e^j (resp., V_i^l) for each Poisson stream N_e^j (resp., N_i^l); their equation is

$$dV_t = -\gamma V_t dt + \sum_j (V_e^j - V_t) a_e^j dN_e^j(t) + \sum_l (V_i^l - V_t) a_i^l dN_i^l \tag{2.26}$$

where $V_e^j \geq 0$ and $V_i^l \leq 0$. One motivation for (2.26) is to regard the Poisson events as the openings (and subsequent closings) of various ion-specific passages through the membrane. During the open period ions of the appropriate type pass into or out of the cell through such a passage in a direction (and at a rate) depending on the sign (and magnitude, respectively) of the difference between an equilibrium potential V_e^j or V_i^l and the membrane potential V_t. Another is to regard the Poisson events as the arrivals of vesicles containing quantities of various types of neurotransmitters, each of which causes hundreds or thousands of ion gates to open and leads to a jump in the membrane voltage of a magnitude and direction depending upon the difference between the membrane voltage potential and the trans-membrane ionic concentration gradient. Note that it is not γ, but rather $\beta := \gamma + \sum_j a_e^j f_e^j + \sum_l a_i^l f_i^l$ which should be interpreted as a "leakage rate" for this model; in fact, γ may even be negative so long as β is positive.

Again (2.26) is of the form (2.1) or (2.23), with $\xi_0 = x_0$, $a_s(x) = -\beta x + \lambda$, $b_s(x) = 0$, and (for example) $U = \{-q, \cdots, p\}$ and

$$f_x(x,u) = \begin{cases} (V_e^j - x)a_e^j & \text{if } u = j, \quad 1 \le j \le p \\ (V_i^l - x)a_i^l & \text{if } u = -l, \ 1 \le l \le q \\ 0 & \text{else} \end{cases}$$

$$\mu(\{u\}) = \begin{cases} f_e^j & \text{if } u = j, \quad 1 \le j \le p \\ f_i^l & \text{if } u = -l, \ 1 \le l \le q \\ 0 & \text{else} \end{cases}$$

The verification of (A) is easy, and we have the following result. For each $k > 1$ let $\{\xi_t^k\}$ be a solution to (2.26) with fixed p, q, $\{V_e^j\}$, $\{V_i^l\}$, and x_0, but with γ, $\{a_e^j\}$, $\{a_i^l\}$, $\{f_e^j\}$, and $\{f_i^l\}$ allowed to depend on an index parameter k. Set

$$\beta^k := \gamma^k + \sum_j a_e^{j,k} f_e^{j,k} + \sum_l a_i^{l,k} f_i^{l,k}$$

$$\lambda^k := \sum_j V_e^j a_e^{j,k} f_e^{j,k} + \sum_l V_i^l a_i^{l,k} f_i^{l,k}$$

$$\delta^k := \lambda^k / \beta^k.$$

Theorem 2.7. Let c_k be any sequence such that, for some real number α_1 and positive numbers α_0, α_2, and β,

$$\lim_{k\to\infty} \sum_j (a_e^{j,k})^2 f_e^{j,k} + \sum_l (a_i^{l,k})^2 f_i^{l,k} = \alpha_2$$

$$\lim_{k\to\infty} c_k \left[\sum_j (V_e^j - \delta^k)(a_e^{j,k})^2 f_e^{j,k} + \sum_l (V_i^l - \delta^k)(a_i^{l,k})^2 f_i^{l,k} \right] = -\tfrac{1}{2}\alpha_1$$

$$\lim_{k\to\infty} c_k^2 \left[\sum_j (V_e^j - \delta^k)^2 (a_e^{j,k})^2 f_e^{j,k} + \sum_l (V_i^l - \delta^k)^2 (a_i^{l,k})^2 f_i^{l,k} \right] = \alpha_0$$

$$\lim_{k\to\infty} \beta^k = \beta,$$

$$\lim_{k\to\infty} \sup_{j,l} \{a_e^{j,k}, a_i^{l,k}\} = 0.$$

Then $V_t^k := c_k(\xi_t^k - \delta^k)$ converges weakly to a solution $\{V_t^*\}$ of the equation

$$dV_t = -\beta V_t dt + \sigma_t(V_t) dW_t \tag{2.27}$$

with $\sigma_t(x) := (\alpha_0 + \alpha_1 x + \alpha_2 x^2)^{1/2}$ and $V_0 := x_0$.

The solution V_t of (2.27) is a non-Gaussian process (since $\alpha_2 > 0$), unlike the Ornstein-Uhlenbeck process obtained in (2.25) as the limit of solutions to (2.22).

We mention as corollaries to the above theorem some known results on diffusion approximations.

Corollary 1. In case λ^k happens to converge to a finite number $\lambda \in \mathbf{R}$, then δ^k must converge to $\delta := \lambda/\beta$ and we may dispense with the rescaling by taking $c_k \equiv 1$ to see that ξ_t^k ($= \delta^k + V_t^k$) itself converges weakly to a solution of

$$dV_t = (\lambda - \beta V_t)dt + \sigma_t(V_t)dW_t.$$

Diffusion equations of this type were considered by Johannesma [1968] as models for the stochastic activity of neurons.

Corollary 2. If we choose c_k such that $c_k \to 0$ and $c_k\delta_k \to 0$ then $\alpha_0 = \alpha_1 = 0$ and (2.27) reduces to

$$dV_t = -\beta V_t dt + \sqrt{\alpha_2}\, |V_t|\, dW_t.$$

Corollary 3. (Boundary behavior). It is easy to show that α_0, α_1, and α_2 above must satisfy $\alpha_0+\alpha_1 x+\alpha_2 x^2 \geq 0$ for all $x \in \mathbf{R}$, and *a fortiori* $\alpha_1^2 \leq 4\alpha_0\alpha_2$. In the case of equality $\alpha_1^2 = 4\alpha_0\alpha_2$ there is a real double root $r = -\alpha_1/2\alpha_2$ to the equation $\sigma^2(x) = 0$ (in fact, $\sigma(x) = |x-r|\sqrt{\alpha_2}$) and the diffusion equation (2.27) becomes singular at $x = r$. In case $r = 0$ the point $x = r$ is an attracting but unattainable point for the diffusion, but if $r > 0$ (and $x_0 < r$) or $r < 0$ (and $x_0 > r$) the point $x=r$ is what Feller called an "entrance boundary," an unattainable boundary point from which the process may start but to which it may not return. This case arises if $|\lambda_k| \to \infty$ and we take $c_k \to 0$ such that $-c_k\lambda_k/\beta$ converges to some non-zero real number r, *e.g.*, $c_k := -\beta r/\lambda_k$. (See Karlin and Taylor [1981] for more details about the boundary behavior of diffusion processes).

In (2.26) the magnitudes of both the excitatory and inhibitory impulses are assumed constant. It is more natural to suppose that the impulse sizes are random. We derive one such result from our main theorem 2.5. Several variants of this kind of result can obviously be similarly obtained. (See a recent paper by Lànskỳ and Lànskà [1985]). Let A_e^j (j=1, 2, $\cdots$) be nonnegative independent random variables with common distribution function F_e, and let A_i^l (l=1,2, $\cdots$) be nonpositive independent random variables with common distribution F_i. Regard F_e (resp. F_i) as the distribution of the random excitatory (resp. inhibitory) synaptic impulses. Assume that

$$\mathbf{E}|A_e^j|^p < \infty \tag{2.28}$$

and

$$\mathbf{E}|A_i^l|^p < \infty$$

for some $p > 2$ and write

$$\mathbf{E}(A_e^j) = a_e, \quad \mathbf{E}(A_i^l) = a_i, \tag{2.29}$$

$$\mathbf{Var}(A_e^j) = \sigma_e^2, \quad \mathbf{Var}(A_i^l) = \sigma_i^2$$

Let N_e and N_i be independent Poisson processes with parameters of f_e and f_i. The random variables A_e^j, A_i^l, N_e, and N_i are all taken to be mutually independent. Then for any Borel subset B of $\mathbf{B}$,

$$\mathbf{N}(B\times[0,t]) := \sum_{j=1}^{N_e(t)} I_B(A_e^j) + \sum_{l=1}^{N_i(t)} I_B(A_i^l)$$

is a Poisson random measure with intensity measure $\mu(da)dt$ where μ is the Borel measure given by $\mu(B) = f_e F_e(B) + f_i F_i(B)$. Instead of the SDE (2.26) let us consider the stochastic integral equation

$$\xi_t = \xi_0 - \beta\int_0^t \xi_s ds + \sum_{j=1}^{N_e(t)} (V_e - \xi_{\tau_j-})A_e^j + \sum_{l=1}^{N_i(t)} (\xi_{\tau_l-} - V_i)A_i^l.$$

Here β is positive and $\{\tau_j\}$, $\{\tau_l\}$ are the jump instants of the processes N_e, N_i respectively. Using the Poisson random measure defined above, this can be recast in the form of a stochastic integral equation of type (2.1):

$$d\xi_t = a_t(\xi_t)dt + \int_{\mathbf{R}} f_t(\xi_{t-}, u)\mathbf{N}(dudt) \tag{2.30}$$

where

$$a_t(x) := -\beta x + (V_e - x)f_e a_e + (x - V_i)f_i a_i, \tag{2.31}$$

and

$$f_t(x,u) := \begin{cases} (V_e - x)u & \text{if } u \geq 0 \\ (x - V_i)u & \text{if } u < 0. \end{cases} \tag{2.32}$$

The conditions (from Theorem 2.1) for the existence of a unique solution of (2.31) are satisfied. Let us now consider the diffusion approximation for a sequence of processes $\{\xi^k\}_{k<\infty}$ where ξ^k is the unique solution of an SIE of the type (2.30) where the coefficient functions $a_t(x)$, $f_t(x, u)$, the measures μ, F_e, F_i, f_e, f_i, $\mathbf{N}$, *etc.*, are now written with a superscript k. The conditions of Theorem 2.5 for weak convergence are easily verified under the following assumptions:

1) $\beta^k \to \beta \quad (\beta > 0)$;
2) $f_e^k a_e^k \to f_e a_e, \quad f_i^k a_i^k \to f_i a_i$;
3) $f_e^k(\sigma_e^k)^2 \to f_e(\sigma_e)^2, \quad f_i^k(\sigma_i^k)^2 \to f_i(\sigma_i)^2$.
4) $V_e^k \to V_e, V_i^k \to V_i$;

We then obtain the following diffusion approximation:

Corollary 4. Under the conditions 1) - 4) above, $\{\xi^k\}_{k<\infty}$ converges weakly to the diffusion process ξ satisfying:

$$d\xi_t = \left[-\beta\xi_t + (V_e - \xi_t)f_e a_e + (\xi_t - V_i)f_i a_i\right]dt + c_t(\xi_t)dW_t$$

where $c_t^2(x) := f_e\sigma_e^2(V_e - x)^2 + f_i\sigma_i^2(x - V_i)^2$ and W is a standard Wiener process.

2.5. The Hodgkin and Huxley equations.

In their seminal papers Hodgkin and Huxley [1952 a,b,c,d] introduced a mathematical model for the flow of current through the surface membrane of the giant axon from a Loligo squid. An important contribution of their work was the separate study of currents due to the passage of sodium, potassium, and chloride ions; the different patterns of membrane voltage dependence for the passage of these three species of ions can explain such diverse neurological phenomena as actions potentials and refractory periods, anode-break excitation and accommodation.

The model represented by the Hodgkin-Huxley equations

$$I = C_m\frac{\partial V}{\partial t} + \bar{g}_K n^4(V - V_K) + \bar{g}_{Na}m^3h(V - V_{Na}) + \bar{g}_{Cl}(V - V_{Cl}) \tag{2.33}$$

$$\frac{\partial n}{\partial t} = \alpha_n(1 - n) - \beta_n n$$

$$\frac{\partial m}{\partial t} = \alpha_m(1 - m) - \beta_m m$$

$$\frac{\partial h}{\partial t} = \alpha_h(1 - h) - \beta_h h$$

is a deterministic, not a stochastic one, and so the theory presented herein is not directly applicable. Nevertheless it is possible (and illuminating) to construct a variety of stochastic models which generalize (2.33); see Stevens [1972] for examples.

In the present (point neuron) setting one could set the net current $I = 0$ and regard the membrane capacitance C_m, the ion-specific reversal potentials V_K, V_{Na}, and V_{Cl} and maximum conductivities $\bar{g}_K$, $\bar{g}_{Na}$, $\bar{g}_{Cl}$ as specified constants. The four-dimensional process $\xi_t = (V,n,m,h)$ could then be modeled as the solution of an $\mathbf{R}^4$-valued stochastic integral equation similar to (2.1), driven by a generalized Poisson process whose events represent the movements of $n-$, $m-$, and $h-$ type ionic gate components into and out of the open configuration. If the increments these events lend to ξ are sufficiently small and if their arrivals are sufficiently frequent then (a vector-valued version of) Theorem 2.6 suggests a multidimensional diffusion model generalizing (2.33).

3. Stochastic Models for Spatially Extended Neurons

We shall denote by X the surface membrane of a neuron, and introduce stochastic models describing the evolution of the membrane potential $u(t, x)$ as a function of time $t \geq 0$ and location $x \in X$. In the preceding section the neuron was modeled as a single point $X = \{x_0\}$, and therefore the membrane potential u could be represented at each time $t > 0$ by the one-dimensional quantity $u(t, x_0)$. Even in the simplest spatially-extended case, that in which we take the neuron to be an infinitely-thin cylinder (*i.e.*, we take X to be an interval $[0, b]$), the space of possible values for the membrane potential $u(t, \cdot)$ at time $t \geq 0$ is infinite dimensional.

In this section we postulate that the membrane potential should exhibit a linear return to equilibrium following any random disturbances. This allows us to employ series expansions and the tools of harmonic analysis to study the behavior of spatially-extended neurons subject to a Gaussian stream or a generalized Poisson stream of random impulses.

Let $u(t, x)$ represent the value of the membrane potential (or, more precisely, the difference between the membrane potential and the resting potential) at the site x of the membrane X. As an important illustration we take X to be an infinitely thin cylinder of length $b > 0$, represented mathematically by the line segment $[0, b]$. The so-called core conductor theory suggests that, in the absence of external impulses, u should solve the cable equation

$$\frac{\partial u}{\partial t} = -\lambda u + \beta \Delta u \qquad t>0,\ 0<x<b \tag{3.1}$$

for some constants α, $\beta>0$, with specified initial value

$$u(0, x) = u_0(x),$$

and with Neumann boundary conditions:

$$\frac{\partial u}{\partial x}(t, 0) = \frac{\partial u}{\partial x}(t, b) = 0.$$

Using standard methods in partial differential equations it can be easily shown that the solution to (3.1) may be represented by $u(t,\cdot) = T_t u_0$ for a continuous contraction semigroup T_t on $H := L^2([0, b], dx)$ given by

$$(T_t f)(x) := \int_0^b G(x,y;t)\, f(y)\, dy.$$

Here $G(x,y;t)$ is the Green's function

$$G(x,y;t) = \sum_{n=0}^{\infty} e^{-\lambda_n t}\, \phi_n(x)\, \phi_n(y) \qquad (t > 0),$$

with eigenvalues and ortho-normal eigenfunctions given by

$$\lambda_n = \alpha + \beta(n\pi/b)^2, \quad \phi_n(x) = (2/b)^{1/2} \cos(n\pi x/b)$$

for $n \geq 1$, and

$$\lambda_0 = \alpha, \qquad \phi_0(x) = (1/b)^{1/2}.$$

The generator $-L$ is given by $-L := -\alpha I + \beta\Delta$ and the solution to (3.1) by $u(t, x) = \int_0^b G(x,y;t)u_0(y)dy$ for $t > 0$ and u_0 in the domain of L.

If the membrane potential receives random impulses at time t and site x, the differential equation in (3.1) may be replaced by

$$\frac{\partial V}{\partial t} = -\lambda V + \beta\Delta V + \dot{Z}_{tx} \tag{3.2}$$

where $\dot{Z}_{tx}$ represents the random impulse (assumed, for the present, to be Gaussian with mean $m(x)$). The above equation is completely heuristic and has to be made rigorous. For a suitable class Φ of "smooth" functions write:

$$\xi_t[\phi] := \int_0^b V(t, x)\, \phi(x)\, dx, \qquad \phi \in \Phi,\ t > 0.$$

Then (again formally using (3.1)),

$$\begin{aligned} \frac{d}{dt}\, \xi_t[\phi] &= \int_0^b \frac{\partial V}{\partial t}\, \phi(x)\, dx \\ &= \int_0^b -L'V(t, x)\, \phi(x)\, dx + \int_0^b \phi(x)\, \dot{Z}_{tx}\, dx. \\ &= \int_0^b -V(t, x)\, L\phi(x)\, dx + \int_0^b \phi(x)\, \dot{Z}_{tx}\, dx. \end{aligned}$$

$$= -\xi_t[L\phi] + \int_0^b \phi(x)m(x)\,dx + \int_0^b \phi(x)\,\dot{W}_{tx}\,dx, \text{ say.}$$

Now define the last integral rigorously as the stochastic integral $\int_0^b \phi(x)d_xW_{tx}$ where W_{tx} is the two parameter Yeh-Wiener process (or the *Brownian sheet*) with zero mean and covariance $\mathbf{E}W_{tx}W_{sy} = \min(t,s)\min(x,y)$. Write

$$W_t[\phi] := \int_0^b \phi(x)\,d_xW_{tx}$$

and

$$m[\phi] := \int_0^b m(x)\,\phi(x)\,dx.$$

Then a rigorous reformulation of (3.2) is

$$d\xi_t = (-L'\xi_t + m)\,dt + dW_t$$

or, in spatially integrated form,

$$d\xi_t[\phi] = (-\xi_t[L\phi] + m[\phi])\,dt + dW_t[\phi], \tag{3.3}$$

with initial value $\xi_0[\phi]$ a Gaussian random variable independent of $\{W_t[\psi]\}_{t<\infty,\ \psi\in\Phi}$.
For each ϕ, $W_t[\phi]$ is a real-valued Wiener process with mean zero and covariance

$$\mathbf{E}\,W_t[\phi]\,W_s[\psi] = \int_0^b \phi(x)\psi(x)\,dx \cdot \min(t,s)$$

$$= \langle\phi,\psi\rangle_H \cdot \min(t,s).$$

For this example, the natural choice for Φ is the linear space $\Phi = \cap\Phi_p$ where, for $p \in \mathbf{R}$

$$\Phi_p := \left\{\phi\in H : \sum_{n=0}^{\infty} (1+\lambda_n)^{2p}\langle\phi,\phi_n\rangle_H^2 < \infty\right\} \tag{3.4}$$

with dual space $\Phi' = \cup\Phi_{-p}$. The family of norms $\|\phi\|_p$ with $\|\phi\|_p^2 := \sum_{n=0}^{\infty}(1+\lambda_n)^{2p}\langle\phi,\phi_n\rangle_H^2$ defines a topology under which Φ is a countably Hilbertian nuclear space. It can then be shown that (3.3) can be written in the form

$$d\xi_t = (-L'\xi_t + m)dt + dW_t\,, \tag{3.5}$$

where $W = (W_t)$ is a Wiener process with continuous sample paths lying in Φ' (in fact, in Φ_{-p} for all $p > 1/4$). The operator L' is continuous and linear on Φ', defined by the relation $L'f[\phi] = f[L\phi]$ for all $\phi\in\Phi$ and $f\in\Phi'$.

3.1. Infinite-dimensional Ornstein-Uhlenbeck processes.

The SDE (3.5) makes sense for any measurable space X, with the Hilbert space H given by $H = L^2(X, d\Gamma)$ for some positive measure Γ, T_t a continuous contraction semigroup on H with compact generator $-L$, Φ given as in (3.4) with λ_n replaced by the nth smallest eigenvalue of L, $m \in \Phi'$ arbitrary, and W_t a Φ'-valued Wiener process with mean

$$\mathbf{E}W_t[\phi] = 0$$

and covariance

$$\mathbf{E}\ W_t[\phi]W_s[\psi] = Q(\phi,\psi)\cdot\min(t,s)$$

for some positive, continuous bilinear form Q on $\Phi\times\Phi$. This SDE is called a Φ'-valued (or spatio-temporal) Ornstein-Uhlenbeck (OU) SDE and its solution, a Φ'-valued OU process.

In the particular example of a cylinder-shaped axon or muscle fiber (which we have discussed at length to motivate our general approach), it has been shown by Walsh [1981] that the solution of (3.5) is given by a two-parameter process $V(t,x)$ such that $\xi_t[\phi] = \int_0^b V(t,x)\phi(x)dx$. The reason for introducing the Φ'-valued SDE for the membrane potential is that if the neuron X cannot be represented by an interval $[0, b]$, *e.g.*, if X is a two-dimensional region, a sphere S^d in $\mathbf{R}^{d+1}$ $(d \geq 2)$ or, more generally, a compact Riemannian manifold in two or more dimensions, the solution of (3.5) can *only* be given as a generalized process *i.e.*, a process taking values in some suitable space Φ' of generalized functions. The general situation is described as follows.

Theorem 3.1. Let ξ_0 be a Φ'-valued random variable independent of the Wiener process (W_t). Then the SDE (3.5) has a unique Φ'-valued solution $\xi = (\xi_t)$. Moreover, there exists a $p>0$ such that $\xi_\bullet \in C(\mathbf{R}_+,\Phi_{-p})$ a.s.

3.2. Discontinuous (Poisson driven) OU processes.

Let $\mathrm{N}(d\eta da dt)$ be a Poisson random measure on $\Phi'\times\mathbf{R}\times\mathbf{R}_+$ with intensity measure $\mu(d\eta da)dt$ and let $\tilde{\mathrm{N}}(d\eta da dt) := \mathrm{N}(d\eta da dt) - \mu(d\eta da)dt$ be its fully-compensated version. The intention is that $\mathrm{N}(\Lambda\times A\times[0, t])$ should represent the number of voltage impulses of size $a \in A \subseteq \mathbf{R}$ arriving at "sites" $\eta \in \Lambda$ at times $s \leq t$. An impulse arriving at a single point $\{x_0\}$ would be represented in this context by the "site" $\eta = \delta_{x_0}$, but we can now admit more general impulses-- those arriving simultaneously at more than one point, those arriving "smeared out" over a region, *etc.* If we represent excitatory and inhibitory synaptic impulses in this way by distributions η on the neuron X, the membrane potential ξ_t satisfies an SDE of the form

$$d\xi_t = (-L'\ \xi_t + m)dt + \int_{\mathbf{R}}\int_{\Phi'} a\ \eta\ \tilde{\mathrm{N}}(d\eta da dt) \tag{3.6}$$

with a given initial value ξ_0 and with $m := \int_{\mathbf{R}}\int_{\Phi'} a\eta\mu(d\eta da)$.

Some explanation of (3.6) is in order. Here, $M_t := \int_0^t \int_{\mathbf{R}}\int_{\Phi'} a\ \eta\ \tilde{\mathrm{N}}(d\eta da ds)$ is a Φ'-valued martingale (which we may take to be right-continuous) such that for each $\phi \in \Phi$,

$$M_t[\phi] = \int_0^t \int_{\mathbf{R}} \int_{\Phi'} a\, \eta[\phi]\, \tilde{N}(d\eta da ds).$$

We require that $\int_{\mathbf{R}} \int_{\Phi'} a^2\, \eta[\phi]^2\, \mu(d\eta da)$ be finite so that $\{M_t[\phi]\}_{0 \le t \le T}$ will be a square integrable martingale. Furthermore, it can be shown that m is an element of Φ'.

In earlier work [Kallianpur and Wolpert 1983], the above integral is taken over X instead of Φ'. The present version is more flexible (and more general) and is justified because any attempt to make a precise measurement say of current injection at a point x will render, in reality, a weighted average of the current injection at points near x; the linear functionals η of Φ' represent just such averages.

Under appropriate conditions the SDE (3.6) has a unique solution and there exists a $q \in \mathbf{R}$ such that $\xi_{\bullet}$ almost surely lies in the Skorokhod space $D(\mathbf{R}_+, \Phi_{-q})$ of Φ_{-q}-valued right continuous functions with left limits.

3.3. Myelinated fiber or axon with a single node of Ranvier.

Let the fiber be denoted by $X = [0, b]$ and let x_0 be the node of Ranvier (alternately, one might think of a current injection at the single point x_0). Let us take the simpler definition of M_t with random impulses arriving at points $x \in X$ rather than generalized sites $\eta \in \Phi'$. We take μ to be of the form $\mu(B \times A) = \delta_{x_0}(B) \cdot \mu_1(A)$ where $\delta_{x_0}(B) := 1_B(x_0)$ and

$$\mu_1(A) = \sum_{j=1}^{p} f_e^j\, 1_A(a_e^j) + \sum_{l=1}^{q} f_i^l\, 1_A(-a_i^l)\ .$$

Here $a_e^j > 0$, $-a_i^l < 0$ are the possible magnitudes of excitatory and inhibitory impulses and f_e^j, f_i^l are the intensity parameters of the independent Poisson processes giving rise to these impulses (it seems natural to take $p = q = 1$ in this problem). It is easy to verify that

$$\begin{aligned} \mathbf{E}\, M_t[\phi]^2 &= t\, Q(\phi, \phi) \\ &:= t \iint a^2 \phi(x)^2\, \mu(dxda) \end{aligned}$$

is given by

$$Q(\phi, \phi) = \sigma^2\, \phi(x_0)^2$$

with

$$\sigma^2 := \sum_{j=1}^{p} f_e^j\, (a_e^j)^2 + \sum_{l=1}^{q} f_i^l\, (a_i^l)^2.$$

Also we have $m[\phi] = \gamma\, \phi(x_0)$ with $\gamma := \sum_j f_e^j\, a_i^j - \sum_{l=1} f_i^l\, a_i^l\ .$

If it is assumed that in the absence of random disturbances the fiber behaves deterministically like the axon discussed at the beginning of Section 3, then the voltage potential at time $t>0$ is the solution of

$$d\xi_t = (-L'\,\xi_t + \gamma\,\delta_{x_0})dt + dM_t, \tag{3.7}$$

where δ_{x_0} denotes the Dirac δ-function at x_0. This can be written in spatially-integrated form as:

$$d\xi_t[\phi] = (-\xi_t[L\phi] + \gamma\phi(x_0))dt + dM_t[\phi].$$

Let us now consider the diffusion approximation. Let ξ^n and M^n be as above, with

$$\lim_{n\to\infty} \max_{j,\,l} \{a_e^{j,n}, a_i^{l,n}\} = 0, \tag{i}$$

$$\lim_{n\to\infty} \sigma_n^2 = \sigma^2 \qquad (0<\sigma^2<\infty) \tag{ii}$$

and

$$\lim_{n\to\infty} \gamma_n = \gamma \qquad (\gamma<\infty). \tag{iii}$$

Let the initial random variables ξ_0^n, independent of M^n, converge in distribution to some limiting distribution, and let ξ_0 have that limiting distribution. Then the approximation (in the sense of weak convergence) to the processes $\xi_\bullet^k$ is given by the OU process $\xi_\bullet$, the unique solution of the equation

$$d\xi_t = (-L'\,\xi_t + \gamma\,\delta_{x_0})\,dt + dW_t.$$

Here $W_\bullet$ is a centered Wiener process, independent of ξ_0, with covariance functional $Q(\phi, \psi) = \sigma^2\phi(x_0)\psi(x_0)$. Furthermore, it can be shown that $\xi_\bullet \in C(\mathbf{R}_+, \Phi_{-q})$ a.s., for some $q>\frac{1}{4}$. In the absence of a myelin sheath, we could allow the Poisson impulses to arrive at random points x chosen uniformly over the axon.

The approximation result stated above is a consequence of the general theorem given below. It is an extension by Christensen [1985] of a result due to Kallianpur and Wolpert [1983]. Christensen's version is more general in the sense that it does not make the assumption that T_t is a *contraction* semigroup, so that the generator A need not be of the form $A = -L$ for a *positive* operator L.

Theorem 3.2. Let there exist positive numbers r_0, r_1, r_2, and c, a positive bilinear form Q defined and continuous on $\Phi\times\Phi$, and an element $m\in\Phi'$ such that:

(1)

$$(m^n[\phi])^2 + Q^n(\phi, \phi) \le c\|\phi\|_{r_1}^2 \qquad \text{for each } n < \infty;$$

(2)

$$\lim_{n\to\infty} Q^n(\phi, \phi) = Q(\phi, \phi)$$

(3)

$$\lim_{n\to\infty} m^n[\phi] = m[\phi]$$

(4) For each n the initial random variable η^n is independent of M^n and $\{\eta^n\}$ converges in law to some Φ_{-r_0}-valued random variable η;

(5)

$$\sup_n \max\{\mathbf{E}\|\eta^n\|_{-r_2}^2, \mathbf{E}\|\eta^n\|_{-r_0}^2\} < \infty$$

(6)

$$\lim_{n\to\infty} \int_{\mathbf{R}}\int_{\Phi'} |a\eta[\phi]|^3\, \mu^n(d\eta da) = 0.$$

Then the Φ'-valued process $\xi^n_\bullet$ solving

$$d\xi^n_t = A'\,\xi^n_t\,dt + m^n\,dt + dM^n_t$$

with $\xi^n_0 = \eta^n$ converges weakly to the OU process $\xi_\bullet$ which is the solution of the SDE

$$d\xi_t = (A'\,\xi_t + m)\,dt + dW_t$$

with $\xi_0 = \eta$, where W is a zero mean Φ'-valued Wiener process with covariance functional Q. Moreover, for each $T>0$, there exists $p_T>0$ such that $\xi^T_\bullet := (\xi_t)_{0\le t\le T}$ satisfies

$$\xi^T_\bullet \in C([0, T];\, \Phi_{-p_T}) \qquad a.s.$$

Remark. If T_t is a contraction semigroup, there is a fixed p such that $\xi_\bullet := (\xi_t)_{t\in \mathbf{R}_+}$ satisfies

$$\xi_\bullet \in C(\mathbf{R}_+, \Phi_{-p}) \qquad a.s.$$

This final assertion can fail if T_t is taken to be a noncontractive semigroup or if W is replaced by a more general martingale.

4. Spatially extended neurons: Nonlinear infinite-dimensional SDE's

We introduce now two classes of Φ'-valued SDE's for spatially extended neurons, one to correspond to the discontinuous (Poisson) and one for the continuous but non-Gaussian diffusion cases.

4.1. Discontinuous SDE's for Φ'-valued processes.

The SDE we consider is a generalization of the equations discussed in Theorem 1.1 in Section 1. For simplicity, however, the term involving the Wiener process is omitted. Let

$$a_t(\mathrm{v}) : \ \mathbf{R}_+ \times \Phi' \to \Phi' \tag{i}$$

and

$$f_t(\mathrm{v}, u) : \ \mathbf{R}_+ \times \Phi' \times U \to \Phi' \tag{ii}$$

be jointly continuous, where U is a topological space and Φ' is endowed with the strong topology.

Let

$$\mathbf{N}(du, dt) \tag{iii}$$

be a Poisson random measure on $\Phi' \times \mathbf{R}_+$ with intensity measure $\mu(du)dt$.

The SDE that is appropriate for us is

$$d\xi_t = a_t(\xi_t)\,dt + \int_U f_t(\xi_{t-}, u)\mathbf{N}(du, dt), \tag{4.1}$$

with ξ_0 a given Φ'-valued random variable independent of $\mathbf{N}$.

For reasons of space it is not possible here to give a precise definition of what is meant by a solution of (4.1) , nor to give conditions to be satisfied by the coefficient functions that ensure the existence of a unique solution. If $\xi = (\xi_t)$ is a solution on some probability space (Ω, F, P) then ξ will have sample paths in the Skorokhod space $D := D(\mathbf{R}_+, \Phi')$ of Φ'-valued right continuous functions with left limits. In seeking diffusion approximations to (4.1) our concern will be to study the weak convergence of a sequence $P^k := \mathbf{P}\,(\xi^k)^{-1}$ of measures induced on D by solutions ξ_k of SDE's (4.1) with coefficient functions a^k, f^k, and measures μ^k.

Note that (4.1), in compensated form, can be written as

$$d\xi_t = \tilde{a}_t(\xi_t)\,dt + \int_U f_t(\xi_{t-}, u)\,\tilde{\mathbf{N}}(dudt) \tag{4.2}$$

where

$$\tilde{a}_t(\xi_t) := a_t(\xi_t) + \int_U f_t(\xi_t, u)\,\mu(du)$$

and

$$\tilde{\mathbf{N}}(dudt) := \mathbf{N}(dudt) - \mu(du)dt.$$

The reversal potential model can be described in this setting; we will generalize Corollary 4 of Theorem 2.7 to the spatially extended neuron. Let A_e^j, A_i^l, F_e, F_i, N_e, N_i, f_e, f_i be as in Corollary 4. Take $U := \Phi' \times \mathbf{R}$. Let η_e and η_i be fixed elements of Φ' called the *reversal potentials* for the excitatory and inhibitory impulses respectively. Let $\mathbf{N}(d\eta\ da\ ds)$ be the Poisson random measure such that, for any Borel sets $\Lambda \subset \Phi'$ and $B \subset \mathbf{R}$,

$$\mathbf{N}(\Lambda \times B \times [0, t]) := \delta_{\eta_e}(\Lambda) \sum_{j=1}^{N_e(t)} 1_B(A_e^j) + \delta_{\eta_i}(\Lambda) \sum_{l=1}^{N_i(t)} 1_B(A_i^l)$$

The intensity measure is then given by

$$\mu(\Lambda \times B) := f_e\, \delta_{\eta_e}(\Lambda)\, F_e(B) + f_i\, \delta_{\eta_i}(\Lambda)\, F_i(B).$$

Let us choose $a_t(v) := -L'v$ for $v \in \Phi'$ and for $(\eta, u) \in \Phi' \times \mathbf{R}$,

$$f_t(v, \eta, u) := \begin{cases} (\eta - v)u & \text{if } u \ge 0, \\ (v - \eta)u & \text{if } u < 0. \end{cases}$$

Then the SDE with reversal potentials is given by

$$\xi_t = \xi_0 + \int_0^t a_s(\xi_s)\,ds + \sum_{j=1}^{N_e(t)} (\eta_e - \xi_{\tau_j-})A_e^j + \sum_{l=1}^{N_i(t)} (\xi_{\tau_l'-} - \eta_i)A_i^l. \tag{4.3}$$

Let us apply (4.3) to the special example considered in Section 3 where $\mathbf{X} = [0,1]$ is the model of an axon or muscle fiber and the white noise impulses are uniformly distributed over the axon, *i.e.*, $\Gamma(dx) = (dx)$ is Lebesgue measure, and T_t is the semigroup of the Neumann problem. Then, since $\xi_t[\phi] = \int_0^1 v(t,x)\phi(x)\,dx$, setting $\eta_e[\phi] = \int_0^1 \eta_e(x)\phi(x)\,dx$ (similarly for η_i) we obtain the equation

$$v(t, x) = v(0, x) - \int_0^t L'v(s, x)ds + \sum_{j=1}^{N_e(t)} A_e^j [\eta_e(x) - v(\tau_j -, x)] + \sum_{l=1}^{N_i(t)} A_i^l [v(\tau_l' -, x) - \eta_i(x)].$$

Here the reversal potentials are allowed to vary with x, *i.e.*, with the site on the membrane at which impulses arrive. The above class of SDE's and the diffusion approximation problem are being studied by G. Kallianpur, S. Ramasubramanian, and G. Hardy.

4.2. Non Gaussian diffusion SDE's.

These are non-Gaussian generalizations of the OU processes considered in Section 1.

An interesting non-Gaussian (non linear) SDE closely related to the OU SDE is the following:

$$d\xi_t = [-L'\xi_t + m_t(\xi_t)]\, dt + dW_t$$

where L' and W are as in Section 3.1. Instead of assuming that m (which stands for the mean of the noise impulses received at time t at site x) is a constant, one can let m depend both on t and the instantaneous state ξ_t. In other words we assume $m_t(v)$: $\mathbf{R}_+ \times \Phi' \to \Phi'$ and in general, $m_t(v)$ is a nonlinear function of t and v. If we further assume that $m_t(v) = P_t'v$ where P_t is a continuous linear map from Φ to Φ and $m_t(v)[\phi] = v[P_t\phi]$, then we have the equation:

$$d\xi_t = (-L'\xi_t + P_t'\xi_t)dt + dW_t. \tag{4.4}$$

In this special form, the SDE occurs in the context of other physical problems *e.g.*, in connection with fluctuation theorems in interacting particle systems. (see Mitoma [1983], Kallianpur and Perez-Abreu [1986]).

Diffusion approximations to SDE's of the form (4.2) turn out, under suitable conditions, to be of the form

$$d\xi_t = A(t, \xi_t)dt + B(t, \xi_t)\, dW_t \tag{4.5}$$

$$\xi_0 = \eta.$$

Here the coefficient functions A, B are mappings

$$A : \mathbf{R}_+ \times \Phi' \to \Phi' \qquad \text{a)}$$

$$B : \mathbf{R}_+ \times \Phi' \to \mathbf{L}(\Phi', \Phi'), \qquad \text{b)}$$

where $\mathbf{L}(\Phi', \Phi')$ denotes the family of all continuous linear operators from Φ' to Φ', $W = (W_t)$ is a Φ'-valued Wiener process with covariance Q, and η is a Φ'-valued initial random variable independent of W. In order to give a precise meaning to (4.5) as a stochastic integral equation, one needs to discuss in some detail the properties of Φ'-valued Wiener processes and of stochastic integrals of the kind $\int_0^t f_s\, dW_s$ where f_s is a stochastic process with values in $\mathbf{L}(\Phi',\Phi')$.

We omit this discussion as well as the somewhat lengthy proof of the result given below, for lack of space and also because it lies outside the main sphere of interest of this article. The work presented here is due to Kallianpur and Wolpert [1985, unpublished].

Theorem 4.1. A unique solution to (4.5) exists if for every $T > 0$ and sufficiently large $m \geq 0$, there exist numbers $r > 2$, $\theta > 0$ and $p \geq m$ such that A, B the initial measure μ_0 for ξ_0 and the covariance functional Q satisfy the following conditions:

(Initial Condition).
$$\int_{\Phi'} \|v\|^r_{-m}\, \mu_0(dv) < \infty. \tag{IC}$$

(Coercivity). Let j_m be the canonical isomorphism between Φ_m and Φ_{-m}. For each $t \leq T$ and $v \in \Phi$

$$2A_t(j_m v)[v] + (r-1)\|Q_{B_t'(v)}\|_{-m,-m} \leq \theta(1+\|j_m v\|^2_{-m}); \tag{CC}$$

here $\|\cdot\|_{-m,-m}$ is the trace norm of the nuclear operator determined by the bilinear form $Q_{B_t'(v)}$:

$$Q_{B_t'(v)}(\phi, \psi) := Q(B_t'(v)\phi, B_t'(v)\psi), \qquad \phi, \psi \in \Phi$$

and $B_t'(v) : \Phi \to \Phi$ is the dual map of $B_t(v)$.

(Linear Growth). For each $t \leq T$ and $v \in \Phi_{-m}$, $A_t(v) \in \Phi_{-p}$ and

$$\| A_t(v) \|^2_{-p} \leq \theta\ (1 + \|v\|^2_{-m}) \tag{LG}$$

$$\|Q_{B_t'(v)}\|^2_{-m} \leq \theta\ (1 + \|v\|^2_{-m}).$$

(Monotonicity). For each $t \leq T$ and u, $v \in \Phi_{-m}$, $A_t(u)$, $A_t(v) \in \Phi_{-p}$ and

$$2\langle u-v, A_t(u)-A_t(v)\rangle_{-p} + (r-1)\|Q_{B_t'(u)-B_t'(v)}\|_{-p,-p} \leq \theta\|u-v\|^2_{-p}. \tag{MC}$$

(Joint Continuity).
$$A\colon [0, T] \times \Phi' \to \Phi' \tag{JC}$$

and

$$B : [0, T] \times \Phi' \to \mathbf{L}(\Phi', \Phi')$$

are jointly continuous. Observe that the indices m and p may depend on T.

Furthermore, the unique solution $\xi = (\xi_t)$ has the property that $\xi^T_\bullet := (\xi_t)_{0 \leq t \leq T}$ belongs to the space of continuous functions $\mathbf{C}([0, T], \Phi_{-p_T})$ a.s.

The conditions listed above are similar to (but not identical with) those used by Krylov and Rozovskii [1979] in their investigation of stochastic evolution equations. It may be mentioned that, in our proof, the monotonicity condition is employed in proving uniqueness. Without it, the remaining conditions imply the existence of a weak solution.

References.

Billingsley, P. [1968]. *Convergence of Probability Measures.* John Wiley & Sons, Inc., New York.

Christensen, S.K. and G. Kallianpur [1985]. Stochastic differential equations for neuronal behavior. *Tech. Rept.* 103, Center for Stochastic Processes, University of North Carolina at Chapel Hill.

Cope, D.K. and H.C. Tuckwell [1979]. Firing rates of neurons with random excitation and inhibition. *J. Theor. Biol.* **8**, 1-14.

Gikhman, I.I. and A.V. Skorokhod [1972]. *Stochastic Differential Equations*. Springer-Verlag, Berlin.

Hodgkin, A.L. and A.F. Huxley [1952a]. Currents carried by sodium and potassium ions through the membrane of the giant axon of *Loligo*. *J. Physiol.* **116**, 449-472.

Hodgkin, A.L. and A.F. Huxley [1952b]. The components of membrane conductance in the giant axon of *Loligo*. *J. Physiol.* **116**, 473-496.

Hodgkin, A.L. and A.F. Huxley [1952c]. The dual effect of membrane potential on sodium conduction in the giant axon of *Loligo*. *J. Physiol.* **116**, 497-506.

Hodgkin, A.L. and A.F. Huxley [1952d]. A quantitative description of membrane current and its application to conduction and excitation in nerve. *J. Physiol.* **117**, 500-544.

Ikeda, N. and S. Watanabe [1981]. *Stochastic Differential Equations and Diffusion Processes*. North-Holland, Amsterdam.

Johannesma, P.I.M. [1968]. Diffusion models for the stochastic activity of neurons. In: *Neural Networks*. Caianiello, E.R. ed. Springer-Verlag, Berlin.

Kallianpur, G. [1983]. On the diffusion approximation to a discontinuous model for a single neuron. *Contributions to Statistics*, Essays in Honour of Norman L. Johnson, ed. by P.K. Sen, North-Holland, 247-257.

Kallianpur, G. and V. Perez-Abreu [1986]. Stochastic evolution equations with values on the dual of a countably Hilbert nuclear space. *Tech. Rept.* 145, Center for Stochastic Processes, University of North Carolina at Chapel Hill.

Kallianpur, G. and R.L. Wolpert [1984]. Infinite dimensional stochastic differential equation models for spatially distributed neurons. *J. Appl. Math. and Optimization.*

Karlin, S. and H.M. Taylor [1981]. *A Second Course in Stochastic Processes*. Academic Press, New York.

Krylov, N.V. and B.L. Rozovskii [1979]. Stochastic evolution equations. Eng. Trans. from *Itogi Nauki i Tekhniki,* **14**, 71-146.

Kubo, R. [1986]. Brownian Motion and Nonequilibrium Statistical Mechanics. *Science* **233**, 330-334.

Lànskỳ, P. and V. Lànskà [1985]. Diffusion approximations of the neuronal model with synaptic reversal potentials. [Preprint].

Liptser, R.S. and A.N. Shiryaev [1984]. Weak convergence of a sequence of semimartingales to a process of diffusion type. *Math. USSR Sbornik,* **49**, 171-194.

Mitoma, I. [1985]. An infinite-dimensional inhomogeneous Langevin's equation. *J. Funct. Anal.* **61**, 342-359.

Noda, M., S. Shimizu, T. Tanabe, T. Takai, T. Kayano, T. Ikeda, H. Takahashi, H. Nakayama, Y. Kanaoka, N. Minamino, K. Kangawa, H. Matsuo, M. Raftery, T. Hirose, S. Inayama, H. Hayashida, T. Mihata, and S. Numa [1984]. Primary structure of *Electrophorus electricus* sodium channel deduced from cDNA sequence. *Nature* **312**, 121-127.

Rall, W. [1978]. Core conductor theory and cable properties of neurons. In: Brookhart J.M., V.B. Mountcastle (eds) *Handbook of Physiology*. Amer. Physiol. Soc., Bethesda, 39-98.

Ricciardi, L.M. and L. Sacerdote [1979]. The Ornstein-Uhlenbeck process as a model for neuronal activity. *Biol. Cybernetics* **35**, 1-9.

Stein, R.B. [1965]. A theoretical analysis of neuronal variability. *Biophys. J.* **5**, 173-194.

Stevens, C.F. [1972]. Inferences about membrane properties from electrical noise measurements. *Biophys. J.* **12**, 1028-1047.

Stroock, D.W. and S.R.S. Varadhan [1979]. *Multidimensional Diffusion Processes*. Springer-Verlag, Berlin.

Walsh, J.B. [1981]. A stochastic model of neural responses. *Adv. Appl. Prob.* **13**, 231-281.

Wan, F.Y.M. and H.C. Tuckwell [1979]. The response of a spatially distributed neuron to white noise current injection. *Biol. Cybernetics* **33**, 39-55.

NOTE ON THE ORNSTEIN-UHLENBECK PROCESS MODEL FOR STOCHASTIC ACTIVITY OF A SINGLE NEURON

Shunsuke Sato

Department of Biophysical Engineering
Faculty of Engineering Science, Osaka University
Toyonaka, Osaka 560 JAPAN

Summary Spontaneous activity of a single neuron is considered using the Ornstein-Uhlenbeck process model. The interspike intervals are viewed as the first-passage-times for the process starting at some initial value through a constant boundary. The moments of the first-passage-time probability density function(p.d.f.), the asymptotic forms of the p.d.f. for large boundary and for large time are obtained.

1. Introduction

Spontaneous activities of single neurons belonging to complex networks such as Purkinje cells are frequently modeled using diffusion processes including the simplest Brownian motion. If the effective neuronal input may be taken as the result of the superposition of 10^4 to 10^5 independent point processes describing the time sequence of PSP's and an arrival of the point process changes on the membrane potential positively or negatively, the random walk models and hence their continuous time and continuous space limits, i.e., diffusion processes seem to be reasonable candidates to account for the membrane potential fluctuation[1]. We do not go into details about the derivations of the diffusion models from this standpoints, since one may consult papers [2] ,[3] for these, except for pointing out that the neuronal firing is considered to occur when the membrane potential achieves some value as threshold which may change with time. Brownian motion model[4] and the Ornstein-Uhlenbeck process model[2] have been thus proposed as the simplest ones. Such diffusion models are now considered to be too oversimplified in explaining the neuronal firing in several respects, nevertheless it is worth to study because these models offer us interesting mathematical problems - namely the first passage time problems whose explicit solutions are still unknown except for the simplest cases. If we replace the membrane potential with diffusion process, and the threshold with a boundary S(t), then the neuronal firing time is viewed as the process' first passage time through the boundary S(t).

In the sequel, we shall concentrate ourselves on the Ornstein-Uhlenbeck model as such neuronal events. In other words, we shall focus on the first passage time problem for the O-U process through a generally time varying boundary S(t).

The first passage time problem for the O-U process has been studied from various points of view: moments[2],[5], asymptotic behaviors[5],[6], numerical solutions[1],[7], etc. Here we give some new results on the moments and the asymptotic behavior in a very brief way using the Laplace transform technique. More precise discussions will be made in a subsequent paper.

2. Preliminaries

Consider the Ornstein-Uhlenbeck process X(t) generated by the stochastic differential equation:

$$dX(t) = -\frac{X(t)}{\theta}dt + \sqrt{\mu}\,dB(t) \qquad (1)$$

where B(t) is the Wiener process and θ, μ are positive constants. The term $\mu dB(t)$ is understood to be the totality of the input which causes the fluctuation of the membrane potential, and θ the membrane time constant by which the membrane potential decays to the steady state value. Denote by $p(x,t|y,s)$ (or $p(x,t|y,0) = p(x,t|y)$, since the process is stationary) the transition p.d.f. of the process. Our problem is then stated as follows: Obtain the first passage time p.d.f. through a generally time varying boundary S(t) for the O.U. process X(t) starting at $x_0 < S(0)$. Denote the p.d.f. by $g(t,S(t)|x_0)$. As is well known, we have the following relation:

For $x \gtrless S(t) \gtrless x_0$,

$$p(x,t|x_0) = \int_0^t p(x,t-u|S(u))g(u,S(u)|x_0)du \qquad (2)$$

The above integral equation on $g(t,S(t)|x_0)$ has been numerically solved by several methods[8],[9], and some interesting features on the first passage time p.d.f. as well as on the asymptotic means and variance were revealed[5],[6],[10].

For a constant boundary case, one may take the Laplace transform technique to approach the problem: In fact, denoting the Laplace transform of $p(x,t|y)$ and $g(t,S|x_0)$ for a constant S by $p^*(\lambda,x|y)$ and $g^*(\lambda,S|x_0)$ respectively, we know that the explicit expression for the g^* is given by[10],[2],[3]

$$g^*(\lambda,S|x_0) = \begin{cases} \exp\left(\dfrac{x_0^2-S^2}{2\mu\theta}\right) \dfrac{D_{-\lambda\theta}(-x_0\sqrt{2/\mu\theta})}{D_{-\lambda\theta}(-S\sqrt{2/\mu\theta})}, & S > x_0, \quad (3a) \\[2ex] \exp\left(\dfrac{x_0^2-S^2}{2\mu\theta}\right) \dfrac{D_{-\lambda\theta}(x_0\sqrt{2/\mu\theta})}{D_{-\lambda\theta}(S\sqrt{2/\mu\theta})}, & 0 < S < x_0, \quad (3b) \end{cases}$$

where $D_\lambda(z)$ is the parabolic cylinder function ([12], vol.II).

In what follows, we shall take $\theta = 1$ and $\mu = 2$ for the sake of simplicity. Eq.(3a) can be written as[5],[6]

$$g^*(\lambda,S|x_0) = \frac{\phi(\lambda,x_0)}{\phi(\lambda,S)} \tag{4}$$

where

$$\phi(\lambda,z) = F\left(\frac{\lambda}{2},\frac{1}{2};\frac{z^2}{2}\right) + \frac{\Gamma(\frac{1+\lambda}{2})}{\Gamma(\frac{\lambda}{2})}\sqrt{2}z\, F\left(\frac{1+\lambda}{2},\frac{3}{2};\frac{z^2}{2}\right) \tag{5a}$$

$$= \sum_{n=0}^{\infty} \frac{(\sqrt{2}z)^n}{n!} \frac{\Gamma(\frac{n+\lambda}{2})}{\Gamma(\frac{\lambda}{2})} \tag{5b}$$

In eq.(5), $F(\alpha,\gamma;z)$ is the Kummer function defined as

$$F(\alpha,\gamma;z) = \sum_{n=0}^{\infty} \frac{(\alpha)_n}{(\gamma)_n} \frac{z^n}{n!}$$

$$(\beta)_n = \beta(\beta+1)\ldots(\beta+n-1) \tag{6}$$

and $\Gamma(\cdot)$ is the gamma function. Note that $\phi(0,z) = 1$.

3. Moments

The moments can be obtained using the Siegert's formula[11]. In fact, the first few moments were calculated via the formula[2],[10].

In this section, we shall compute the moments by making use of $g^*(\lambda,S|x_0)$. Let us denote by $t_n(S|x_0)$ the n-th moment of the first passage time p.d.f.:

$$t_n(S|x_0) = \int_0^{\infty} t^n g(t,S|x_0)dt \tag{7}$$

Since we know the Laplace transform $g^*(\lambda,S|x_0)$ of the p.d.f., $t_n(S|x_0)$, n=0,1,2,... are obtained via the formula:

$$t_n(S|x_0) = (-1)^n \frac{\partial^n}{\partial \lambda^n} g^*(\lambda,S|x_0)\bigg|_{\lambda=0} \tag{8}$$

$$n = 0,1,2,\ldots$$

Thus differentiating both sides of the trivial variant of eq.(4) with respect to λ and putting $\lambda = 0$, we have

$$\sum_{k=0}^{n} \binom{n}{k} (-1)^k t_k(S|x_0)\phi^{(n-k)}(0,S) = \phi^{(n)}(0,x_0) \tag{9}$$

where

$$\phi^{(k)}(0,z) = \frac{\partial^k}{\partial \lambda^k} \phi(\lambda,z)\bigg|_{\lambda=0}, \quad k = 0,1,\ldots \tag{10}$$

Especially for $x_0 = 0$,

$$\sum_{k=0}^{n} \binom{n}{k} (-1)^k t_k(S|0) \phi^{(n-k)}(0,S) = \delta_{n,0} \tag{11}$$

where δ_{ij} is Kronecker's delta. Equation (9) ((10)) can be recursively solved with respect to $t_n(S|x_0)$ ($t_n(S|0)$).

For instances,

$$\begin{aligned}
t_0(S|x_0) &= 1 \\
t_1(S|x_0) &= \phi_1(S) - \phi_1(x_0) \\
t_2(S|x_0) &= 2[\phi_1(S)]^2 - \phi_2(S) \\
&\quad - 2\phi_1(S)\phi_1(x_0) + \phi_2(x_0) \\
t_3(S|x_0) &= 6[\phi_1(S)]^3 - 6\phi_1(S)\phi_2(S) + \phi_3(S) \\
&\quad - \{6[\phi_1(S)]^2 - 3\phi_2(S)\}\phi_1(x_0) \\
&\quad + 3\phi_1(S)\phi_2(x_0) - \phi_3(x_0) \\
&\cdots \quad \cdots \quad \cdots
\end{aligned} \tag{12}$$

where we have put $\phi_k(z) = \phi^{(k)}(0,z)$.

Expressions for $\phi^{(1)}(0,z)$, $\phi^{(2)}(0,z)$ and $\phi^{(3)}(0,z)$ in the forms of power series in z are given in [2], [5] and [10]. It is not so hard to obtain the expressions to $\phi^{(k)}(0,z)$ for $k \geqq 4$. To this end, let us put

$$\rho_n(\lambda) = \frac{\Gamma(\frac{n+\lambda}{2})}{\Gamma(\frac{\lambda}{2})} \tag{13}$$

From the definition(5b) of $\phi(\lambda,z)$,

$$\phi^{(k)}(0,z) = \sum_{n=1}^{\infty} \frac{(\sqrt{2}z)^n}{n!} \rho_n^{(k)}(0), \qquad k=1,2,\ldots \tag{14}$$

It is easy to see that

$$\rho_n^{(1)}(0) = \frac{\Gamma(\frac{n}{2})}{2} \tag{15a}$$

$$\rho_n^{(k+1)}(0) = \frac{k+1}{k} \sum_{j=1}^{k} \binom{k}{j} \rho_n^{(j)}(0)\, \xi_n^{(k-j)}(0) \tag{15b}$$

$$k=1,2,\ldots$$

where

$$\xi_n(\lambda) = [\psi(\frac{n+\lambda}{2}) - \psi(1+\frac{\lambda}{2})]/2 \tag{16}$$

with $\psi(z)$ being the Di-gamma function, i.e.,

$$\psi(z) = \frac{1}{\Gamma(z)} \frac{d}{dz} \Gamma(z) \tag{17}$$

Relations (14) and (15) enable us to calculate $\phi^{(k)}(0,z)$.

Now let us consider asymptotic moments, namely moments for large S. Recall the expression (5a) of $\phi(\lambda,z)$. Using the asymptotic expansion of $F(\alpha,\gamma;z)$ for large z [12];

$$F(\alpha,\gamma;z) = \frac{\Gamma(\gamma)}{\Gamma(\alpha)} e^z z^{\alpha-\gamma}[1 + (z^{-1})] \tag{18}$$

We obtain

$$\phi(\lambda,z) = \frac{2e^{\lambda \lg(z/\sqrt{2})}}{\Gamma(\frac{\lambda}{2})} / g(z) [1 + O(z^{-1})] \tag{19}$$

where

$$g(z) = \frac{z}{\sqrt{2\pi}} \exp[- \frac{z^2}{2}] \tag{20}$$

Accordingly

$$\frac{\partial}{\partial\lambda}\phi(\lambda,z) = \frac{2e^{\lambda \lg\frac{z}{\sqrt{2}}}}{\Gamma(z)}[\lg\frac{z}{\sqrt{2}} - \frac{1}{2}\psi(\frac{\lambda}{2})]/g(z)[1 + O(z^{-1})]$$

Hence

$$\phi^{(1)}(0,z) = g^{-1}(z)[1 + O(z^{-1})] \tag{21}$$

For large z, $\phi^{(k)}(0,z)$, k=0,1,2,... are of order $(q(z)^{-1})$, because, roughly speaking, the evaluation of the k-th derivative of $[2e^{\lambda \lg(z/\sqrt{2})}/\Gamma(\lambda/2)]$ at $\lambda = 0$ gives us the term of order $(\lg(z/\sqrt{2}))^k$. Now one may show without difficulty that

$$t_1(S|x_0) \sim 1/q(s)$$
$$t_2(S|x_0) \sim 2/[q(S)]^2 \qquad (22)$$
$$t_3(S|x_0) \sim 6/[q(S)]^3$$
$$\cdots \quad \cdots \quad \cdots$$

which in turn gives us the central moments: $\mu_1(S)$, $\mu_2(S)$, and $\mu_3(S)$, ... And finally we obtain

$$M = 1/q(S) \qquad ;\ \text{mean}$$
$$V = 1/[q(S)]^2 \qquad ;\ \text{variance} \qquad (23)$$
$$\Sigma = 2 \qquad ;\ \text{skewness}$$

for large S.

Table of M, V, and Σ for $\lambda = 1$ and $\mu = 2$ and for various S and x_0 was given in [10]. One may find in the table that the skewness approaches 2 as S becomes large.

4. Asymptotic behavior of $g(t,S|x_0)$

As indicated by eq.(4), if we know zeros of $\phi(\lambda,z)$, g^* can be inverted. We shall discuss the zeros firstly. Let us rewrite eq.(4) as

$$g^*(\lambda,S|x_0) = \frac{\Phi(\lambda,x_0)}{\Phi(\lambda,S)} \qquad (24)$$

where

$$\Phi(\lambda,z) = \frac{1}{\Gamma(\frac{1+\lambda}{2})} F(\frac{\lambda}{2},\frac{1}{2};\frac{z^2}{2}) + \frac{\sqrt{2}\,z}{\Gamma(\frac{\lambda}{2})} F(\frac{1+\lambda}{2},\frac{3}{2};\frac{z^2}{2}) \qquad (25a)$$

$$= \sum_{n=0}^{\infty} \frac{(\sqrt{2}z)^n}{n!} \frac{\Gamma(\frac{n+\lambda}{2})}{\Gamma(\frac{\lambda}{2})\Gamma(\frac{1+\lambda}{2})} \qquad (25b)$$

Note that $\Phi(\lambda,z)$ is analytical everywhere as a function of λ and z and the zeros of $\Phi(\lambda,z)$ with respect to λ coincide with those of $\phi(\lambda,z)$. Note also that for $p = 0,1,\ldots,$

$$\Phi(-p,z) = \frac{(-1)^p}{2^{p/2}\sqrt{\pi}} H_p(z) \tag{26}$$

where $H_p(z)$ is the Hermite polynomial of order p:

$$H_p(z) = (-1)^p \exp(\frac{z^2}{2}) \frac{d^p}{dz^p} \exp(-\frac{z^2}{2}) \tag{27}$$

In view of (25b) and (26), one may easily see that approximate solutions of $\Phi(\lambda,z) = 0$ near z=0 are given by

$$\lambda = \lambda_p(z) = -2p-1 + \frac{(2p+1)!!}{(2p)!!}\sqrt{\frac{2}{\pi}}z, \quad p = 0,1,2,... \tag{28}$$

On the other hand, we note that ,for large z,

$$\Phi^{(k)}(-p,z) = \frac{(-1)^p}{2^p} \frac{kp!}{\sqrt{\pi}} \frac{(lg\frac{z}{\sqrt{2}})^{k-1}}{(\frac{z}{\sqrt{2}})^p} / g(z) [1 + O(\alpha^{-1})] \tag{29}$$

where $\alpha = lg(z/\sqrt{2})$ and g(z) is the same function as defined in (20). In fact, from (25a) and (18), one may see that for a large but fixed z,

$$\Phi(\lambda,z) = [\theta(\lambda)/g(z)][1+O(z^{-1})] \tag{30}$$

where

$$\theta(\lambda) = \frac{2e^{\alpha\lambda}}{\Gamma(\frac{1+\lambda}{2})\Gamma(\frac{\lambda}{2})} \tag{31}$$

Note that for small λ and for a non-negative integer p, $\theta(-p+\lambda)$ can be written as

$$\theta(-p+\lambda) = (-1)^p \frac{e^{-\alpha p}}{2^p} e^{\alpha\lambda} \omega_p(\lambda) \tag{32}$$

where the function

$$\omega_p(\lambda) = \frac{\lambda(1-\lambda)...(p-\lambda)}{\Gamma(1+\frac{\lambda}{2})\Gamma(\frac{1+\lambda}{2})} \tag{33}$$

is infinitely differentiable near $\lambda = 0$. Now it is easy to see that for large z (and hence for large α)

$$\theta^{(k)}(-p) = (-1)^p \frac{e^{-\alpha p}}{2^p} \frac{kp!}{\sqrt{\pi}} \alpha^{k-1} [1 + O(\alpha^{-1})] \tag{34}$$

Then the relation (29) follows. Now expanding $\Phi(-p+\lambda, z)$ as

$$\Phi(-p+\lambda, z) = \Phi(-p, z) + \Phi^{(1)}(-p, z)\lambda + \Phi^{(2)}(-p, z)\frac{\lambda^2}{2} + \cdots$$

and making use of eq.(29), we obtain approximate solutions of $\Phi(\lambda, z) = 0$ for large z as follows:

$$\lambda = \lambda_p(z) = -p - \frac{z^p H_p(z)}{p!} g(z), \quad p = 0,1,2,\ldots \tag{35}$$

Note also that

$$0 < -\lambda_0(S) \ll 1 < -\lambda_1(S) < 2 < -\lambda_2(S) < \cdots$$

Namely for large S, $\lambda_0(S) \sim g(S)$ is very close to zero while $|\lambda_p(S)| > 1$ for p=1,2,... Therefore we may conclude that for large S

$$g[t, S|0] \sim q(S)e^{-q(S)t} \tag{36}$$

This asymptotic form for large S also provides us the asymptotic mean, variance, and skewness, ... which are identical with those given in (23).

We should point out here that there exist curves $\lambda = \lambda_p(z)$, p=0,1,2,... such that $\Phi(\lambda_p(z), z) = 0$ for any z, and that the curves $\lambda = \lambda_p(z)$ behave as the rhs of (28) for small z and as the rhs of (35) for large z. Hence $g(t, S|x_0)$ is expressible as the sum of exponential functions:

$$g(t, S|x_0) = \sum_p A_p(S|x_0) e^{\lambda_p(S)t} \tag{37}$$

Let us consider the asymptotic behavior of $g(t,S|x_0)$ for both large t and small t. Sato[5] showed that for large t, the $g(t,S|x_0)$ is proportional to exp(-$\lambda(S)t$) where $-\lambda(S)$ is the smallest zero in modulus of $\phi(\lambda,S)$ as a function of λ. Here one should note that the function $-\lambda(S)$ is $\lambda_0(S)$ in our context, since the zeros of $\phi(\lambda,S)$ are identical with those of $\Phi(\lambda,S)$ for a given S. In view of (37), it is easy to see that for large t $g(t,S|x_0)$ can be approximated as

$$g(t,S|x_0) \sim A_0(S|x_0)e^{\lambda_0(S)t} \tag{38}$$

Note also that both $A_0(S|x_0)$ and $\lambda_0(S)$ approach g(S) as S becomes large.

On the other hand, for large λ, $g^*(\lambda,S|x_0)$ becomes

$$g^*(\lambda,S|x_0) = \begin{cases} e^{-\sqrt{\lambda}(S-x_0)}, & S > x_0 \\ e^{-\sqrt{\lambda}(x_0-S)}, & x_0 > S > 0 \end{cases} \tag{39}$$

Hence we may conclude that for small time t, $g(t,S|x_0)$ is of order

$$\exp[-\frac{(S-x_0)^2}{2t}] \tag{40}$$

as expected.

We should point out finally that more information on $g(t,S|x_0)$ is obtained through the nature of zeros of the function $\Phi(\lambda,z)$ defined in eq.(25).

References

[1] L.M.Ricciardi, L.Sacerdote and S.Sato: Diffusion approximation and first passage time problem for a model neuron. II. Outline of a computation method, Mathematical Biosciences, 64,29-44(1983)

[2] R.Capocelli and L.M.Ricciardi: Diffusion approximation and first passage time problem for a model neuron, Kybernetik,8,214-223(1971)

[3] G.Sampath and S.K.Srinivasan: Stochastic Models for Spike Trains of Single Neurons, Lecture Notes in Biomathematics 16, Springer-Verlag, Berlin 1977

[4] G.L.Gerstein and B.Mandelbrot: Random walk models for the spike activity of a single neuron, Biophysical J.,4,41-68(1964)

[5] S.Sato: On the moments of the firing interval of the diffusion approximated model neuron, Mathematical Biosciences, 39,53-70(1978)

[6] S.Sato: Evaluation of the first passage time probability to a square root boundary for the Wiener process, J. Applied Probability,14,850-856(1977)

[7] L.Favella, M.T.Reineri, L.M.Ricciardi and L.Sacerdote: First passage time problems and related computational methods, Cybernetics and Systems,13,95-128(1982)

[8] J.Durbin: Boundary crossing probabilities for the Brownian motion and Poisson processes and techniques for computing the power of the Kolmogorov-Smirnov test, J. Applied Probability, 8,431-453(1971)

[9] K.S.Anderssen,F.R. De Hoog and R.Weiss: On the numerical solution of Brownian motion processes, J. Applied Probability, 10,409-418(1973)

[10] G.Cerbone, L.M.Ricciardi and L.Sacerdote:Mean variance and skewness of the first passage time for the Ornstein-Uhlenbeck process, Cybernetics and Systems,12,395-429(1981)

[11] A.J.F.Siegert: On the first passage time probability function, Physical Review,81,617-623(1951)

[12] A.Erdelyi:Higher Transcendental Functions, vol. I, vol. II, McGraw-Hill, New York,1953

IV. FLUCTUATION IN LIVING CELLS

FLUCTUATION IN LIVING CELLS: EFFECT OF FIELD FLUCTUATION AND ASYMMETRY OF FLUCTUATION

Fumio Oosawa, Masateru Tsuchiya and Tomoko Kubori
Department of Biophysical Engineering, Osaka University
Osaka 560, Japan

Summary

The electric potential in living cells of paramecium shows large spontaneous fluctuation, which consists of basic fluctuation and spikelike fluctuation. The spikelike fluctuation triggers transient reversal of ciliary beating and causes discontinuous change of the swimming direction. A positive shift of the basic potential increases the probability of the spikelike fluctuation. The spike is generated by opening of electric field-sensitive channels in the cell membrane. A differential equation is proposed to describe the probabilistic behavior of these channels in a fluctuating electric field. The fluctuating field increases the average rates of open-close transitions of channels and shifts the average opening probability towards 1/2. The open-close fluctuation in an assembly of the channels has asymmetry with respect to time reversal. Free energy is continuously consumed for generation of the spikelike fluctuation. The proposed equation which contains fluctuating quantities in exponential terms has a definite physical basis and is useful for the analysis of stochastic processes in a fluctuating field.

1. Introduction

Living cells do not always show deterministic behavior but sometimes show probabilistic behavior. Paramecium cells, for example, swim straight and change the swimming direction discontinuously. The time interval of the discontinuous change of swimming direction has nearly an exponential distribution, suggesting that it happens as a result of stochastic processes in the cell. The average time interval or the average frequency of directional changes is regulated depending on the environmental condition, and this regulation makes possible the chemotaxis and thermotaxis of paramecium cells.[1)]

Paramecium cells have a large number of cilia on their cell surface and swim by beating these cilia. The discontinuous change of swimming direction is caused by transient reversal of the beating direction of cilia, which is initiated by depolarization of the electric potential in the cell.[2] Recently, it was found that the electric potential in the cell has a large spontaneous fluctuation and a spikelike fluctuation induces the reversal of ciliary beating.[3] The fluctuation is not simply a thermal one but produced by consuming free energy.

In this paper, we describe the characteristic features of the potential fluctuation in paramecium cells and propose a differential equation to express the process of amplification of fluctuation. This equation is generally useful to describe a state fluctuation of molecules in a fluctuating field. Nonlinear effects of the fluctuating field give remarkable characters to the solution of the equation. The results of the computer analyses of the equation are compared with experimental data.

2. The Potential Fluctuation in Living Cells of Paramecium

The electric potential in a living cell of paramecium can be measured by inserting a microelectrode into the cell fixed on a glass plate under an optical microscope. The potential is about - 30 mV on the average, but it has a large spontaneous fluctuation even without any external stimuli, as shown in Fig. 1.[3]

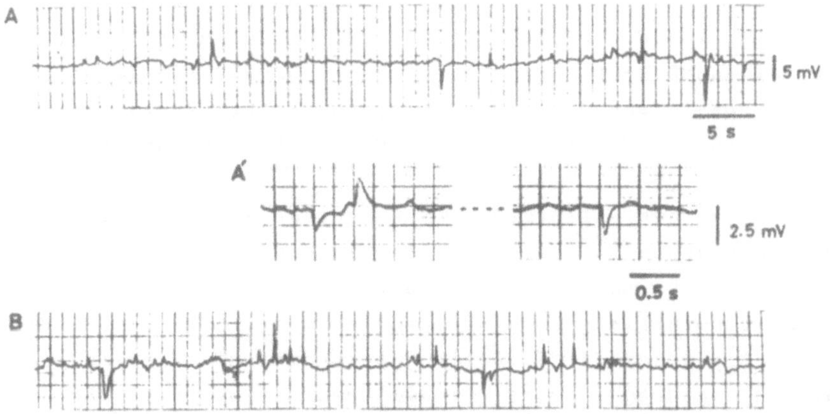

Fig. 1. A record of the fluctuating electric potential in a paramecium cell in a stationary state.

The fluctuation apparently consists of two components, conventionally named basic fluctuation and spikelike fluctuation. The latter is distinguishable from the former by a sharp rising phase and the height of a spike often attains a few mV.

The basic fluctuation has a Gaussian distribution, the half height width of which is from one to a few mV. Its power density spectrum is flat up to a few kHz and then goes down. The value of the potential in the basic fluctuation where a spike begins to rise was measured in a record of the fluctuating potential, and its histogram was obtained.[4)] Then, the probability of generation of the spike was calculated as a function of the potential in the basic fluctuation. The probability is nearly zero at the average potential and begins to increase rapidly at a few mV higher than the average.

The electric potential inside the cell is determined by concentrations of various ions inside and outside and permeabilities of these ions across the membrane. In the case of paramecium cells, an inward current of calcium ions (Ca^{2+}) and an outward current of potassium ions (K^{+}) flow across the membrane. The dependence of the basic fluctuation on the concentrations of ions outside indicated that the fluctuation of the permeability of K^{+} is a main origin of the potential fluctuation. If channels for these ions in the membrane fluctuate between two states, an opened state and a closed state, the current fluctuates and the potential fluctuates.

Besides those channels which are responsible for generation of the basic fluctuation, paramecium cells have another type of channels for Ca^{2+} in the membrane of cilia. They are sensitive to the electric field in the membrane in such a way that the depolarization of the potential inside the cell promotes the opening of the channel.[2)] If a certain number of those channels are opened simultaneously, the potential shows a sharp rise. Thus, the spikelike fluctuation is produced by the response of the field-sensitive channels to the basic fluctuation.

If the average potential or the average amplitude of the basic fluctuation changes with a change in the environmental condition, the probability of the spikelike fluctuation changes. Upon a sudden drop of the environmental temperature, for example, paramecium cells increase the frequency of discontinuous changes of swimming direction. The temperature drop induces a small depolarization of the average potential and an increase of the amplitude of basic fluctuation, which result in an increase in the probability of spikelike fluctuation, as shown in Fig. 2.[4)] Spikes are generated frequently, but still at random intervals.

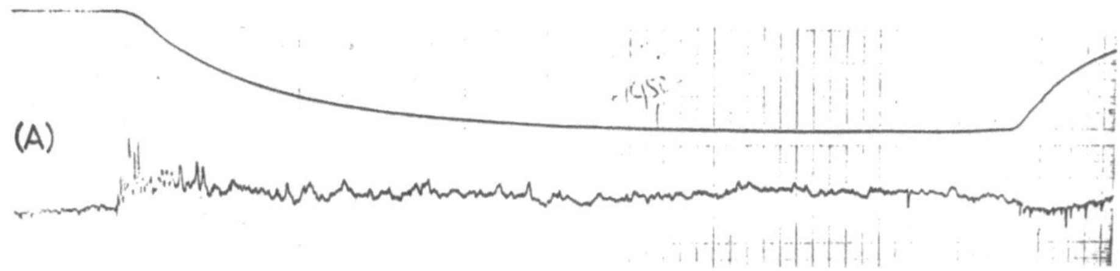

Fig. 2. A record of the fluctuating potential in a paramecium cell upon a temperature drop from 25 ^{o}C to 20 ^{o}C.

3. The Equation to Describe the State Fluctuation of Channels

Here, we focus our attention to the probabilistic relation between the basic fluctuation and the spikelike fluctuation, and construct a rate equation to describe the state fluctuation of channels which are sensitive to the electric field.

Suppose that a channel molecule in a membrane can assume two states, an opened state (o) and a closed state (c). The molecule fluctuates between two states with rate constants of transitions from o to c and from c to o, k_+ and k_-. If there are N molecules independent of each other, the number of molecules in the state o, n, changes with time according to the following equation;

$$dn(t)/dt = - k_+ n + k_-(N - n) \tag{1}$$

This equation describes the average behavior of the assembly of N independent molecules. If we define the probability that one of the molecules is in the state o as p;

$$dp(t)/dt = - k_+ p + k_-(1 - p) \tag{2}$$

The ratio n/N or the probability p tends to $k_-/(k_+ + k_-) = p_o$ after a sufficiently long time. This is true if k_+ and k_- are really constants.

Now, let us suppose that the free energy of the molecule in two states depends on the electric field E. Such situation happens if the molecule has different electric dipoles in two states. The ratio of rate constants must be related to the equilibrium constant K and the free energy difference between two states, $\delta\mu \cdot E$ by the equation;

$$k_-/k_+ = K = \exp(+ \delta\mu \cdot E/kT) \tag{3}$$

where k is the Boltzmann constant and T is the absolute temperature. Therefore, we give the following forms to rate constants;

$$k_+ = k_{+o} \exp(-(1/2)\, \delta\mu \cdot E/kT) \tag{4.1}$$

$$k_- = k_{-o} \exp(+(1/2)\, \delta\mu \cdot E/kT) \qquad (4.2)$$

We apply the same forms to rate constants when the field E is not constant but fluctuates with time. The concept of the rate constant is established after statistical averaging of short-range interaction of the molecule with surrounding molecules which makes possible fast exchange of energy. We consider the fluctuation of electric field, which is mostly much slower than the fluctuation of short-range interaction. Then, rate constants fluctuate with fluctuating field E. The above equation is written as

$$dp(t)/dt = -k_{+o}\exp(-\beta E(t))\, p(t) + k_{-o}\exp(+\beta E(t))(1 - p(t)) \qquad (5)$$

where $\beta = (1/2)\, \delta\mu/kT$. Here we assume that E(t) in this equation is a fluctuating component of the field and its time average $\langle E \rangle$ is zero.

It must be noticed that the expression of rate constants as an exponential function of the field E is consistent with the experimental data on the probability of generation of the spikelike fluctuation. The equation (5) is the same as proposed previously to discuss the effect of the field fluctuation on the state of macromolecules.[5)]

4. Behaviors of the Solution of the Proposed Equation

If there is no fluctuation of the field E, the solution of the equation (5), p(t), tends to a constant value $k_{-o}/(k_{+o} + k_{-o}) = p_o$ and the rate of approach to this value is given by $(k_{+o} + k_{-o})$. If the field E fluctuates, p is not constant but fluctuates even after a long period. If the fluctuation of E is of a Gaussian type, the average of k_+ and k_- is always larger than k_{+o} and k_{-o}, respectively, because

$$\langle k_+ \rangle = k_{+o} \langle \exp(-\beta E(t)) \rangle = k_{+o}\exp((\beta^2/2)\langle E^2 \rangle) \qquad (6.1)$$

$$\langle k_- \rangle = k_{-o} \langle \exp(+\beta E(t)) \rangle = k_{-o}\exp((\beta^2/2)\langle E^2 \rangle) \qquad (6.2)$$

The fluctuation of the field makes the transition of the molecule between two states more frequent. This is one of the nonlinear effects of the field fluctuation.

Defining the deviation of rate constants from their averages as

$$\delta k_+ = k_+ - \langle k_+ \rangle \qquad (7.1)$$

$$\delta k_- = k_- - \langle k_- \rangle \qquad (7.2)$$

the equation (5) is rewritten as

$$\begin{aligned} dp(t)/dt &= -(\langle k_+ \rangle + \delta k_+)(p_o + P) + (\langle k_- \rangle + \delta k_-)(1 - p_o - P) \\ &= -\delta k_+(p_o + P) - (\langle k_+ \rangle + \langle k_- \rangle)P + \delta k_-(1 - p_o - P) \qquad (8) \end{aligned}$$

where P(t) is the deviation of the probability p from its value without fluctuation of k's;

$$P(t) = p(t) - p_o \tag{9.1}$$

$$p_o = \langle k_-\rangle/(\langle k_+\rangle + \langle k_-\rangle) = k_{-o}/(k_{+o} + k_{-o}) \tag{9.2}$$

The last equation was derived from (6.1) and (6.2). The solution of (8) can be formally obtained, but it is more convenient to express the solution in a power series of the fluctuating component of rate constants, δk_+ and δk_- putting:

$$p(t) = p_o + P_1(t) + P_2(t) + \ldots \tag{10}$$

The first order term $P_1(t)$ must satisfy the equation;

$$dP_1(t)/dt = -\delta k_+ p_o + \delta k_-(1 - p_o) - (\langle k_+\rangle + \langle k_-\rangle)P_1 \tag{11}$$

The solution is given by

$$P_1(t) = \exp(-(\langle k_+\rangle + \langle k_-\rangle)t)\int^t \exp(+(\langle k_+\rangle + \langle k_-\rangle)t')$$
$$(-\delta k_+(t')p_o + \delta k_-(t')(1 - p_o))\,dt' \tag{12}$$

Then, the second order term $P_2(t)$ must satisfy the equation;

$$dP_2(t)/dt = -(\langle k_+\rangle + \langle k_-\rangle)P_2 - (\delta k_+ + \delta k_-)P_1 \tag{13}$$

The solution is given by

$$P_2(t) = \exp(-(\langle k_+\rangle + \langle k_-\rangle)t)\int^t \exp(+(\langle k_+\rangle + \langle k_-\rangle)t')$$
$$(-(\delta k_+(t') + \delta k_-(t'))P_1(t')\,dt'$$
$$= \exp(-(\langle k_+\rangle + \langle k_-\rangle)t)\int^t\int^{t'} \exp(+(\langle k_+\rangle + \langle k_-\rangle)t'')$$
$$(-(-\delta k_+(t'')p_o + \delta k_-(t'')(1-p_o))(\delta k_+(t') + \delta k_-(t'))dt'dt'' \tag{14}$$

The time average of P_1 is zero because the time averages of δk_+ and δk_- are zero. On the other hand, the average of $P_2(t)$ does not vanish. If the correlation between the fluctuating fields at t' and t" depends only on the time difference $\tau = t' - t''$, we find

$$\langle \delta k_+(t')\cdot\delta k_+(t'')\rangle = k_{+o}{}^2\exp((\beta^2/2)\langle E^2\rangle)(\exp((\beta^2/2)\langle E(0)E(\tau)\rangle)-1) \tag{15}$$

and similar expressions for the products of δk's at different times. Then, the time average of $P_2(t)$ is given by

$$\langle P_2\rangle = k_{+o}k_{-o}(k_{+o} - k_{-o})/(k_{+o} + k_{-o})^2$$
$$\int \exp(-(\langle k_+\rangle + \langle k_-\rangle)\tau)2\sinh((\beta^2/2)\langle E(0)E(\tau)\rangle)\,d\tau \tag{16}$$

Thus, the time average of the probability p is shifted from p_o by the fluctuation of the field. If $k_{+o} > k_{-o}$, p_o is smaller than 1/2 and $\langle P_2 \rangle$ is positive. If $k_{+o} < k_{-o}$, p_o is larger than 1/2 and $\langle P_2 \rangle$ is negative. Therefore, the probability p is moved by the fluctuation of the field towards 1/2.

The average amplitude of the fluctuation of the probability p around its average is estimated by

$$\langle (p - \langle p \rangle)^2 \rangle = \langle p^2 \rangle - \langle p \rangle^2 = P_1{}^2 + \ldots. \tag{17}$$

From (12)

$$\langle (p - \langle p \rangle)^2 \rangle = k_{+o}{}^2 k_{-o}{}^2 / (k_{+o} + k_{-o})^3$$
$$\int \exp(-(\langle k_+ \rangle + \langle k_- \rangle)\tau) 4\sinh((\beta^2/2)\langle E(0)E(\tau)\rangle)\, d\tau \tag{18}$$

If the field fluctuation has a principal frequency ω, the effect of fluctuation on p decreases with increasing frequency ω in the form of $1/(1 + (\omega/\omega_o)^2)$, where $\omega_o = 1/(\langle k_+ \rangle + \langle k_- \rangle)$. If the field fluctuation is much faster than the average rates of transition of molecules, they can respond only to the average field. Even in this case however, the fluctuation increases the average frequency of transitions. These results are illustrated in Fig. 3 and Fig. 4.

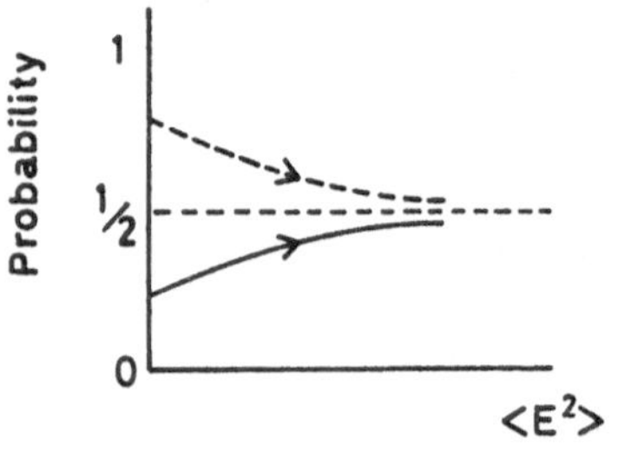

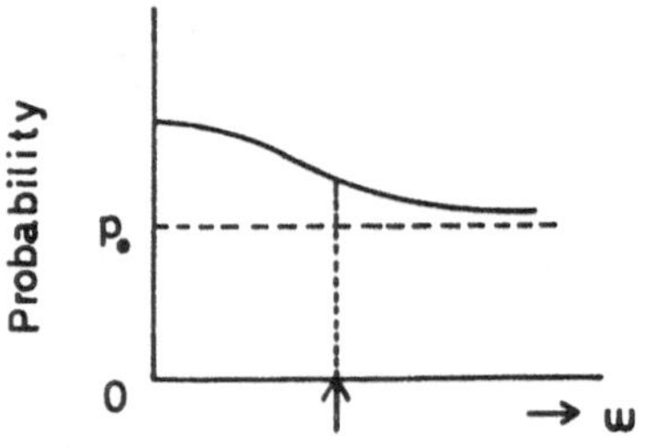

Fig. 3. The behavior of the state probability p with increasing amplitude of the fluctuating field.

Fig. 4. The behavior of the state probability p with increasing frequency of the fluctuating field.

5. Demonstration of the Probability Fluctuation by Computer Simulation

In the above section, we derived the approximate solution of the equation (5) up to the second order of the fluctuating field. If the field fluctuation becomes large, it is difficult to follow the behaviors of the probability p analytically. Computer simulation is more useful. Putting an appropriate time interval Δt, the probability p at $t_{i+1} = t_i + \Delta t$ is calculated from p at t_i according to (5) with suitable values of k_{+o} and k_{-o} and fluctuating field $E(t_i)$

with a coefficient β. To generate $E(t_i)$ with arbitrary correlation times we assume a conventional relation;

$$E(t_{i+1}) = (1 - A)^{1/2}E(t_{i-1}) + (A(2 - A))^{1/2}G(t_i) \quad 1 \geq A \geq 0 \qquad (19)$$

where G is a random number having a Gaussian distribution around zero generated in a computer. If A is zero, the field has no fluctuation. If A is unity, E represents a white noise with no time correlation. With the increase of A from zero to unity, the time correlation of E becomes shorter. The results of computation are shown in Fig. 5 and Fig. 6. The fast approach of the probability towards the average and its fluctuation around the average are remarkable. The analytical treatment in the previous section gave good approximation.

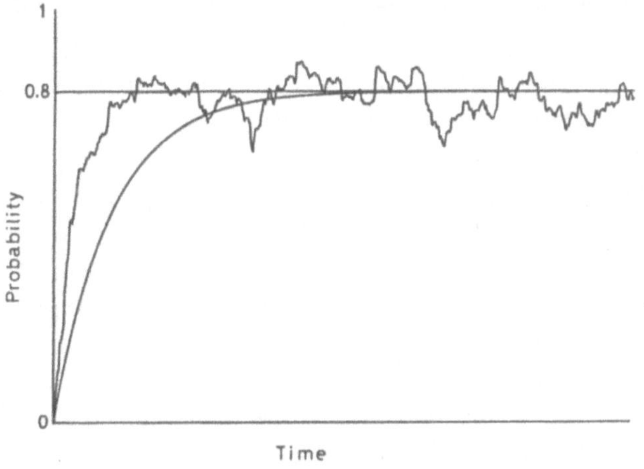

Fig. 5. The behavior of the fluctuating probability p generated by a computer; $k_{+o} = 0.2$, $k_{-o} = 0.8$, the time interval 0.01, $\langle E^2 \rangle = 1$ and $\beta = 1$, with A = 0 and 0.5, to show approach to a stationary state.

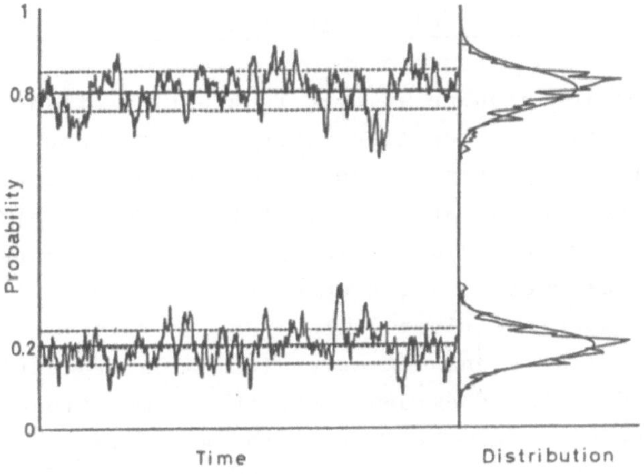

Fig. 6. The behavior of the fluctuating probability p generated by a computer in a stationary state.

Let us suppose a single channel molecule making transitions between two states. Without using the probability p, we can describe the state of the molecule changing with time by assigning number 1 to the opened state and 0 to the closed state. If the molecule is in the state 1 at t_i, we consider in the next time interval the possibility of transition from 1 to 0. The rate constant gives the probability of the transition in unit time and the state of the molecule at t_{i+1} is determined probabilistically. This process can be performed in the computer, using the value of rate constants defined previously. After computation, the state at t_{i+1} is found to be 1 or 0. By repeating the same process, we can make a record of the state of the molecule for a certain period.

Next, we can suppose an assembly of N channel molecules. For each molecule, we can make a record of the state changing with time, by the above method. By summing up the records for N molecules, we obtain a record of the state of the assembly which is expressed by the number of molecules in the opened state, n. If the total number of molecules N is sufficiently large, the behavior of n agrees with that of p determined by the equation (1).

If the field fluctuates, we have to notice the following point. If all N molecules are in the same fluctuating field $E(t_i)$ at each time t_i, the summation of the records for N molecules constructed by the computer must become equivalent to the calculation of n or Np according to (5). If N molecules are in the same average field with different fluctuations, the summation of the records gives a quite different result. In other words, the equation (5) describes the behavior of an assembly of a large number of molecules, all of which are in the same fluctuating field.

6. Asymmetry of the State Fluctuation with respect to Time Reversal

Living cells of paramecium produce a large fluctuation of the intracellular electric potential. The fluctuation in a thermodynamic equilibrium must be symmetric with respect to time reversal. However, the fluctuation in a non-equilibrium stationary state can be asymmetric. Actually, in a record of the fluctuating potential of a paramecium cell, we can find the asymmetry, which means that free energy is consumed in the cell to produce the fluctuation.

Let us suppose again a single channel molecule making transitions between two states, 1 and 0. It is evident that the fluctuation between two values cannot produce asymmetry with respect to time reversal. This is true even if the rate constants or the transition probabilities have fluctuations. What does happen in an assembly of N molecules, where the state of the assembly is represented by integers between N and 0 according to the number of molecules in the state 1? If the field is constant and therefore the transition probabilities are constant, the asymmetry does not appear in the fluctuation of the state of the assembly. The state approaches to an equilibrium and the fluctuation becomes purely thermal. On the other hand, if the field fluctuates, the asymmetry can occur.

In a record of the state of the assembly for a certain period, we can find the following event. The number representing the state takes a value X_k at time t and another value X_j at $t + \tau$; where X_k and X_j are between N and 0. By scanning the record, we can count the number of times M where this event actually happened; M is a function of X_k and X_j and the time different τ . Then, we can construct a matrix $M(X_k, X_j; \tau)$ with X_k and X_j as two components at a fixed value of τ . The asymmetry of fluctuation of X(t) with respect to time reversal is equivalent **to** the asymmetry of the matrix M. That is, if $M(X_k, X_j; \tau) \neq M(X_j, X_k; \tau)$, the fluctuation is asymmetric. The degree of asymmetry may be evaluated by the following quantity Φ;

$$\Phi(X_k, X_j : \tau) = |M(X_k, X_j; \tau) - M(X_j, X_k; \tau)| / (M(X_k, X_j; \tau) + M(X_j, X_k; \tau)) \tag{20}$$

Fig. 7 shows an example of the matrix $\Phi(X_k, X_j; \tau)$ obtained from a record of the state of an assembly of N molecules generated by a computer. All molecules are assumed to be in the same fluctuating field $F(t_i)$. The asymmetry becomes remarkable with the progress of computation for a long period. As a reference, the matrix obtained from a record of the same assembly in a constant field is shown in Fig. 8. The asymmetry disappears with the progress of computation.

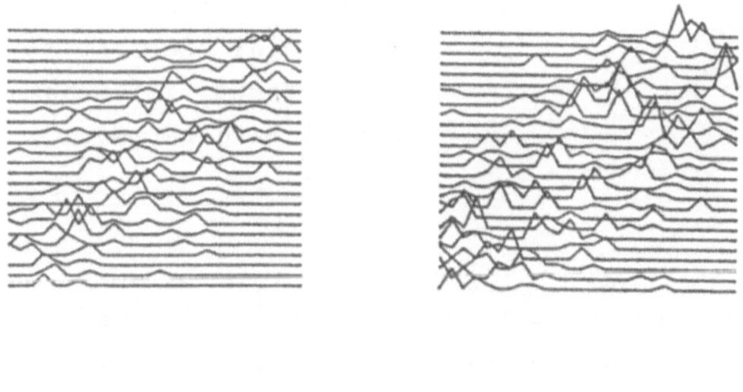

Fig. 7. The matrix Φ to show asymmetry of fluctuation, which becomes remarkable with the progress of computation. (left $i \leq 2000$, right $i \leq 15000$)

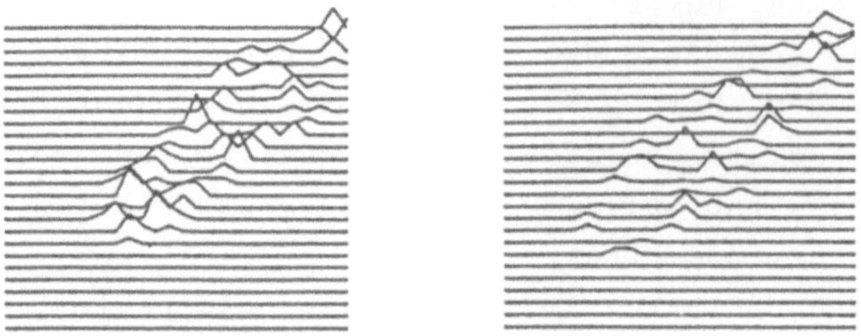

Fig. 8. The matrix Φ for the state of independent molecules where an apparent asymmetry decays with the progress of computation.

Suppose a number of channel molecules distributed in an area of a membrane. The electric field on each molecule fluctuates with time. If the field fluctuation has a long spatial correlation, many channel molecules are in the same fluctuating field. The transitions of these molecules have an apparent correlation. Then, a large fluctuation of the electric current takes place. In this condition, the fluctuation has asymmetry with respect to time reversal. A flow of free energy occurs from the fluctuating field to the channel molecules. If the field fluctuation has no spatial correlation, the molecules make transitions independently, and the fluctuation of the state of the assembly has no asymmetry.

To compare the results of computation with experimental data, we have undertaken to measure the current fluctuation in an artificial membrane into which ion channels are incorporated.[6] From a record obtained in a membrane having about fifty channels incorporated, a matrix Φ was constructed. The asymmetry appeared, as shown in Fig. 9.

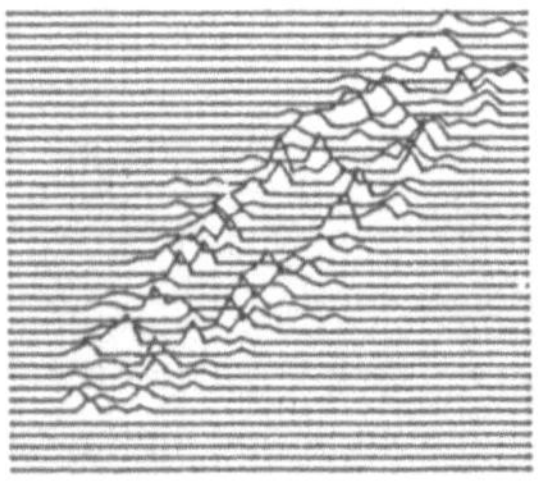

Fig. 9. A matrix Φ constructed from a record of the fluctuating current in an artificial membrane to which about fifty channels were incorporated.

As described previously, the potential fluctuation in a paramecium cell has an asymmetry. It is not easy, however, to obtain a record of the fluctuating potential for a period sufficiently long to construct the matrix Φ.

7. Discussions

In this paper, we have proposed a differential equation which includes exponential functions of fluctuating quantities to describe the state of molecules in a fluctuating field. The equation has a definite physical meaning and a mathematically interesting form. Usually, a Langevin equation has been applied to describe the state of molecules in a fluctuating environment. A random force appears as an additive term in the equation. On the other hand, in the proposed equation, the effect of the fluctuating field is not simply additive.

A mathematically generalized and refined treatment of our equation has been performed by Professor T. Hida in Nagoya University. The behavior of the solution of our equation in the limit of the field fluctuation with short time correlation has been analysed by Professor H. Watanabe in Kyushu University. The mathematical analyses on our equation under various conditions are expected to be developed further.

The shift of the average probability of the state of molecules by the fluctuating field, together with the asymmetry of fluctuation of the state, is associated with a flow of free energy from the field to the molecules. This flow suggests the presence of the reaction from the molecules to the field. The equation (5) we proposed expresses the action of the fluctuating field on the molecules. We have to construct another equation to express a change of the field caused by the fluctuation of the molecules. The current through the channels must change the potential near the channels. In the treatment of the equation (5) we assumed that the fluctuating field is given externally whatever the states of the molecules are.

In the case of paramecium cells, the above assumption is equivalent to the assumption that the spikelike fluctuation of the potential is affected by the basic fluctuation probabilistically, but the basic fluctuation is not affected by the spikelike fluctuation. This is acceptable in paramecium cells which have a large number of field insensitive channels responsible for basic fluctuation. The fluctuating potential is spread in the cell and the basic fluctuation has a spatial correlation which is suitable to generate spikelike fluctuations of small and variable magnitudes at random intervals. If the contribution of field sensitive channels is too large, the spike once generated becomes always large. Paramecium cells have a nice combination of field insensitive channels and field sensitive channels to regulate the spikelike fluctuation.

In the next step, we have to develop a more general treatment of interaction between the fluctuating field and the fluctuating state of molecules.

References

1) Y. Nakaoka and F. Oosawa; J. Protozoology, 24, 575 (1977)
   F. Oosawa and Y. Nakaoka; J. Theor. Biol., 66, 747 (1977)

2) Y. Naitoh and R. Eckert; Cilia and Flagella, ed. by O. Sleigh, Acad. Press (1974)

3) T. Majima; Biophys. Chem., 11, 101 (1980)

4) H. Toyotama; Doctor thesis, Osaka Univ.

5) F. Oosawa; J. Theor. Biol., 52, 175 (1975)

6) Data obtained in the laboratory of M. Kasai

SOME ASPECTS OF OOSAWA'S EQUATION

Hisao Watanabe

Department of Applied Science
Faculty of Engineering
Kyushu University
Fukuoka 812, Japan

Summary. Professor Oosawa [1] proposed an ordinary stochastic differential equation arising from the study of fluctuation in living cells. In this report, we consider Gaussian approximations to the above equation by using the averaging methods.

F. Oosawa [1] has proposed the study of the following ordinary stochastic differential equation

$$(1) \qquad \frac{dn_{\lambda,\beta}(t)}{dt} = -(ae^{-\beta E_\lambda(t)} + be^{\beta E_\lambda(t)})n_{\lambda,\beta}(t) + be^{\beta E_\lambda(t)}$$

where β, a and b are positive constants and $E_\lambda(t)$ is a Gaussian stochastic process with mean zero and correlation function $e^{-\lambda|t|}$ $(\lambda > 0)$, i.e. the so-called Ornstein-Uhlenbeck process. Of course, (1) can be easily solved, however it is not easy to visualize the behavior of trajectories of $n_{\lambda,\beta}(t)$ from the mathematical expression of the solution. Here, we show a result of some analysis about (1). We put

$$(2) \qquad \begin{cases} a(t,\omega) = -(ae^{-\beta E_1(t)} + be^{\beta E_1(t)}) \\ b(t,\omega) = be^{\beta E_1(t)} \\ F(t,x,\omega) = a(t,\omega)x + b(t,\omega). \end{cases}$$

As is well known, the relation $E_\lambda(t) = E_1(\lambda t)$ holds with probability one. Then (1) can be written in the form:

$$(3) \qquad \frac{dn_{\lambda,\beta}(t)}{dt} = F(\lambda t\ ,\ n_{\lambda,\beta}(t),\omega).$$

Furthermore, if we put $\lambda = 1/\varepsilon$ and $n_{\lambda,\beta}(t) = n^\varepsilon(t)$, then $n^\varepsilon(t)$ satisfies the following ordinary differential equation

$$(3)' \quad \begin{cases} \frac{dn^{\varepsilon}(t)}{dt} = F(\frac{t}{\varepsilon}, n^{\varepsilon}(t), \omega) \\ n^{\varepsilon}(0) = x \in R^{d}. \end{cases}$$

We now observe the asymptotic expansion for $n^{\varepsilon}(t)$ as $\varepsilon \to 0$. There are many researches on this kind of problems (see the references in [2]). Here we analyse in line with H. Watanabe [2]. The conditions required in Theorem in [2] are satisfied for $n^{\varepsilon}(t)$. The results are as follows: Let $E(F(t,x,\omega)) = \overline{F}(x)$. Let $n^{0}(t)$ the solution of the following equation

$$\begin{cases} \frac{dn^{0}(t)}{dt} = \overline{F}(n^{0}(t)) \\ n^{0}(0) = x \in R^{d}. \end{cases}$$

Then, $(n^{\varepsilon}(t) - n^{0}(t))/\sqrt{\varepsilon}$ weakly converges to the Gaussian stochastic process which is determined by the following stochastic differential equation

$$y^{0}(t) = w^{0}(t) + \int_{0}^{t} F'(n^{0}(\tau))y^{0}(\tau)d\tau,$$

where $w^{0}(t)$ is a Gaussian process with independent increments, mean zero and covariance

$$E(w^{0}(t)^{2}) = \int_{0}^{t} A(n^{0}(\tau))d\tau$$

$$G(x) = \int_{0}^{\infty} E(\tilde{F}(\tau,x,\omega)\tilde{F}(0,x,\omega)d\tau$$

and $\tilde{F} = F - E(F)$.

More explicitly, $n^{0}(t) = c + de^{-ft}$, where $c = a/(a+b)$, $d = (n^{0}(0) - a/(a+b))$ and $f = e^{\beta^{2}/2}(a+b)$.

$$y^{0}(t) = \int_{0}^{t} e^{-\overline{a}(t-s)}dw^{0}(s),$$

$$\overline{a} = E(a(t,x,\omega)) = -e^{\beta^{2}/2}(a+b)$$

$$G(x) = Ax^{2} + Bx + C$$

$$A = e^{\beta^{2}}(a^{2}D(\beta^{2}) + 2abD(-\beta^{2}) + b^{2}D(\beta^{2}))$$

$$B = -2e^{\beta^{2}}(abD(-\beta^{2}) + a^{2}D(\beta^{2}))$$

$$C = e^{\beta^{2}}a^{2}D(\beta^{2})$$

$$D(x) = \int_{0}^{x} (e^{v}-1)/vdv.$$

Furthermore, we have

$$E(y^0(t)^{2n}) = 1\cdot 3\cdot \cdots (2n-1)(\sigma^2(t))^n$$

$$\sigma^2(t) = \int_0^t e^{-2\bar{a}(t-s)} D(n^0(s))ds$$

$$= \frac{e^{\beta^2/2}}{(a+b)^3}(ab)^2(D(\beta^2) - D(-\beta^2)) + 0(e^{-\beta t}) \qquad (t \to \infty).$$

Formally, we have the following expression

$$n^{\varepsilon}(t) \sim n^0(t) + \frac{1}{\sqrt{\lambda}}\, y^0(t) \qquad \text{for large } \lambda .$$

We can see from computer simulation that such a formal relation holds even if λ is not large.

[1] F. Oosawa, M. Tsuchiya and T. Kubori, Fluctuation in living cells: Effect of field fluctuation and asymmetry of fluctuation, (In these Proceedings).

[2] H. Watanabe, Fluctuations in certain dynamical systems with averaging, Stochastic processes and their applications, 21 (1985), 147-157.

V. MATHEMATICAL METHODS RELATED TO OTHER PROBLEMS IN BIOLOGY, EPIDEMIOLOGY, POPULATION DYNAMICS, ETC.

PROBLEMS OF EPIDEMIC MODELLING

J. Gani
Statistics and Applied Probability Program
University of California
Santa Barbara, CA 93106, USA

This note gives a brief review of some aspects of epidemic modelling which I have found of interest. The field is now very broad, and it is difficult to provide more than a partial flavor of recent developments. We shall concentrate on three topics: epidemic data fitting, matrix-geometric methods for general epidemics, and the duration of an epidemic in an immigration type model. These will provide a sample of current research problems.

1. Epidemic data fitting

In the classical deterministic epidemic models for viral diseases developed by Kermack and McKendrick (1927) the spread of infection in a population of $x(t)$ susceptibles, $y(t)$ infectives and $z(t)$ removals where $x(t)+y(t)+z(t) = N$ fixed, is governed by the differential equations

$$\frac{dx}{dt} = -\beta xy, \qquad \frac{dy}{dt} = \beta xy - \gamma y, \qquad \frac{dz}{dt} = \gamma y, \tag{1.1}$$

where β,γ are the infection and removal rates respectively. The stochastic version of the general epidemic for $X(t)$ susceptibles, $Y(t)$ infectives and $Z(t)$ removals relies on the analysis of the bivariate Markov chain $\{X(t), Y(t); t\geq 0\}$ for which the relevant infinitesimal transition probabilities are $q_{(x,y),(x-1,y+1)} = \beta xy$ and $q_{(x,y),(x,y-1)} = \gamma y$. In his treatise, Bailey (1975) has reported in some detail on estimation methods for the parameters β and γ of various diseases.

More recently, in their stimulating review paper, Dietz and Schenzle (1985) have outlined the history of household epidemic statistics and described, among other material, the analysis of 664 cases of the common cold by Heasman and Reid (1961). The model used here was a chain binomial, of which the standard Reed-Frost version provided a rather inadequate fit. In such a model, if X_t,Y_t are susceptibles and infectives at the discrete times $t = 0,1,2,\ldots,$ then

(1.2)

$$P\{X_{t+1} = x_{t+1},\ Y_{t+1} = y_{t+1} | X_t = x_t,\ Y_t = y_t\} = \binom{x_t}{y_{t+1}}(1-(1-p)^{y_t})^{y_{t+1}}(1-p)^{y_t x_{t+1}},$$

where p is the probability of contact with an infective. Heasman and Reid obtained the estimate $\hat{p} = 0.114$ for the contact probability; this was refined by Becker (1981) who found $\hat{p} = 0.116$ and Schenzle (1982) who obtained $\hat{p} = 0.107$ from pooled data.

Schenzle (1982) had pointed out that Heasman & Reid's pooled frequencies could not be satisfactorily interpreted by fitting alternative chain models, and a return to the original data of Brimblecombe et al. (1958) seemed necessary if the epidemic was to be modelled appropriately. Of the eight models considered, that which appeared to provide the best fit was a Reed-Frost chain in which the cross-infection

Table 1. Schenzle's changing infection rate
Reed-Frost model fitted to common cold data

Chain type	Observed frequencies	Expected frequencies
1	423	422.3
11	131	130.1
111	36	43.0
1111	14	13.8
112	8	6.8
12	24	20.2
121	11	11.5
11111	4	3.4
1112	2	1.7
1121	2	3.0
113	2	0.5
1211	3	1.9
122	1	2.4
13	3	2.3
131	0	1.0
14	0	0.1
Total	664	664.0

rate changed during the course of the epidemic (see Table 1) so that

(1.3) $$1-p = q = q_0 - at \qquad t = 0,1,2,3,$$

where $a < \frac{1}{3} q_0$. Using maximum likelihood methods, Schenzle found $\hat{q}_0 = 0.893$ and $\hat{a} = 0.03$, but expressed some doubts as to the meaningfulness of the model. Certainly the alternative Reed-Frost model, in which q was itself considered as a

Beta random variable (the BaRF model of Schenzle (1982)) provided a far better fit than the ordinary Reed-Frost, or the Becker (1981) models in which the probabilities p_i of exposure to i infectives were arbitrary parameters to be estimated from the data. Gani and Mansouri have recently verified the goodness of a similar fit in a technical report (1986).

What appears to have emerged from this data fitting exercise is the difficulty of ascertaining the appropriateness of the models on the basis of the imperfect data currently available. More details about the data and its collection are required, as Dietz and Schenzle (1985) point out, if one is to draw firm epidemiological conclusions from the models used.

2. Matrix-geometric methods

About six years ago, Saunders (1980) considered an alternative infection mechanism for the general stochastic epidemic $\{X(t), Y(t); t \geq 0\}$ having the infinitesimal transition probabilities

$$(2.1) \qquad q_{(x,y),(x-1,y+1)} = \frac{\beta xy}{(x+y)^\alpha} = f_{xy} \qquad \alpha > 0 \quad ,$$

rather than the usual βxy, and the same $q_{(x,y),(x,y-1)} = \gamma y$ as before. In this case, after a simple time transformation, the forward Kolmogorov equations for the probabilities $p_{xy}(t) = P\{X(t) = x, Y(t) = y | X(0) = x, y(0) = a\}$ become

$$(2.2) \qquad p'_{xy} = \frac{(x+1)(y-1)}{(x+y)^\alpha} p_{x+1,y-1} - \left(\frac{xy}{(x+y)^\alpha} + \rho y\right)p_{xy} + \rho(y+1)p_{x,y+1}$$

$$0 \leq x \leq n, \qquad 0 \leq y \leq n+a, \qquad 0 \leq x+y \leq n+a,$$

where ρ is the relative removal rate γ/β.

The standard p.g.f. methods are now unavailing; Gani and Purdue (1984) have shown, however, that these equations can be solved recursively using matrix-geometric methods. If we write

$$\underset{\sim}{P}_x(t) = \begin{bmatrix} p_{x0}(t) \\ p_{x1}(t) \\ \cdots \\ p_{x,n+a-x}(t) \end{bmatrix}$$

for the (n+a-x+1)-vector of probabilities for which there are x susceptibles, then

$$(2.3) \qquad \underset{\sim}{P}_n' = \{-(B_n+A_n) + \Delta_n A_n\} \underset{\sim}{P}_n$$

where

$$B_n = \begin{bmatrix} 0 & & & \\ & f_{n1} & & \\ & & \cdots & \\ & & & f_{na} \end{bmatrix}, \quad A_n = \begin{bmatrix} 0 & & & \\ & \rho & & \\ & & \cdots & \\ & & & \rho a \end{bmatrix}, \quad \Delta_n = \begin{bmatrix} 0 & 1 & & \\ & 0 & 1 & \\ & & \cdots & \\ & & & 0 \end{bmatrix}.$$

Similarly,

$$(2.4) \qquad \underset{\sim}{P}_x' = \{-(B_x+A_x)+\Delta_x A_x\} \underset{\sim}{P}_x + B_{x+1}^{+} \underset{\sim}{P}_{x+1}^{+} \qquad x = 0,1,\ldots, x-1 ,$$

where

$$B_x = \begin{bmatrix} 0 & & & \\ & f_{x1} & & \\ & & \cdots & \\ & & & f_{x,n+a-x} \end{bmatrix}, \quad A_x = \begin{bmatrix} 0 & & & \\ & \rho & & \\ & & \cdots & \\ & & & \rho(n+a-x) \end{bmatrix}, \quad \Delta_x = \begin{bmatrix} 0 & 1 & & \\ & 0 & 1 & \\ & & \cdots & \\ & & & 0 \end{bmatrix},$$

and B_{x+1}^{+}, $\underset{\sim}{P}_{x+1}^{+}$ are the augmented matrices

$$B_{x+1}^{+} = \begin{bmatrix} 0 & \\ & B_{x+1} \end{bmatrix}, \qquad \underset{\sim}{P}_{x+1}^{+} = \begin{bmatrix} 0 \\ \underset{\sim}{P}_{x+1} \end{bmatrix}$$

so that the appropriate dimensions are observed in (2.4). Taking Laplace transforms of (2.3) and (2.4), the following recursive result are obtained

$$\hat{p}_{ny}(s) = \int_0^\infty e^{-st} p_{ny}(t)dt = \rho^{a-y} \frac{a!}{y!} \prod_{r=y}^{a} (s+f_{nr}+r\rho)^{-1} \qquad y = 0,1,\ldots,a,$$

(2.5)

$$\hat{p}_{xy}(s) = \int_0^\infty e^{-st} p_{xy}(t)dt = \sum_{r=y-1}^{n+a-x-1} \frac{(r+1)!}{y!} \rho^{r+1-y} \frac{f_{x+1,r}\, \hat{p}_{x+1,r}(s)}{\prod_{\ell=y}^{r+1} (s+f_{x\ell}+\ell\rho)}$$

$$x = 1,\ldots, n-1, \qquad y = 1,\ldots, n+a-x.$$

Analogous methods have also yielded results in the case of the epidemic with carriers, considered by Booth, Gani, Malice, Mansouri and Maravankin (1986). Results of this type are particularly useful in deriving the probabilities

$\Pi_{x0} = \lim_{t\to\infty} p_{x0}(t) = \lim_{s\to 0} s\hat{p}_{x0}(s)$ of x survivors after the epidemic has subsided.

3. Duration of an epidemic with immigration

The following epidemic model has recently attracted the attention of Marie-Pierre Malice (1986) and myself. Let $\{S_i\}_{i=0}^{\infty}$ be the number of susceptibles in a population at the start of the year i, with $\{X_i\}_{i=0}^{\infty}$ being the newborn susceptibles (immigrants) during that year. Suppose that only a proportion $0 < Z_i < 1$ of the susceptibles S_{i-1} remains uninfected at the end of year i-1, then assuming for simplicity that all infants are born simultaneously at the start of year i,

$$S_0 = X_0 \tag{3.1}$$

$$S_i = X_i + Z_i S_{i-1} \qquad i = 1,2,\dots .$$

Let us assume that the $\{Z_i\}_{i=0}^{\infty}$ are i.i.d. random variables, which are also independent of the $\{X_i\}_{i=0}^{\infty}$ but such that each Z_i may depend on S_{i-1}. We see that the $\{S_i\}_{i=0}^{\infty}$ form a Markov chain.

For example $U_i = Z_i S_{i-1}$ could be the binomial r.v. $B(S_{i-1},p)$ so that

$$P\{Z_i S_{i-1} = j\} = \binom{S_{i-1}}{j} p^j q^{S_{i-1}-j} . \tag{3.2}$$

Then we could write the p.g.f.

$$L_i(\theta) = E(\theta^{S_i}) = E(\theta^{X_i})E(\theta^{Z_i S_{i-1}})$$

$$= \chi(\theta)E((p\theta+q)^{S_{i-1}}) \tag{3.3}$$

$$= \chi(\theta)L_{i-1}(p\theta+q) .$$

It can be shown here, that as $i \to \infty$, a limiting p.g.f. $L(\theta)$ exists which satisfies the functional relation

$$L(\theta) = \chi(\theta)L(p\theta+q) . \tag{3.4}$$

Its solution, outlined in Kuczma (1968), is of the form

$$L(\theta) = \prod_{n=0}^{\infty} \chi(p^n\theta+1-p^n) \quad . \tag{3.5}$$

We may now ask questions such as "when does the epidemic cease?"

This will clearly occur when $Z_i = 1$, namely when all the susceptibles S_{i-1} survive over a unit time period; if $Z_i = 0$ so that all susceptibles are removed, we shall assume that the epidemic continues since contact may still occur between infectives and the newborn susceptibles.

Let us write the p.g.f.s of $S_0, S_1, \ldots, S_{i-1}$ when the epidemic continues up to time i; these are

$$\begin{aligned} \underline{L}_0(\theta) &= \theta^{S_0} = L_0(\theta) \\ \underline{L}_1(\theta) &= \{(p\theta+q)^{S_0}-(p\theta)^{S_0}\}\chi(\theta) = \{\underline{L}_0(p\theta+q) - \underline{L}_0(p\theta)\}\chi(\theta) \\ \underline{L}_i(\theta) &= \{\underline{L}_{i-1}(p\theta+q) - \underline{L}_{i-1}(p\theta)\}\chi(\theta) \qquad i = 2,\ldots \quad . \end{aligned} \tag{3.6}$$

Now, if the epidemic ceases at time T, $Z_T = 1$, and the p.g.f. of S_T will then be $\underline{L}_{T-1}(p\theta)\chi(\theta)$. Thus we are able to write the joint p.g.f of the time T at which the epidemic stops and the susceptibles S_T as

$$W(\alpha,\theta) = E(\alpha^T\theta^{S_T}) = \sum_{T=1}^{\infty} \alpha^T \{\underline{L}_{T-1}(p\theta)\}\chi(\theta) \tag{3.7}$$

where the $\underline{L}_{T-1}(\theta)$ are given by (3.6).

It can be seen that the distribution of T is honest, since from (3.6)

$$\begin{aligned} \underline{L}_1(1) &= 1-\underline{L}_0(p) \\ \underline{L}_i(1) &= \underline{L}_{i-1}(1)-\underline{L}_{i-1}(p) \qquad i = 2,\ldots \quad . \end{aligned}$$

Hence adding both sides of the equations, we conclude that

$$\sum_{i=1}^{\infty} \underline{L}_i(1) = 1 + \sum_{i=1}^{\infty} L_i(1) - \sum_{i=0}^{\infty} \underline{L}_i(p)$$

or $$\sum^{\infty} \underline{L}_i(p) = 1.$$

An interesting example arises when S_0 itself has a Poisson distribution identical with that of the $\{X_i\}$, with p.g.f. $e^{\lambda(\theta-1)}$. It is then easy to show that

$$
\begin{aligned}
&\underline{L}_0(\theta) = e^{\lambda(\theta-1)} \\
(3.8)\qquad &\underline{L}_1(\theta) = e^{\lambda(1+p)(\theta-1)}(1-e^{-\lambda(1-p)}) \\
&\underline{L}_i(\theta) = e^{\lambda \frac{1-p^{i+1}}{1-p}(\theta-1)} \prod_{k=1}^{i} (1-e^{-\lambda(1-p^k)}) \qquad i = 2,\ldots,
\end{aligned}
$$

so that

$$
\begin{aligned}
W(\alpha,\theta) &= \sum_{T=1}^{\infty} \alpha^T e^{\lambda(\frac{1-p^T}{1-p})(p\theta-1)} \prod_{k=1}^{T-1} (1-e^{-\lambda(1-p^k)}) e^{\lambda(\theta-1)} \\
(3.9)\qquad &= \sum_{T=1}^{\infty} \alpha^T e^{\lambda(\frac{1-p^{T+1}}{1-p})(\theta-1)} e^{-\lambda(1-p^T)} \prod_{k=1}^{T-1} (1-e^{-\lambda(1-p^k)}) .
\end{aligned}
$$

Note that the probability that the epidemic ceases at T is now given explicitly by

$$
(3.10)\qquad e^{-\lambda(1-p^T)} \prod_{k=1}^{T-1} (1-e^{-\lambda(1-p^k)}) ,
$$

or the product of the conditional probabilities $1-e^{-\lambda(1-p^k)}$ of not ceasing at times $k = 1, \ldots, T-1$, and $e^{-\lambda(1-p^T)}$ of ceasing at T. We see that the susceptibles S_T follow a Poisson distribution with p.g.f. $e^{\lambda(\frac{1-p^{T+1}}{1-p})(\theta-1)}$ when the duration of the epidemic is T.

4. Concluding remarks

Dietz & Schenzle (1985) have already indicated many of the unresolved problems of epidemic theory which remain to be tackled; these include data-fitting and discrimination between models, age-specific infection models, recurrence and periodicity of epidemics, the geographical spread of diseases, and the interaction of genetics and epidemiology. Nåsell (1985), following Macdonald (1957), has pointed out that parasitic and helminthic diseases are now far more prevalent than viral ones, and their modelling is vastly more complicated and challenging. While Dietz and Schenzle (1985) are perhaps a little pessimistic as to the value of mathematical epidemiology, so long as these diseases are not eradicated, there will continue to be a role, however modest, for the mathematical theory of infectious diseases.

References

Bailey, N.T.J. (1975) The Mathematical Theory of Infectious Diseases. Griffin, London.

Becker, N. (1981) A general chain binomial model for infectious diseases. Biometrics 37, 251-258.

Booth, J., Gani, J., Malice, M.-P., Mansouri, H. and Maravankin, G. (1986) A general solution for the epidemic with carriers. Statist. Prob. Letters 4, 9-15.

Brimblecombe, F.W.S., Cruickshank, R., Masters, P.L., Reid, D.D. and Stewart, G.T. (1958) Family studies in respiratory infections. Brit. Med. J. 1, 119-128.

Dietz, K. and Schenzle, D. (1985) Mathematical models for infectious disease statistics. In A Celebration of Statistics, A.C. Atkinson and S.E. Fienberg, (Editors). Springer-Verlag, New York, 167-204.

Gani, J. and Mansouri, H.. (1986) An improved fit in the chain binomial model for the common cold. UCSB Technical Report, 1-8.

Gani, J. and Purdue P. (1984) Matrix-geometric methods for the general stochastic epidemic. IMA J. Maths Appl. Med. Biology 1, 333-342.

Heasman, M.A. and Reid, D.D. (1961) Theory and observation in family epidemics of the common cold. Brit. J. Prev. Soc. Med. 15, 12-16.

Kermack, W.O. and McKendrick, A.G. (1927) Contributions to the mathematical theory of epidemics. Proc. Roy. Soc. A 115, 700-721.

Kuczma, M. (1968) Functional Equations in a Single Variable. Polish Scientific

Macdonald, G. (1957) The Epidemiology and Control of Malaria. Oxford Univ. Press, London.

Malice, Marie-Pierre (1986) Some epidemic models for non-homogeneous populations. Ph.D. Thesis, Department of Statistics, University of Kentucky.

Nåsell, I. (1985) Hybrid Models of Tropical Infections. Lecture Notes in Biomathematics, Springer-Verlag, Berlin.

Saunders, I.W. (1980) A model for myxomatosis. Math. Biosciences 48, 1-15.

Schenzle, D. (1982) Problems in drawing epidemiological inferences by fitting epidemic chain models to lumped data. Biometrics 38, 843-847.

MARKOV SEMIGROUPS ASSOCIATED WITH ONE-DIMENSIONAL LÉVY OPERATORS
—— REGULARITY AND CONVERGENCE ——

Akira Negoro
Faculty of Liberal Arts, Shizuoka University
Shizuoka 422, Japan
and
Masaaki Tsuchiya
College of Liberal Arts, Kanazawa University
Kanazawa 920, Japan

Summary. Many diffusion operators appearing in the diffusion approximation to discrete models are degenerate. For example, the diffusion operator $\frac{1}{2}x(1-x)(d/dx)^2 + [u-(u+v)x](d/dx) \quad (0 < x < 1)$ arises as a diffusion approximation for the Wright-Fisher model with mutation and migration. To obtain an error estimate for such diffusion approximation, it is useful to show the smoothness of solutions of the diffusion equations. Ethier has obtained important results for the smoothness problem, especially in the one-dimensional case. Motivated by his work, we will study the smoothness problem for certain degenerate integro-differential operators appearing in the theory of Markov processes. These operators include diffusion operators and are called Lévy operators (in this note, we treat the case without boundary). Our result can be used to get some limit theorem for stochastic processes with discontinuous paths. We will discuss the generation of the semigroups by one-dimensional Lévy operators and the differentiability preserving properties of the semigroups. Convergence problems for the semigroups are also treated.

1. Introduction

As is well known, many interesting degenerate diffusion equations appear in investigation on population genetics and for such investigation it is important to study smoothness properties of solutions of the equations (cf. [2]). In the one-dimensional case, Ethier [3] has obtained a definitive result on the differentiability of solutions and one of the present authors studied the analyticity of time-homogeneous solutions ([12], [13]).

Here we are concerned with the smoothness problem for Lévy operators. Solving such a problem is important to construct Markov processes with discontinuous paths.

The first time we obtained our result, as in the seminar talk, we owed the generation of the semigroups to Watanabe's unpublished work on stochastic differential equations; so we treated the Lévy operators in more restricted form at that time. Here the generation of the semigroups is carried out along the same line as [8], but the smoothness assumption on the coefficients of the Lévy operators is weaker than that of [8]. Moreover, the uniqueness of semigroups associated with a Lévy operator is also shown in the scheme of the martingale problem for the Lévy operator. The detailed proofs will be given in [6].

2. The martingale problems for Lévy operators

First, we will introduce some notations. Let R be the real line. Let C be the space of continuous real functions on R. C_c, C_0 and C_b stand for the subspaces of C consisting of functions which, respectively, have compact support in R, vanish at infinity and are bounded on R. Assume that these spaces are normed by the essential supremum norm, denoted by $\|\cdot\|_0$. For a positive integer n, denote by C^n the space of n times continuously differentiable real functions on R. Moreover we set

$$C_c^n = C^n \cap C_c \ ;$$

$$C_0^n = \{f \in C^n\colon f^{(k)} \in C_0,\ k = 0,1,\cdots,n\} \ ;$$

$$C_b^n = \{f \in C^n\colon f^{(k)} \in C_b,\ k = 0,1,\cdots,n\} \ ;$$

$$D_b^n = \{f \in C^{n-1}\colon f^{(k)} \in C_b,\ k = 0,1,\cdots,n-1, \text{ and } f^{(n-1)} \text{ is Lipschitz continuous}\}.$$

Define the norm $\|\cdot\|_n$ on these function spaces by $\|f\|_n = \sum_{k=0}^{n} \|f^{(k)}\|_0$.

Let $a(x)$, $b(x)$ and $c(x)$ be bounded Borel functions on R, let $a(x) \geqq 0$ and let $\nu(x,dy)$ be a kernel such that for each Borel set E in R, $\nu(x,E)$ is a Borel function of x and for each $x \in R$, $\nu(x,dy)$ is a positive measure on R satisfying $\nu(x,\{0\}) = 0$ and $\int_R y^2/(1+y^2)\nu(x,dy) < \infty$. Then we define a Lévy operator L by

$$\begin{aligned} Lf(x) &= a(x)f^{(2)}(x) + b(x)f^{(1)}(x) + c(x)f(x) \\ &\quad + \int_R [f(x+y)-f(x)-I_{\{|y|\leqq 1\}}(y)f^{(1)}(x)y]\nu(x,dy) \qquad (2.1) \end{aligned}$$

and denote by L_0 the operator L with $c = 0$.

Now let us consider the martingale problem for L_0 (the L_0-martingale problem). We refer to [11] for the basic result on the martingale problems for Lévy operators. Let $W = D([0,\infty) \to R)$ be the Skorohod space, that is, the space of right continuous functions w on $[0,\infty)$ into R having left limits. For $w \in W$, we denote by $x(t,w)$ the position of w at the time t. Let $\mathcal{B}_t$ and $\mathcal{B}$ be the usual σ-algebras on W generated by $\{x(s): 0 \leqq s \leqq t\}$ and $\{x(s): 0 \leqq s < \infty\}$, respectively. For $f \in C_b^2$, let

$$L_f(t) = \int_0^t L_0 f(x(s))ds,$$

$$M_f(t) = f(x(t)) - f(x(0)) - L_f(t).$$

Then a probability measure P on $(W, \mathcal{B})$ is called <u>a solution to the L_0-martingale problem</u> starting at x, if M_f is a P-martingale with the filtration $\{\mathcal{B}_t\}$ and $P[x(0) = x] = 1$. We denote by $\langle M_f \rangle$ the predictable quadratic variation process for the martingale M_f.

<u>Proposition 2.1. Suppose that</u> $a(x)$, $b(x)$ <u>and</u> $\int_R y^2/(1+y^2)\nu(x,dy)$ <u>are bounded in</u> x. <u>Then any solution</u> P <u>to the L_0-martingale problem satisfies the following</u>:

(i) <u>for each</u> $f \in C_b^2$

$$\langle M_f \rangle(t) = L_{f^2}(t) - 2\int_0^t f(x(s))dL_f(s) \qquad (P\text{-}\underline{a.s.});$$

(ii) $P[x(t) \neq x(t-)] = 0$ <u>for each</u> $t \geqq 0$.

<u>Remark.</u> We can get the same conclusion for probability measures on W satisfying one of the equivalent conditions of Theorem (1.1) in [11].

Now for a, b, c and ν, we set the following condition:

(H.1) (i) $a, b, c \in C_b$.

(ii) For each $x \in R$, $\nu(x,dy)$ is absolutely continuous with respect to a common positive measure $\nu(dy)$ on R such that $\nu(\{0\}) = 0$ and $\int_R y^2/(1+y^2)\nu(dy) < \infty$, that is, $\nu(x,dy) = d(x,y)\nu(dy)$. Furthermore, for each $y \in R$, $d(\cdot,y)$ is continuous and uniformly bounded.

Under the condition (H.1), we may assume that $0 \leqq d \leqq 1$ and we will assume that this inequality holds in what follows. Under the condition (H.1), the Lévy operator L is rewritten as

$$Lf(x) = a(x)f^{(2)}(x) + b(x)f^{(1)}(x) + c(x)f(x)$$
$$+ \int_R [f(x+y)-f(x)-I_{\{|y|\leq 1\}}(y)f^{(1)}(x)y]d(x,y)\nu(dy) \qquad (2.1)$$

and we say that L is the Lévy operator made of the data $[a, b, c, d; \nu]$ The condition (H.1) also yields the existence of solutions to the L_0-martingale problem (see [11, Theorem (2.2)]). Then in the same way as [3, Proposition 1], we have

Proposition 2.2. *Assume that* (H.1) *and the uniqueness of solutions to the L_0-martingale problem hold. Let P_x be the solution to the L_0-martingale problem starting at x. Then the Feynman-Kac formula*

$$T(t)f(x) = E^{P_x}[f(x(t))\exp(\int_0^t c(x(s))ds] \tag{2.3}$$

defines a strongly continuous non-negative semigroup $\{T(t)\}$ on C_0 whose infinitesimal generator is an extension of L acting on C_c^2. Moreover, $\{T(t)\}$ is the only semigroup with such properties.

So we say that $\{T(t)\}$ given by (2.3) is the semigroup associated with L or the data $[a, b, c, d; \nu]$.

Conversely, we have the following fact (cf. [14, Proposition 1]).

Proposition 2.3. *Assume that* (H.1) *holds. If L_0 acting on C_0^2 (or C_c^2) is closable and its closure generates a strongly continuous semigroup on C_0, then the uniqueness of solutions to the L_0-martingale problem holds.*

3. Generation of the semigroups and their differentiability preserving properties

In the rest of the paper, we assume that the condition (H.1) always holds. For the data $[a, b, c, d; \nu]$, let

$$\nu_\varepsilon(dy) = I_{\{|y|>\varepsilon\}}(y)\nu(dy)$$

and let L_ε and $L_{\varepsilon,0}$ be the Lévy operators made of $[a, b, c, d; \nu_\varepsilon]$ and $[a, b, 0, d; \nu_\varepsilon]$, respectively. Furthermore, set $d^{(k)}(x,y) = (\partial/\partial x)^k d(x,y)$ and $\| d(\cdot,y) \|_n = \sum_{k=0}^{n} \| d^{(k)}(\cdot,y) \|_0$. Then we introduce the second condition:

$(H.2)_n$ For a positive integer n, $a \in C_b^{2\vee n}$, $b, c \in C_b^n$, $d(\cdot,y) \in C_b^n$ for each y and

$$\int_R \frac{y^2}{1+y^2} \| d(\cdot,y) \|_n \nu(dy) < \infty.$$

Under the conditions (H.1) and $(H.2)_n$ ($n \geqq 1$), using the method of Ethier [3], we see that L_ε acting on C_c^2 generates a unique strongly continuous semigroup $\{T_\varepsilon(t)\}$ on C_0 and it satisfies

$$T_\varepsilon(t): C_0^n \to C_0^n \qquad (t \geqq 0),$$

$$\| T_\varepsilon(t) \|_n \leqq \exp(\lambda_{\varepsilon,n} t) \qquad (t \geqq 0)$$

for some positive constant $\lambda_{\varepsilon,n}$ and the restriction of $\{T_\varepsilon(t)\}$ to C_0^n is strongly continuous in the norm $\| \cdot \|_n$.

To obtain a uniform estimate for the norm $\| T_\varepsilon(t) \|_n$ with respect to ε, we need the third condition:

(H.3) $$\int_{|y| \leqq 1} |y| \, \| d^{(1)}(\cdot,y) \|_0 \nu(dy) < \infty.$$

Then we set

$$\lambda_n = \max_{0 \leqq j \leqq n} \{ \sum_{k=j}^{n} [\| e_{kj} \|_0 + \frac{1}{2}\binom{k}{j-2} \int_{|y| \leqq 1} y^2 \| d^{(k-j+2)}(\cdot,y) \|_0 \nu(dy)] + 2j \int_{|y| \leqq 1} |y| \, \| d^{(1)}(\cdot,y) \|_0 \nu(dy) \}, \qquad (3.1)$$

where

$$e_{kj} = \left| \binom{k}{j-2} a^{(k-j+2)}(x) + \binom{k}{j-1} b^{(k-j+1)}(x) + \binom{k}{j} c^{(k-j)}(x) \right| + 2\binom{k}{j} \int_{|y|>1} \| d^{(k-j)}(\cdot,y) \|_0 \nu(dy)$$

and assume that $\binom{k}{-2} = \binom{k}{-1} = 0$. Then in the same way as Norman [7], we have a fundamental lemma.

Lemma 3.1. Assume that (H.1), $(H.2)_n$ $(n \geqq 1)$ and (H.3) hold. Then for every $f \in C_0^n$

$$\| T_\varepsilon(t) f \|_n \leqq \exp(\lambda_n t) \| f \|_n \qquad (t \geqq 0).$$

When we replace the space C in $(H.2)_n$ by the space D, we denote the condition by $(H.2')_n$, that is,

$(H.2')_n$ For a positive integer n, assume that $a \in D_b^{2\vee n}$, $b, c \in D_b^n$, $d(\cdot,y) \in D_b^n$ for each y and

$$\int_R \frac{y^2}{1+y^2} \| d(\cdot,y) \|_n \nu(dy) < \infty.$$

For the data $[a, b, c, d; \nu]$, we denote by μ_n the positive constant defined as in (3.1) replacing $\| e_{kj} \|_0$ by f_{kj}, where

$$f_{kj} = \binom{k}{j-2} \| a^{(k-j+2)} \|_0 + \binom{k}{j-1} \| b^{(k-j+1)} \|_0 + \binom{k}{j} \| c^{(k-j)} \|_0$$
$$+ 2\binom{k}{j} \int_{|y|>1} \| d^{(k-j)}(\cdot,y) \|_0 \nu(dy).$$

Then using Lemma 3.1, we can show that for $\lambda > \mu_2$ the range of $\lambda - L_0$ acting on C_0^2 is dense in C_0. Therefore the operator L_0 with domain C_0^2 satisfies the conditions of Theorem 1.2 in [10] (see also [2, Theorem A.6]). So, with the help of Proposition 2.3, we have

Theorem 3.2. Under the conditions (H.1), $(H.2')_2$ and (H.3), the uniqueness of solutions to the L_0-martingale problem holds.

Next we have the differentiability preserving property of the semigroup $\{T(t)\}$ associated with L, using Lemma 3.1, the standard argument (see [7]) and some delicate calculations.

Theorem 3.3. Under (H.1), $(H.2')_n$ $(n \geqq 2)$ and (H.3), we get

$$T(t): D_b^n \to D_b^n \qquad (t \geqq 0),$$

$$\| T(t) \|_n \leqq \exp(\mu_n t) \qquad (t \geqq 0).$$

Remark. Assume that (H.1), $(H.2)_{n+2}$ $(n \geqq 0)$ and (H.3) hold. Then

$$T(t): C_0^n \to C_0^n \qquad (t \geqq 0),$$

$$\| T(t) \|_n \leqq \exp(\lambda_n t) \qquad (t \geqq 0)$$

and the restriction of $\{T(t)\}$ to C_0^n is strongly continuous in the norm $\| \cdot \|_n$.

4. Convergence of Lévy operators and the associated semigroups

Here we will consider the relation between the convergence of Lévy operators and that of the associated semigroups. For this purpose we will treat the Lévy operators in the following form:

$$Lf(x) = a(x)f^{(2)}(x) + b(x)f^{(1)}(x) + c(x)f(x)$$
$$+ \int_R [f(x+y)-f(x)- \frac{y^2}{1+y^2}f^{(1)}(x)y]d(x,y)\nu(dy). \qquad (4.1)$$

The second form (4.1) is derived from the first form (2.2) by modifying b suitably. In this section, we assume that all the Lévy operators are represented in the second form.

Let L_m $(m = 1,2,\cdots)$ and L be the Lévy operators made of data $[a_m, b_m, c_m, d_m; \nu_m]$ $(m = 1,2,\cdots)$ and $[a, b, c, d; \nu]$, respectively. Furthermore, suppose that L_m $(m = 1,2,\cdots)$ and L satisfy (H.1) and $0 \leqq d_m \leqq 1$, $0 \leqq d \leqq 1$. Then we say that $L_m \to L$ as $m \to \infty$, if

(i) $\lim_{\varepsilon \downarrow 0} \limsup_{m\to\infty} \| \frac{1}{2}\int_{|y|\leqq\varepsilon} y^2 d_m(\cdot,y)\nu_m(dy) + a_m - a \|_0 = 0;$

(ii) $\| b_m - b \|_0 \to 0$ as $m \to \infty$;

(iii) $\| c_m - c \|_0 \to 0$ as $m \to \infty$;

(iv) $\| d_m(\cdot,y) - d(\cdot,y) \|_0 \to 0$ as $m \to \infty$ uniformly in y on any compact set in $R\backslash\{0\}$;

(v) $d(x,y) \in C[R\times(R\backslash\{0\})]$;

(vi) $\lim_{m\to\infty} \int_R f(y)\nu_m(dy) = \int_R f(y)\nu(dy)$

for every bounded continuous function f vanishing in some neighborhood of 0.

N.B. By Kondō's advice, the condition (v) is improved as above. In the first draft, we assumed that $d(x,\cdot) \in C^1(R\backslash\{0\})$ and $(\partial/\partial y)d(x,y)$ is bounded.

It should be noticed that these conditions cover those for the convergence of infinitely divisible distributions (cf. [4], [9]).

Lemma 4.1. *If $L_m \to L$ as $m \to \infty$, then $\| L_m f - Lf \|_0 \to 0$ for every $f \in C_0^2$.*

Combining Lemma 4.1 with the results in [1] and [11], we have

Theorem 4.2. *Let P_m be a solution to the $L_{m,0}$-martingale problem $(m = 1,2,\cdots)$ and satisfy $\lim_{\ell\to\infty} \sup_m P_m[|x(0)| \geqq \ell] = 0$. Assume that $L_{m,0} \to L_0$ as $m \to \infty$. Then $\{P_m\}$ is tight and any limit point P_∞ in the weak topology is a solution to the L_0-martingale problem.*

Using Proposition 2.1(ii), Proposition 2.3 and Theorem 4.2, we can get

Corollary 4.3. *Assume that $L_m \to L$ as $m \to \infty$ and that the uniqueness of solutions to the $L_{m,0}$-martingale problem $(m = 1,2,\cdots)$ and the L_0-martingale problem hold, respectively. Let $\{T_m(t)\}$ and $\{T(t)\}$*

be the semigroups associated with L_m and L, respectively. Then

$$\lim_{m\to\infty} T_m(t)f(x) = T(t)f(x)$$

for every $t \geqq 0$, $f \in C_b$ and $x \in R$.

5. Stochastic differential equations of jump-type

In Theorem 3.3, we assume that $n \geqq 2$ for the condition $(H.2)_n$. If we use Watanabe's unpublished work on stochastic differential equations of jump-type, we can get more sharp result on the differentiability preserving properties of the semigroup.

He gave a new formulation of stochastic differential equations associated with Lévy operators and obtained the existence and uniqueness theorem for solutions of the equations as follows. The stochastic differential equation associated with L_0 is given by

$$\begin{aligned} dx(t) &= \sqrt{2a}(x(t))dB(t) + b(x(t))dt \\ &+ \int_{|y|>1}\int_{z=0}^{1} yI_{[0,d(x(t-),y)]}(y)p(dt,dydz) \qquad (5.1) \\ &+ \int_{|y|\leqq 1}\int_{z=0}^{1} yI_{[0,d(x(t-),y)]}(y)q(dt,dydz), \end{aligned}$$

where B is a one-dimensional Brownian motion, p is an $(R\setminus\{0\})\times[0,1]$-valued stationary point process with characteristic measure $\nu(dy)dz$ and

$$q(dt,dydz) = p(dt,dydz) - dt\nu(dy)dz.$$

We refer to [5] for Poisson point processes.

Proposition 5.1. (Watanabe [15]) Assume that (H.1) holds and that $\nu(dy) = K/y^2$ $(y \neq 0)$ with a positive constant K in some neighborhood of 0. Furthermore, assume that $\sqrt{a}$, b, $d(\cdot,y) \in D_b^1$ (i.e., Lipschitz continuous) and $\int_R y^2/(1+y^2) \| d^{(1)}(\cdot,y) \|_0 \nu(dy) < \infty$. Then the stochastic differential equation (5.1) has a unique strong solution.

Since the consequence of Proposition 5.1 yields the uniqueness of solutions to the L_0-martingale problem (note that the uniqueness holds without (H.3)), we see that the conclusion of Theorem 3.3 is valid in the case where $n = 1$, under the following assumptions:

(i) (H.1) holds;

(ii) $\nu(dy)$ satisfies the condition mentioned in Proposition 5.1;

(iii) $(H.2')_1$ holds;

(iv) (H.3) holds.

Acknowledgments

The authors express their deep gratitude to Professor Shinzo Watanabe who gave them permission to reproduce part of his unpublished work. The authors are also grateful to Professor Ryōji Kondō for his helpful advice.

References

1. P. Billingsley: Convergence of Probability Measures, J. Wiley, New York, 1968.
2. S. N. Ethier: An error estimate for the diffusion approximation in population genetics, Ph. D. Thesis, Univ. Wisconsin, 1975.
3. S. N. Ethier: Differentiability preserving properties of Markov semigroups associated with one-dimensional diffusions, Z. Wahrsch. Verw. Gebiete 45 (1978), 225-238.
4. B. V. Gnedenko and A. N. Kolmogorov: Limit Distributions for Sums of Independent Random Variables, revised ed., Addison-Wesley, Reading, 1968 (English translation from Russian, 1949).
5. N. Ikeda and S. Watanabe: Stochastic Differential Equations and Diffusion Processes, North-Holland/Kodansha, Amsterdam/Tokyo, 1981.
6. A. Negoro and M. Tsuchiya: (in preparation).
7. M. F. Norman: A "psychological" proof that certain Markov semigroups preserve differentiability, SIAM-AMS Proc. 13(1981), 197-211.
8. K. Sato: Integration of the generalized Kolmogorov-Feller backward equations, J. Fac. Sci. Univ. Tokyo Sec. I, 9 (1961), 13-27.
9. K. Sato: Infinitely Divisible Distributions, Seminar on Probability Vol. 52, 1981 (in Japanese).
10. K. Sato and T. Ueno: Multi-dimensional diffusion and the Markov process on the boundary, J. Math. Kyoto Univ. 4 (1965), 529-605.
11. D. W. Stroock: Diffusion processes associated with Lévy generators, Z. Wahrsch. Verw. Gebiete 32 (1975), 209-244.
12. M. Tsuchiya: Resolvents for one-dimensional diffusion operators with real analytic coefficients, Ann. Sci. Kanazawa Univ. 20 (1983), 13-17.
13. M. Tsuchiya: Analyticity preserving properties of resolvents for degenerate diffusion operators in one dimension, Proc. Amer. Math. Soc. 90 (1984), 91-94.
14. M. Tsuchiya: Martingale problems and semigroups, Ann. Sci. Kanazawa Univ. 21 (1984), 19-22.
15. S. Watanabe: Stochastic differential equations of jump-type, 1974 (unpublished note).

ON SOME CONDITIONS FOR DIFFUSION PROCESSES TO STAY ON THE BOUNDARY OF A DOMAIN

Norio Okada
Department of Mathematics
Josai University
1-1 Keyakidai Sakado
Saitama, 350-02 Japan

Summary

In population genetics, it is frequently done to approximate discrete models by diffusion models. From a mathematical point of view, this diffusion approximation problem is usually treated as the problem of convergence of discrete models (suitably normalized and interpolated) to a diffusion process on a bounded closed domain. In many cases it is easy to get from the discrete models an explicit form of the limiting differential operator. But, in order to prove the convergence of the stochastic processes, it is necessary to prove the uniqueness of the diffusion process associated with the differential operator. This uniqueness problem is often a hard mathematical problem due to degeneracy of the operator on the boundary. Sometimes it is helpful to prove certain regularity properties for diffusion processes (not assumed to be unique) associated with the given operator. Especially in the problem of convergence of discrete models without mutation and migration, it is important to show that sample paths of the diffusion processes cannot enter the interior from the boundary.

In this paper we consider this property for diffusion processes on a general bounded closed domain whose behavior in the interior is determined by a given diffusion operator. As an application of our results, we get this property for the diffusion process corresponding to the discrete models without mutation and migration. Consequently its uniqueness follows easily.

1. Introduction

Let G be a bounded domain in R^d with a boundary ∂G and $\overline{G} = G \cup \partial G$. Let $C = C([0,\infty),\overline{G})$ be the space of $\overline{G}$-valued continuous functions defined on $[0,\infty)$, $x(t,\omega) = \omega(t)$ for $\omega \in C$ and $\mathcal{N}_t$ and $\mathcal{N}$ be the σ-fields generated by $\{x(s)\colon 0 \leq s \leq t\}$ and $\{x(s)\colon s \geq 0\}$, respectively. For each $i,j = 1,\dots,d$, let $a_{ij}(x)$ and $b_i(x)$ be continuous functions in G such that the matrix $a(x) = (a_{ij}(x))_{i,j=1,\dots,d}\colon G \to R^d \otimes R^d$ is symmetric and positive definite and define the diffusion operator L in G by

$$L = \frac{1}{2}\sum_{i,j=1}^{d} a_{ij}(x)\frac{\partial^2}{\partial x_i \partial x_j} + \sum_{i=1}^{d} b_i(x)\frac{\partial}{\partial x_i} .$$

Let $(x(t),C,P_x)$ be a conservative diffusion process with state space $\overline{G}$ such that its behavior in the interior G is determined by L. In this paper we consider an analytic condition under which sample paths of such a diffusion process $(x(t),C,P_x)$ cannot enter the interior G from the boundary ∂G.

In Section 2 we state our results. In Section 3 we introduce some applications of our results, one of which appears in the diffusion approximation problem in population genetics. In Section 4 we prove our results stated in Section 2.

2. Results

For each $x,y \in \overline{G}$ and a subset A of $\overline{G}$, let $\rho(x,y)$ denote the Euclidean distance between x and y and $\rho(x,A) = \inf\{\rho(x,z): z \in A\}$. For a given set A, we let $\overline{A}$ and A° denote the closure and the interior of A, respectively, $\partial A = \overline{A} - A^\circ$ and $C_b(A)$ denote the space of bounded and continuous functions on A. Further we let $C^2(A)$ denote the space of functions on A which can be extended to twice continuously differentiable functions in an open neighborhood of A.

Let $\tau(\partial G) = \inf\{t \geqq 0: x(t) \in \partial G\}$ and, for each $\varepsilon > 0$, $\tau_\varepsilon = \inf\{t \geqq 0: x(t) \in B_\varepsilon(\partial G)\}$, where $B_\varepsilon(\partial G) = \{y \in \overline{G}: \rho(y,\partial G) \leqq \varepsilon\}$. We say that $(x(t),C,P_x)$ is an L(G)-diffusion process if $(x(t),C,P_x)$ is a conservative strong Markov process with state space $\overline{G}$ and $\{f(x(t\wedge\tau_\varepsilon)) - \int_0^{t\wedge\tau_\varepsilon} Lf(x(s))ds, \mathcal{N}_t : t \geqq 0\}$ is a P_x-martingale for all $f \in C^2(\overline{G})$ and $\varepsilon > 0$.

Now we put the following analytic condition.

[Condition 1]. There is a closed set V and, for each $n = 1,2,3,\ldots$, there are open sets Δ_n and Γ_n and a positive function $w_n(x)$ in $C^2(\Delta_n - V) \cap C_b(\overline{\Delta}_n - V^\circ)$ which satisfy the following (i)-(v):

(i) $G \supset \Delta_n \supset \overline{\Gamma}_n$ and $\Gamma_n \supset V$ for each $n = 1,2,3,\ldots$ and $V^\circ \neq \phi$.

(ii) $Lw_n \leqq \alpha w_n$ in $\Delta_n - V$ for some positive constant α.

(iii) $\inf_{n\geqq 1} \min_{y\in\partial V} w_n(y) \geqq \beta$ for some positive constant β.

(iv) $\min_{y\in\partial\Delta_n} w_n(y) \geqq \max_{y\in\partial\Gamma_n} w_n(y)$.

(v) $\limsup_{n\to\infty} \max_{y\in\partial\Gamma_n} w_n(y) = 0$.

In the one-dimensional case, [Condition 1] is equivalent to that ∂G is natural or exit.

Then we have the following results.

<u>Theorem 1</u>. <u>Suppose that [Condition 1] holds. Then we have</u>

$P_x[x(t) \in \partial G$ *for all* $t \geqq \tau(\partial G)] = 1$ *for all* $x \in \bar{G}$ *if* $(x(t), C, P_x)$ *is an* $L(G)$-*diffusion process*.

Corollary 1. *We have* $\bigcup_{n=1}^{\infty} \Gamma_n = G$ *for* $\{\Gamma_n\}$ *satisfying* [*Condition* 1].

Under some regularity conditions on ∂G and the coefficients $a_{ij}(x)$ and $b_i(x)$ $(i,j=1,\ldots,d)$, we conjecture that, if $P_x[x(t) \in \partial G$ for all $t \geqq \tau(\partial G)] = 1$ for all $x \in \bar{G}$ hold for any $L(G)$-diffusion process $(x(t), C, P_x)$, then we have [Condition 1]. But we cannot prove it yet. We shall treat further arguments related to this problem elsewhere.

3. *Examples*

In this section, we introduce two examples such that [Condition 1] holds.

Example 1. Assume that ∂G is the regular C^3-boundary and, for each $i,j = 1,\ldots,d$, $a_{ij}(x)$ and $b_i(x)$ are uniformly Lipschitz continuous in G. Obviously $a_{ij}(x)$ and $b_i(x)$ have Lipschitz continuous extensions to $\bar{G} = G \cup \partial G$ and we denote these extensions by the same letters $a_{ij}(x)$ and $b_i(x)$. Since ∂G is the regular C^3-boundary, $\rho(x) = \rho(x, \partial G)$ is in $C^2(B_\varepsilon(\partial G))$ for some $\varepsilon > 0$ sufficiently small. Further we assume that $\sum_{i,j=1}^{d} a_{ij}\, \partial\rho/\partial x_i\, \partial\rho/\partial x_j(x) = 0$ and $L\rho(x) = 2^{-1}\sum_{i,j=1}^{d} a_{ij}\, \partial^2\rho/\partial x_i \partial x_j(x) + \sum_{i=1}^{d} b_i\, \partial\rho/\partial x_i(x) \leqq 0$ for all $x \in \partial G$. Then we have [Condition 1].

In fact it follows from the assumptions that there are a closed set V and a positive constant α such that $G \supset V \supset G - B_\varepsilon(\partial G)$, $\rho \in C^2(\bar{G}-V) \cap C_b(\bar{G}-V^\circ)$ and $\rho(x) \leqq 1$, $\sum_{i,j=1}^{d} a_{ij}\, \partial\rho/\partial x_i\, \partial\rho/\partial x_j(x) \leqq \alpha\rho(x)$ and $L\rho(x) \leqq \alpha\rho(x)$ for all $x \in \bar{G} - V$. Now let $c = \inf\{\rho(x,y) : x \in \partial G,\ y \in V\}$ and, for each $n = 1,2,3,\ldots$, let $\Gamma_n = \{x \in G : \rho(x) > c/(n+1)\}$ and $w_n(x) = \{\rho(x) \log \rho(x) - \rho(x) \log(c/(n+1)) - \rho(x) + c/(n+1) + 2\}/\log(n+1)$. Then $w_n(x)$ is a positive function in $C^2(G-V) \cap C_b(G-V^\circ)$ satisfying $w_n(x) = 2/\log(n+1)$ for all $x \in \partial\Gamma_n$, $w_n(x) \geqq 2/\log(n+1)$ for all $x \in G - V^\circ$, $w_n(x) \geqq c$ for all $x \in \partial V$ and $\alpha w_n(x) - Lw_n(x) \geqq \alpha\{1 + c/(n+1) - \rho(x)\}/\log(n+1) > 0$ for all $x \in \bar{\Gamma}_n - V$. Consequently, for each $n = 1,2,3,\ldots$, we can choose an open set Δ_n in such a way that $\bar{\Gamma}_n \subset \Delta_n \subset G$ and $\alpha w_n \geqq Lw_n$ in $\Delta_n - V$. Thus these V, Δ_n, Γ_n and $w_n(x)$ satisfy [Condition 1].

Example 2. Let $\bar{G} = K = \{x = (x_1,\ldots,x_d) \in R^d : x_i \geqq 0$ for each $i = 1,\ldots,d$ and $x_{d+1} = 1 - \sum_{i=1}^{d} x_i \geqq 0\}$, $a_{ij}(x) = x_i(\delta_{ij} - x_j)$ on K and $b_i(x) = 0$ on $F_i = \partial K \cap \{x_i = 0\}$ for each $i,j = 1,\ldots,d$ and $\sum_{i=1}^{d} b_i(x) = 0$ on $F_{d+1} = \partial K \cap \{x_{d+1} = 0\}$, where δ_{ij} is Kronecker's delta. Moreover we suppose that $b_i(x)$, $i = 1,\ldots,d$, is Hölder continuous of order γ for some $\gamma > 0$ in K. The diffusion operator L in K corresponding to these a_{ij} and b_i is the multi-allelic Wright-Fisher model without mutation and migration in population genetics (cf. Crow and Kimura (1970) and Sato (1976b)).

In this case, we have similar conditions to [Condition 1] as follows. For each $i = 1,2,\ldots,d+1$ and $n = 1,2,3,\ldots$, let $\Gamma_n^i = \{x_i > 1/(n+2)\}$ and $V^i = \{x_i \geq 1/2\}$. From the assumptions on $b_i(x)$, there is a positive constant λ such that $|b_i(x)| \leq \lambda x_i^\gamma$ for all $x \in K$ and each $i = 1,2,\ldots,d+1$, where $b_{d+1}(x) = \sum_{i=1}^d b_i(x)$. Now, for each $i = 1,2,\ldots,d+1$ and $n = 1,2,3,\ldots$, we define $w_n^i(x) = \{\int_{1/(n+2)}^{x_i} \exp(-4\gamma^{-1}\lambda y^\gamma)dy \int_{1/(n+2)}^{y} z^{-1}\exp(4\gamma^{-1}\lambda z^\gamma)dz + 1\}I_n^{-1}$, where $I_n = \int_{1/(n+2)}^{1/2} \exp(-4\gamma^{-1}\lambda y^\gamma)dy \int_{1/(n+2)}^{y} z^{-1}\exp(4\gamma^{-1}\lambda z^\gamma)dz$. Then we have that $w_n^i \in C^2(\{x_i > 0\})$, $w_n^i(x) \geq 1$ for all $x \in \partial V^i$, $w_n^i(x) = I_n^{-1}$ for all $x \in \partial\Gamma_n^i$, $w_n^i(x) \geq I_n^{-1}$ for all $x \in \{x_i > 0\}$ and $\lim_{n\to\infty} I_n = \infty$. Moreover we have that $Lw_n^i < w_n^i$ in $K \cap (\overline{\Gamma}_n^i - V^i)$. Consequently we can choose a positive constant c_n in such a way that $c_n \in (0,1/(n+2))$, $Lw_n^i \leq w_n^i$ in $K \cap (\Delta_n^i - V^i)$ and $\min\{w_n^i(y)\colon y \in K \cap \partial\Delta_n^i\} \geq \max\{w_n^i(y)\colon y \in K \cap \partial\Gamma_n^i\}$ for each $i = 1,2,\ldots,d+1$ and $n = 1,2,3,\ldots$, where $\Delta_n^i = \{x_i > c_n\}$.

Now let $\tau(F_i) = \inf\{t \geq 0\colon x(t) \in F_i\}$ and $(x(t),C,P_x)$ be an $L(G)$-diffusion process. Further we assume that $\{f(x(t\wedge\sigma)) - \int_0^{t\wedge\sigma} Lf(x(s))ds, \mathcal{N}_t\colon t \geq 0\}$ is a P_x-martingale for all $f \in C^2(\overline{G})$, where $\sigma = \wedge_{i=1}^{d+1} \sigma(i)$, $\sigma(i) = \inf\{t \geq 0\colon x(t) = v(i)\}$ and $v(i) = (\delta_{1i},\delta_{2i},\ldots,\delta_{di})$. The existence of such a diffusion process follows easily. Then applying an argument similar to that given in the proof of Theorem 1 to $w_n^i(x)$ with Γ_n^i, Δ_n^i and V^i, we have that $P_x[x(t) \in F_i$ for all $t \geq \tau(F_i)] = 1$ for all $x \in \overline{G}$ and each $i = 1,2,\ldots,d+1$. Consequently we have that $P_x[x(t) \in \bigcap_{k=1}^d F_{i(k)}$ for all $t \geq \vee_{k=1}^d \tau(F_{i(k)})] = 1$ for any $i(1),i(2),\ldots,i(d) \in \{1,2,\ldots,d+1\}$ and $x \in \overline{G}$. Combining these properties with ellipticity of the matrix $(a_{ij}(x))_{i,j=1,\ldots,d}$ in K° and by induction, we get the uniqueness of a probability measure P_x on $(C,\mathcal{N})$ such that $P_x[x(0) = x] = 1$ and $\{f(x(t\wedge\sigma)) - \int_0^{t\wedge\sigma} Lf(x(s))ds, \mathcal{N}_t\colon t \geq 0\}$ is a P_x-martingale for all $f \in C^2(\overline{G})$. This uniqueness is necessary for guaranteeing the diffusion approximation of the discrete model without mutation and migration, for the details of which we refer to Ethier (1975), Guess (1973), Okada (1979) and Sato (1976a,1978).

4. Proofs of our results

Proof of Theorem 1. By the strong Markov property, it suffices to show that $P_x[x(t) \in \partial G$ for all $t \geq 0] = 1$ for each $x \in \partial G$.

We fix n for a while and let $x \in \partial G$ and E_x denote the expectation by P_x. For V given in [Condition 1], let $\tau(V) = \inf\{t \geq 0\colon x(t) \in V\}$. Moreover, for each $p = 1,2,3,\ldots$, let $\xi_p = \inf\{t \geq \eta_{p-1}\colon x(t) \in \overline{\Gamma}_n\}$ and $\eta_p = \inf\{t \geq \xi_p\colon x(t) \in \overline{G} - \Delta_n\}$, where $\eta_0 = 0$. It is obvious that $\lim_{p\to\infty} \xi_p = \infty$ and $x(\tau(V)) \in \partial V$ if $\tau(V) < \infty$. Then noting these facts we have from (iii) of [Condition 1] that

$$\beta E_x[e^{-\alpha\tau(V)}] \leqq \min_{y\in\partial V} w_n(y) E_x[e^{-\alpha\tau(V)}] \leqq E_x[e^{-\alpha\tau(V)} w_n(x(\tau(V)))]$$

$$= \lim_{p\to\infty} E_x[e^{-\alpha(\tau(V)\wedge\xi_p)} w_n(x(\tau(V)\wedge\xi_p))] \ . \tag{1}$$

Moreover

$$E_x[e^{-\alpha(\tau(V)\wedge\xi_p)} w_n(x(\tau(V)\wedge\xi_p))]$$

$$= \sum_{i=2}^{p} E_x[\{e^{-\alpha(\tau(V)\wedge\xi_i)} w_n(x(\tau(V)\wedge\xi_i)) - e^{-\alpha(\tau(V)\wedge\eta_{i-1})}$$

$$w_n(x(\tau(V)\wedge\eta_{i-1}))\} + \{e^{-\alpha(\tau(V)\wedge\eta_{i-1})} w_n(x(\tau(V)\wedge\eta_{i-1}))$$

$$- e^{-\alpha(\tau(V)\wedge\xi_{i-1})} w_n(x(\tau(V)\wedge\xi_{i-1}))\}]$$

$$+ E_x[e^{-\alpha(\tau(V)\wedge\xi_1)} w_n(x(\tau(V)\wedge\xi_1))]$$

$$= \sum_{i=2}^{p} \{E_x[\{\tau(V) > \eta_{i-1}\} : e^{-\alpha(\tau(V)\wedge\xi_i)} w_n(x(\tau(V)\wedge\xi_i))$$

$$- e^{-\alpha\eta_{i-1}} w_n(x(\eta_{i-1}))] + E_x[\{\tau(V) > \xi_{i-1}\} : e^{-\alpha(\tau(V)\wedge\eta_{i-1})}$$

$$w_n(x(\tau(V)\wedge\eta_{i-1})) - e^{-\alpha\xi_{i-1}} w_n(x(\xi_{i-1}))]\}$$

$$+ E_x[e^{-\alpha(\tau(V)\wedge\xi_1)} w_n(x(\tau(V)\wedge\xi_1))] \ . \tag{2}$$

In the last expression in (2), first noting that $x(\xi_i) \in \partial\Gamma_n$ if $\xi_i < \infty$, $x(\eta_{i-1}) \in \partial\Delta_n$ if $\eta_{i-1} < \infty$ and $\xi_i \leqq \tau(V)$ for $\eta_{i-1} < \tau(V)$, we have from (i$\ddot{\text{V}}$) of [Condition 1] that

$$E_x[\{\tau(V) > \eta_{i-1}\} : e^{-\alpha(\tau(V)\wedge\xi_i)} w_n(x(\tau(V)\wedge\xi_i)) - e^{-\alpha\eta_{i-1}} w_n(x(\eta_{i-1}))]$$

$$= E_x[\{\tau(V) > \eta_{i-1}\} : e^{-\alpha\xi_i} w_n(x(\xi_i)) - e^{-\alpha\eta_{i-1}} w_n(x(\eta_{i-1}))]$$

$$\leqq \{\max_{y\in\partial\Gamma_n} w_n(y) - \min_{y\in\partial\Delta_n} w_n(y)\} E_x[\{\tau(V) > \eta_{i-1}\} : e^{-\alpha\xi_i}] \leqq 0 \ . \tag{3}$$

Next noting that $\xi_1 \leqq \tau(V)$ and $x(\xi_1) \in \partial\Gamma_n$ if $\xi_1 < \infty$, we have that

$$E_x[e^{-\alpha(\tau(V)\wedge\xi_1)} w_n(x(\tau(V)\wedge\xi_1))] = E_x[e^{-\alpha\xi_1} w_n(x(\xi_1))]$$

$$\leqq \max_{y\in\partial\Gamma_n} w_n(y) \ . \tag{4}$$

Now we shall estimate the following I_i $(i \geqq 2)$, which is the second term in the last expression in (2):

$$I_i = E_x[\{\tau(V) > \xi_{i-1}\}\colon e^{-\alpha(\tau(V)\wedge\eta_{i-1})} w_n(x(\tau(V)\wedge\eta_{i-1})) - e^{-\alpha\xi_{i-1}} w_n(x(\xi_{i-1}))] .$$

For each $i = 1,2,3,\ldots$ and $\varepsilon > 0$, let η_i^ε, η^ε and $\tau(V_\varepsilon)$ as follows:

$$\eta_i^\varepsilon = \inf\{t \geqq \xi_i\colon x(t) \in B_\varepsilon^n \cup (\bar{G}-\Delta_n)\} ,$$

$$\eta^\varepsilon = \inf\{t \geqq 0\colon x(t) \in B_\varepsilon^n \cup (\bar{G}-\Delta_n)\}$$

and

$$\tau(V_\varepsilon) = \inf\{t \geqq 0\colon x(t) \in V_\varepsilon\} ,$$

where $B_\varepsilon^n = \{y\colon \rho(y,\partial\Delta_n) \leqq \varepsilon\}$ and $V_\varepsilon = \{y\colon \rho(y,V) \leqq \varepsilon\}$. For each $i = 1,2,3,\ldots$, let θ_i be the shift operator on C such that $x(s,\theta_i(\omega)) = x(s+\xi_i(\omega),\omega)$ for $\xi_i(\omega) < \infty$ and $x(s,\theta_i(\omega)) = x$ for $\xi_i(\omega) = \infty$. It is obvious that $\eta^\varepsilon \leqq \tau_\varepsilon$, $\eta_i^\varepsilon \uparrow \eta_i$ and $\tau(V_\varepsilon)\uparrow\tau(V)$ as $\varepsilon\downarrow 0$, $\eta_i^\varepsilon(\omega) = \eta^\varepsilon(\theta_i(\omega)) + \xi_i(\omega)$ and $\tau(V_\varepsilon)(\omega) = \tau(V_\varepsilon)(\theta_i(\omega)) + \xi_i(\omega)$ for $\tau(V_\varepsilon)(\omega) \geqq \xi_i(\omega)$. Then noting these facts, we have by the Lebesgue bounded convergence theorem and the strong Markov property that

$$\begin{aligned} I_i &= \lim_{\varepsilon\downarrow 0} E_x[\{\tau(V_\varepsilon) > \xi_{i-1}\}\colon e^{-\alpha(\tau(V_\varepsilon)\wedge\eta_{i-1}^\varepsilon)} w_n(x(\tau(V_\varepsilon)\wedge\eta_{i-1}^\varepsilon)) \\ &\qquad - e^{-\alpha\xi_{i-1}} w_n(x(\xi_{i-1}))] \\ &= \lim_{\varepsilon\downarrow 0} E_x[\{\tau(V_\varepsilon) > \xi_{i-1}\}\colon e^{-\alpha\xi_{i-1}} E_{x(\xi_{i-1})}[e^{-\alpha(\tau(V_\varepsilon)\wedge\eta^\varepsilon)} \\ &\qquad w_n(x(\tau(V_\varepsilon)\wedge\eta^\varepsilon)) - w_n(x(\xi_{i-1}))]] . \qquad (5) \end{aligned}$$

Moreover applying the martingale property and the Lebesgue bounded convergence and the optional sampling theorems to $f(t,x) = e^{-\alpha t} w_n(x)$, we have from (ii) of [Condition 1] that

$$\begin{aligned} &E_y[e^{-\alpha(\tau(V_\varepsilon)\wedge\eta^\varepsilon)} w_n(x(\tau(V_\varepsilon)\wedge\eta^\varepsilon))] \\ &= \lim_{t\uparrow\infty} E_y[f(\tau(V_\varepsilon)\wedge\eta^\varepsilon\wedge t\wedge\tau_\varepsilon, x(\tau(V_\varepsilon)\wedge\eta^\varepsilon\wedge t\wedge\tau_\varepsilon))] \end{aligned}$$

$$= \lim_{t\uparrow\infty} E_y[f(0,x(0)) + \int_0^{\tau(V_\varepsilon)\wedge\eta^\varepsilon\wedge t\wedge\tau_\varepsilon} (\frac{\partial f}{\partial s} + Lf)(s,x(s))ds]$$

$$= \lim_{t\uparrow\infty} \{w_n(y) + E_y[\int_0^{\tau(V_\varepsilon)\wedge\eta^\varepsilon\wedge t\wedge\tau_\varepsilon} e^{-\alpha s}(Lw_n - \alpha w_n)(x(s))ds]\}$$

$$\leqq w_n(y) \quad \text{for each } y \in \partial\Gamma_n . \tag{6}$$

Noting $x(\xi_{i-1}) \in \partial\Gamma_n$ if $\xi_{i-1} < \infty$, it therefore follows from (5) and (6) that

$$I_i \leqq 0 \quad \text{for each } i = 2,3,4,\dots . \tag{7}$$

Now we obtain from (1), (2), (3), (4) and (7) that

$$\beta E_x[e^{-\alpha\tau(V)}] \leqq \max_{y\in\partial\Gamma_n} w_n(y) \quad \text{for each } x \in \partial G \text{ and } n = 1,2,3,\dots .$$

Hence we get from ($\dot{V}$) of [Condition 1] that

$$E_x[e^{-\alpha\tau(V)}] = 0 \tag{8}$$

and so

$$P_x[\tau(V) < \infty] = 0 \quad \text{for each } x \in \partial G . \tag{9}$$

Since a(x) is positive definite in G, (9) holds for any bounded closed set V such that $G \supset V$ and $V^\circ \neq \phi$. Hence we conclude immediately that $P_x[x(t) \in \partial G$ for all $t \geqq 0] = 1$ for each $x \in \partial G$ and the proof is complete.

Q.E.D.

<u>Proof of Corollary</u> 1. If there is a $x \in G - \bigcup_{n=1}^\infty \Gamma_n$, it follows from (8) in the proof of Theorem 1 that $E_x[e^{-\alpha\tau(V)}] = 0$. But we have $E_x[e^{-\alpha\tau(V)}] > 0$ for each $x \in G$ since a(x) is positive definite in G. Consequently we get $\bigcup_{n=1}^\infty \Gamma_n = G$ for $\{\Gamma_n\}$ satisfying [Condition 1]. Q.E.D.

References

Crow, J.F. and Kimura, M. (1970): An Introduction to Population Genetics Theory. Harper and Row, New York.

Ethier, S.N. (1975): An error estimate for the diffusion approximation in population genetics. Ph. D. Thesis, University of Wisconsin.

Guess, H.A. (1973): On the weak convergence of Wright-Fisher models. Stochastic Process. Appl. 1: 287-306.

Okada, N. (1979): On convergence to diffusion processes of Markov chains related to population genetics. Adv. Appl. Probab. 11: 673-700.

Sato, K. (1976a): Diffusion processes and a class of Markov chains related to population genetics. Osaka J. Math. 13: 631-659.

Sato, K. (1976b): A class of Markov chains related to selection in population genetics. J. Math. Soc. Japan 28: 621-637.

Sato, K. (1978): Convergence to a diffusion of a multi-allelic model in population genetics. Adv. Appl. Probab. 10: 538-562.

The point interaction approximation for diffusion in regions with many small holes.

R. Figari

Department of Theoretical Physics, University of Naples, Naples, Italy.

G. Papanicolaou

Courant Institute, New York University, New York.

J. Rubinstein

Institute for Mathematics and its Applications, Unversity of Minnesota, Minneapolis, Minnesota.

1. Introduction.

Let $u(x,t)$ be the temperature at position x in R^3 and at time $t \geq 0$. For $N=1,2,3,...$ let $w_1^N, w_2^N, ..., w_N^N$ be a sequence of points in R^3 and let D^N be the domain in R^3 defined by

$$D^N = \bigcap_{j=1}^{N} \left\{ x \mid \ |x-w_j^N| > \frac{\alpha}{N} \right\} \tag{1}$$

where α is a fixed positive constant. The temperature u satisfies the initial-boundary value problem

$$\frac{\partial u}{\partial t} = \Delta u \quad in \quad D^N \ , t>0 \tag{2}$$

$$u(x,0)=f(x) \ \text{ for } x \ in \ D^N \text{ and } u(x,t)=0 \ on \ \partial B_j^N \text{ for } t>0 \ , j=1,2,3,...,N \tag{3}$$

Here $f(x)$ is a smooth, positive function of compact support representing the initial temperature distribution and B_j^N is the sphere centered at w_j^N with radius α/N.

We are interested in the behavior of the solution u when N is large and the sequence of sphere centers w_j^N tends to a continuum. That is for every smooth function $\phi(x)$

$$\frac{1}{N} \sum_{j=1}^{N} \phi(w_j^N) \rightarrow \int V(x) \phi(x) dx \quad as \ N \rightarrow \infty \tag{4}$$

where $V(x)$ is the continuum sphere center density, assumed smooth and with compact support.

We are also interested in the analysis of related problems as for example the case of spherical inclusions that melt. This means that the radii of the spheres depend on time, are denoted by $\alpha_j^N(t)/N$ and we have the additional boundary condition

$$\frac{d\alpha_j^N(t)}{dt} = \frac{-1}{N} \frac{1}{4\pi \alpha_j^N(t)/N^2} \int_{|x-w_j^N| = \alpha_j^N(t)/N} \frac{\partial u(x,t)}{\partial n} dS(x) \ , \ j=1,2,3, \cdots ,N \tag{5}$$

Here n is the unit normal on the spheres pointing into the interior of the region D^N. At time zero the scaled radii are equal to $\alpha_0 > 0$

$$\alpha_j^N(0) = \alpha_0 \tag{6}$$

The boundary condition (5) is a simplified form of the usual one in free boundary problems: the rate of displacement of the boundary is proportional to the heat flux crossing the surface. It is simplified because the melting spheres do not change shape and their radii change in proportion to the average heat flux absorbed.

Our purpose here is to analyze problem (2-4) in the continuum limit $N \to \infty$ by a relatively simple and direct method, the point interaction approximation. The radii of the spherical inclusions are already scaled in the above problems to be proportional to $1/N$. That this is appropriate scaling for a continuum limit can be seen easily by calculating the heat absorbed by a single sphere and requiring that N times this quantity be of order one as $N \to \infty$. The point interaction approximation is an intermediate step between (2-4) (or (2-6)) and the continuum limit which has features of both but is much simpler than (2-3) since the effect of the spheres is replaced by an appropriate point source term. The continuum approximation of (2-3) is the solution $\overline{u}$ of the initial value problem

$$\frac{\partial \overline{u}(x,t)}{\partial t} = \Delta \overline{u}(x,t) - 4\pi\alpha V(x)\overline{u}(x,t) \quad x \ in \ R^3 \ , t>0 \tag{7}$$

$$\overline{u}(x,0) = f(x)$$

The point interaction approximation for diffusion in a region with fixed spheres is described in section 2. The proof is given in section 3.

Boundary value problems in regions with many small holes have been analyzed before in a variety of contexts and by several methods. Khruslov and Marchenko [1] use potential theoretic methods and give results in considerable generality regarding the possible distribution of the inclusion centers $\{w_j^N\}$, compatible with (4). Kac [2] studied (2), (3) when the points $\{w_j^N\}$ are independent identically distributed random variables over a region. He used properties of the Wiener sausage. Rauch and Taylor [3] formulated the results of Kac in a more analytic way and generalized them. Papanicolaou and Varadhan [4] studied (2-3) for nonrandom configurations of centers $\{w_j^N\}$ by probabilistic methods and obtained a strong form of convergence to the continuum limit. Ozawa [5] first considered the analysis of boundary value problems in regions with many small holes via a point interaction approximation. A study of the error in the continuum limit and a central limit theorem for it are given by Figari, Orlandi and Teta [6].

The point interaction approximation is a natural tool to analyze a variety of interesting problems in the continuum or homogenization limit. In the physical literature it goes back to Foldy's paper [7 see also 8,9] on sound propagation in a bubbly liquid and perhaps earlier. In almost all papers that followed Foldy's, the point interaction approximation is not treated as an important approximation in itself and averaging is carried out over the sphere center locations $\{w_j^N\}$. The closure problem that arises is then treated in a variety of ways depending on other parameters in the problem. In nonlinear cases, as with melting spheres and bubbles, the closure problems are much more involved. But averaging is not necessary. The continuum limit holds for deterministic sequences satisfying (4) and subject to some other conditions that hold for "most" realizations in the random case. The closure difficulties are thus avoided for many linear and nonlinear problems.

2. Point interaction approximation for diffusion in regions with many fixed inclusions.

We shall analyze the Laplace transform version of (1.2)

$$(-\Delta + \lambda)\, u^N(x) = f(x) \quad , \quad x \ in \ D^N \ , \lambda > 0 \tag{1}$$

$$u^N(x) = 0 \quad , \quad |x - w_j^N| = \frac{\alpha}{N}$$

Let G be the free space Green's function

$$G(x,y) = \frac{e^{-\sqrt{\lambda}\,|x-y|}}{4\pi\,|x-y|} \tag{2}$$

Using Green's theorem we may rewrite (1) in integral form

$$u^N(x) = \int_{D^N} G(x,y)\,f(y)\,dy - \sum_{j=1}^{N} \int_{\partial B_j^N} G(x,y)\,\frac{\partial u^N(y)}{\partial n}\,dS(y) \tag{3}$$

where x is in D^N and n denotes the unit outward normal to the spheres ∂B_j^N.

Now let x tend to the surface of the ith sphere in (3). Using the Dirichlet boundary condition, we rewrite (3) in the form

$$\int_{\partial B_i^N} G(x,y)\,\frac{\partial u^N(y)}{\partial n}\,dS(y) + \sum_{\substack{j=1 \\ j \neq i}}^{N} \int_{\partial B_j^N} G(x,y)\,\frac{\partial u^N(y)}{\partial n}\,dS(y) \tag{4}$$

$$= \int_{D^N} G(x,y) f(y) dy$$

Let

$$\frac{1}{N}\,Q_j^N = \int_{\partial B_j^N} \frac{\partial u^N(y)}{\partial n}\,dS(y) \qquad , \ j = 1,2,\dots,N \tag{5}$$

be the charges induced on the spheres, suitably normalized. Since $f \geq 0$, the Q_j^N are nonnegative.

The spheres B_j^N have radius of order N^{-1} so they are small. We may then consider an approximate form of (4) where we place x at the center w_j^N of the ith sphere in the first term on the left and in the sum. We may also let the y in G in the sum in (4) go to the center w_j^N. Let us denote the approximate charges by q_j^N. Then

$$\frac{1}{4\pi\alpha}\,q_i^N + \frac{1}{N}\sum_{\substack{j=1 \\ j \neq i}}^{N} G(w_i^N,w_j^N)\,q_j^N = \int G(w_i^N,y) f(y) dy \qquad i = 1,2,\dots,N \tag{6}$$

Note that we have also extended the integration on the right to all of R^3.

System (6) is what we call the point interaction approximation (PIA). The main point is to show that, under suitable conditions on the sequence of sphere centers $\{w_j^n\}$,

$$\lim_{N \to \infty} \sup_{1 \leq j \leq N} |\, Q_j^N - q_j^N \,| = 0 \tag{7}$$

That is, the exact charges Q_j^N are well approximated by the the approximate carges q_j^N obtained from the PIA. Once this has been shown it is easy to pass to the continuum limit in (6) using the hypothesis (1.4).

Let $q(x)$ be the solution of the integral equation

$$\frac{1}{4\pi\alpha}\,q(x) + \int G(x,y)V(y)q(y)dy = \int G(x,y) f(y) dy \tag{8}$$

with x in R^3. If we define

$$u(x) = \frac{q(x)}{4\pi\alpha} \tag{9}$$

we see that (8) is the integral equation version of the Laplace transform of (1.7)

$$(-\Delta + \lambda)u(x) + 4\pi\alpha V(x)u(x) = f(x) \quad , \lambda > 0 \,. \tag{10}$$

Using the regularity of the solution u of (10) and standard methods familiar from numerical analysis, along with hypothesis (1.4), we can show that

$$\lim_{N \to \infty} \sup_{1 \leq j \leq N} |\, q_j^N - q(w_j^N) \,| = 0 \tag{11}$$

That is, (8) is the continuum limit of the PIA (6). Combining (7) and (11) we arrive at the desired convergence of the charges

$$\lim_{N\to\infty} \sup_{1\le j\le N} \mid Q_j^N - q(w_j^N) \mid = 0 \tag{12}$$

Once the charges have been shown to converge in the sense of (12) it is easy to show that $u^N(x)$, the solution of (1) converges to $u(x)$ the solution (10), outside a small set of points x near the surfaces of the spheres. We shall therefore concentrate here on proving (7) i.e. in proving the validity of the point interaction approximation.

3. Proof of validity of the point interaction approximation.

For the proof we need some assumptions regarding the sequence of sphere centers $\{w_j^n\}$ in addition to (1.4). We will assume that

$$\inf_{i\ne j} \mid w_i^N - w_j^N \mid \ \ge \frac{1}{N^{1-\nu}} \quad \text{for some} \quad 0<\nu<\frac{1}{3} \tag{1}$$

$$\frac{1}{N^2}\sum_{\substack{i,j=1\\ i\ne j}}^{N} \frac{1}{\mid w_i^N - w_j^N \mid^{3-\varepsilon}} \le C \qquad \text{for some} \quad \varepsilon>0 \tag{2}$$

$$\frac{1}{N^3}\sum_{\substack{i,j,k=1\\ i\ne j\ne k}}^{N} \frac{1}{\mid w_i^N - w_j^N \mid^2}\,\frac{1}{\mid w_k^N - w_i^N \mid^2} \le C \tag{3}$$

These conditions are valid, for example, for sequences of independent identically distributed random sphere centers. They are valid in probability that is, there is a set of sphere center configurations that satisfy (1), (2) and (3) with probability arbitrarily close to one, uniformly in N.

Let us now consider again the integral equation (2.4) where x is on ∂B_i^N. We average over the ith sphere

$$\begin{aligned}&\frac{1}{4\pi(\frac{\alpha}{N})^2}\int_{\partial B_i^N}\int_{\partial B_i^N} G(x,y)\,\frac{\partial u^N(y)}{\partial n}\,dS(y)dS(x)\\ &+\sum_{\substack{j=i\\ j\ne i}}^{N}\frac{1}{4\pi(\frac{\alpha}{N})^2}\int_{\partial B_i^N}\int_{\partial B_j^N} G(x,y)\,\frac{\partial u^N(y)}{\partial n}\,dS(y)dS(x)\\ &=\int_{\partial B_i^N}\int_{D^N} G(x,y)f(y)dy\,.\end{aligned} \tag{4}$$

To simplify (4) we use the elementary identity.

$$\frac{1}{4\pi(\frac{\alpha}{N})^2}\int_{\partial B_i^N} G(x,y)dS(x) = \frac{1}{4\pi\,(\frac{\alpha}{N})}\,\frac{1-e^{-2\sqrt{\lambda}\,\alpha/N}}{2\sqrt{\lambda}\,\alpha/N} \tag{5}$$

when y is on ∂B_i^N also. We use also the mean value theorem for any solution $h(x)$ of $(-\Delta+\lambda)h(x)=0$

$$\frac{1}{4\pi r^2}\int_{|x|=r} h(x)dS(x) = \frac{\sinh\sqrt{\lambda}r}{\sqrt{\lambda}r}\,h(0) \tag{6}$$

Using (5) and (6), simplifying and recalling the definition (2.5) of the charges we obtain the following equations

$$\begin{aligned}&\frac{\sqrt{\lambda}\,\alpha/N}{\sinh(\sqrt{\lambda}\,\alpha/N)}\,\frac{1-e^{-2\sqrt{\lambda}\alpha/N}}{2\sqrt{\lambda}\,\alpha/N}\,\frac{1}{4\pi\alpha}\,Q_i^N\\ &+\frac{1}{N}\sum_{\substack{j=1\\ j\ne i}}^{N} G(w_i^N,w_j^N)\,Q_j^N = \int_{D^N} G(w_i^N,y)f(y)dy + \eta_i^N\,,\\ &\qquad i=1,2,\ldots,N\end{aligned} \tag{7}$$

where

$$\eta_i^N = \sum_{\substack{j=1 \\ j \neq i}}^{N} \int_{\partial B_j^N} \left[G(w_i^N, y) - G(w_i^N, w_j^N) \right] \frac{\partial u^N(y)}{\partial n} \, dS(y) . \tag{8}$$

Lemma 1.

$$\sup_{1 \le i \le N} | \eta_i^N | \le \frac{C}{N^{1+\nu}} \sum_{\substack{j=1 \\ j \neq i}}^{N} G(w_i^N, w_j^N) \, Q_j^N . \tag{9}$$

Proof: We simply note that for y on ∂B_j^N

$$\frac{e^{-\sqrt{\lambda}\alpha/N} \; | w_i^N - w_j^N |}{| w_i^N - w_j^N | + \frac{\alpha}{N}} \le \frac{G(w_i^N, y)}{G(w_i^N, w_j^N)} \le \frac{e^{\sqrt{\lambda}\alpha/N} \; | w_i^N - w_j^N |}{| w_i^N - w_j^N | - \frac{\alpha}{N}}$$

From this and hypethesis (1) the estimate (9) follows easily.

Now we return to equations (7) and use the estimate (9) along with the positivity of the Q_j^N. We see that for N large the error η_i^N can be absorbed into the sum on the left of (7) without changing signs. This and the fact that $f \in C_0^\infty(R^3)$ give us the a-priori estimate

$$0 \le Q_i^N \le C \tag{10}$$

where all constants C that appear (possibly different constants) are independent of N. We also have the estimate

$$0 \le \frac{1}{N} \sum_{\substack{j=1 \\ j \neq i}}^{N} G(w_i^N, w_j^N) \, Q_j^N \le C . \tag{11}$$

Combining (10) and (9) we have now an estimate for the error

$$\sup_{1 \le i \le N} | \eta_i^N | \le \frac{C}{N^\nu} \qquad \nu > 0 . \tag{12}$$

If we also denote by $a_N(\lambda)$ ($\lambda > 0$ fixed) the coefficient in front of $\frac{1}{4\pi\alpha} Q_i^N$ in (7) then clearly

$$a_N \to 1 \qquad \text{as} \qquad N \to \infty \tag{13}$$

Put

$$f_i^N = 4\pi\alpha \int_{D^N} G(w_i^N, y) dy \quad , \quad i = 1,2,\ldots,N \tag{14}$$

and let q_i^N satisfy the PIA (2.6). We write this system in the form

$$(I + A^N) q^N = f^N \tag{15}$$

where $I = (\delta_{ij})$ is the identity matrix and

$$A_{ij}^N = \frac{4\pi\alpha}{N} G(w_i^N, w_j^N) \quad i \neq j \tag{16}$$

$$A_{ij}^N = 0 \qquad i = j$$

The vectors q^N and f^N have components q_i^N and f_i^N. Let $|| \ \ ||$ stand for the l^2 vector (or matrix) norm on R^N.

Lemma 2. For $\lambda > 0$ large enough.

$$\sup_N || A^N || < 1 \tag{17}$$

Proof. Clearly

$$\| A^N \|^2 \le \frac{4\pi\alpha}{N^2} \sum_{\substack{i,j=1 \\ i \ne j}}^{N} G(w_i^N, w_j^N)^2 \tag{18}$$

and this is controlled by (3) and (1.4). In addition, we can use the exponential farther in G that has the parameter λ and we can make the right side of (18) small by choosing λ large.

Thus, (15) is invertible uniformly in N and we may write

$$q^N = (I + A^N)^{-1} f^N \tag{19}$$

Clearly

$$0 \le q_i^N \le C \quad , \quad i = 1, 2, \ldots, N \tag{20}$$

and since the f_i^N are also uniformly bounded we have that

$$\sum_{j=i}^{N} \left[\frac{1}{\sqrt{N}} f_i^n \right]^2 \le C \tag{21}$$

Hence from (17) we deduce that

$$\frac{1}{N} \sum_{j=i}^{N} (q_i^N)^2 \le C \tag{22}$$

To estimate the difference between Q_j^N and q_j^N we need an additional estimate on the errors η_i^N.

Lemma 3.

$$\sum_{i=1}^{N} | \eta_i^N |^2 \le \frac{C}{N} \tag{23}$$

Proof. From (8) and (10) we see that

$$| \eta_i^N | \le \frac{C}{N^2} \sum_{\substack{j=1 \\ j \ne i}} \frac{1}{| w_i^N - w_j^N |^2}$$

We note that this does not follow from the estimate (9). One has to consider the η_i^N from (8) directly. From (2.4) we get

$$\sum_{i=1}^{N} | \eta_i^N |^2 \le \frac{C}{N^4} \sum_{i=1}^{N} \sum_{\substack{j=1 \\ j \ne i}}^{N} \sum_{\substack{k=1 \\ k = i}}^{N} \frac{1}{| w_j^N - w_i^N |^2} \, \frac{1}{| w_k^N - w_i^N |^2}$$

$$= \frac{C}{N} \left\{ \frac{1}{N^3} \sum_{\substack{i,j,k=1 \\ j \ne i \ne k}}^{N} \frac{1}{| w_i^N - w_j^N |^2} \, \frac{1}{| w_k^N - w_i^N |^2} \right.$$

$$\left. + \frac{1}{N^3} \sum_{\substack{j,k=1 \\ j \ne k}}^{N} \frac{1}{| w_j^N - w_k^N |^4} \right\}$$

The first sum on the right is controled by hypothesis (3). In the second sum we note that because of hypothesis (1) and (2)

$$\frac{1}{N^3} \sum_{\substack{j,k=1 \\ j \ne k}}^{N} \frac{1}{| w_i^N - w_k^N |^4} \le C \frac{(N^{1-\gamma})^{1+\varepsilon}}{N} \, \frac{1}{N^2} \sum_{\substack{j,k=1 \\ j \ne k}}^{N} \frac{1}{| w_j^N - w_k^N |^{3-\varepsilon}} \le C$$

This estimate completes the proof of the lemma.

We can now estimate the difference $| Q_j^N - q_i^N |$ between the exact charges and the approximate charges of the PIA. In fact by subtracting (15) from (7) we see that

$$(I + A^N)(Q^N - q^N) = (1 - a^N)Q^N + \eta^N \tag{25}$$

Now $| 1 - a^N | \leq C/N$ for λ fixed and $0 \leq Q_i^N \leq C$. Thus the l^2 norm of the right side of (25) is less than a constant times $N^{-1/2}$, in view of lemma 3. From lemma 2 and this observation we conclude that

$$\sum_{j=1}^{N} (Q_j^N - q_j^N)^2 \leq \frac{C}{N} \tag{26}$$

This implies that

$$\sup_{1 \leq j \leq N} | Q_j^N - q_j^N | \leq \frac{C}{N^{1/2}} \tag{27}$$

We summarize the above in the following theorem.

Theorem

Under hypotheses (1), (2), (3) and (1.4) the charges Q_j^N of problem (2.1), defined by (2.5), and the approximate charges q_j^N satisfying the PIA (2.6) (or (15)) are uniformly close as $N \to \infty$ in the sense of (27).

As we indicated in section 2, the elementary estimate (2.11) gives us the validity of the continuum approximation (2.12) for the charges and hence for the full solution of (2.1) and (2.10).

Acknowledgment

The work of George Papanicolaou was supported by the National Science Foundation and the Office of Naval Research. The work of Rodolfo Figari was partially supported by the Office of Naval Research.

Jacob Rubinstein's current address is Department of Mathematics, Stanford University, Stanford California.

References

[1] E. I. Khruslov and V. A. Marchenko, Boundary value problems in regions with fine-grained boundaries, Naukova Dumka, Kiev, 1974.

[2] M. Kac, Probabilistic methods in some problems of scattering theory, Rocky Mountain J. Math. 4, 1974, 511-538.

[3] J. Rauch and M. Taylor, Potential and scattering theory on wildly perturbed domains, J. Funct. Anal. 18, 1975, 27-59

[4] G. Papanicolaou and S.R.S. Varadhan, Diffusion in regions with many small holes. In Stochastic Differential Systems (ed. B. Grigeliouis). Lecture Notes in Control and Information Theory 25, 190-206, Springer.

[5] S. Ozawa., On an elaboration of M. Kac's Theorem concerning eigenvalues of the Laplacian in a region with randomly distributed small obstacles, Comm. Math. Phys. 91, 1983, 473-487.

[6] R. Figari, E. Orlandi and J. Teta, The Laplacian in regions with many small obstacles: fluctuations around the limit operator 41, 1985, 465-488.

[7] L. L. Foldy, The multiple scattering of waves, Phys. Rev. 67, 1945, 107-119.

[8] R. Caflisch, M. Miksis, G. Papanicolaou and L. Ting, Effective equations for wave propagation in bubbly liquids, J. Fluid Mech. 153, 1985, 259-273 and also 160, 1-14.

[9] J. Rubinstein, NYU Dissertation, 1985.

UNIMODALITY AND BOUNDS OF MODES FOR DISTRIBUTIONS OF GENERALIZED SOJOURN TIMES

Ken-iti Sato

Department of Mathematics
College of General Education
Nogoya University, Nagoya, Japan

Summary. The distribution of the generalized sojourn time T for a birth-and-death process up to the first passage time to the state n, starting at the state m $(m < n)$, is considered. The generalized sojourn time is the sum of the sojourn times at the states i, over $i = 0,1,\ldots,n-1$, with a state-dependent signed weight. A main new result of the paper is that the distribution of T is unimodal. Explicit description of the distribution is given by using exponential distributions on the positive and the negative axis. Bounds of the mode are derived from this description. Other bounds of the modes of general unimodal distributions are given in terms of absolute moments and central absolute moments. Infinite divisibility of T is also proved. These results are extended to generalized sojourn times of diffusion processes, which arise in models of neurobiology and population genetics.

1. Introduction.

We consider distributions of some random quantities related to a birth-and-death process. The birth-and-death process $X(t)$, $t \geq 0$, is a mathematical model for random evolution of the number of individuals of a colony. The structure of the evolution is given by

$$(1.1)\quad \begin{aligned} &P(X(t+\Delta t)=i+1 \mid X(t)=i) = \alpha_i \Delta t + o(\Delta t) \quad \text{for } i \geq 0, \\ &P(X(t+\Delta t)=i-1 \mid X(t)=i) = \beta_i \Delta t + o(\Delta t) \quad \text{for } i \geq 1, \\ &P(X(t+\Delta t)=i \mid X(t)=i) = 1 - (\alpha_i+\beta_i)\Delta t + o(\Delta t) \quad \text{for } i \geq 1, \\ &P(X(t+\Delta t)=0 \mid X(t)=0) = 1 - \alpha_0 \Delta t + o(\Delta t). \end{aligned}$$

In mathematical terms, $X(t)$, $t \geq 0$, is a Markov process taking values in nonnegative integers with time-homogeneous transition probability (1.1). The parameters α_i and β_i are the birth rate and the death rate, respectively, per unit time given that the present population is i. (The α_0 should be considered as the rate of immigration when the population is extinct.) We assume that $\alpha_i > 0$ for $i \geq 0$ and $\beta_i > 0$ for $i \geq 1$. The sample path of $X(t)$ is a step function with jumps of size +1 or -1. Let σ^{mn} be the first time (random) at which $X(t)=n$, given that $X(0)=m$. That is, σ^{mn} is the time required for the population to reach size n, given that the initial size is m. The process can be regarded as a model of a random motion of a particle moving on the set of nonnegative integers. Thus σ^{mn} is called the first passage time to n from the initial state m. Given a function $f(i)$ on the set of nonnegative integers, let us consider a random variable T defined by

$$T = \int_0^{\sigma^{mn}} f(X(t))dt. \tag{1.2}$$

Denote by τ_i^{mn} the length of time spent at the state i before the first passage time σ^{mn}. This quantity is called the sojourn time at the state i. If $m < n$, then the quantity T is written as

$$T = \sum_{i=0}^{n-1} f(i)\tau_i^{mn}, \tag{1.3}$$

that is, T is the sojourn time with a state-dependent weight $f(i)$. The $f(i)$ may be positive, negative, or zero. We call T a generalized sojourn time. In this paper we will study some properties of the distribution of T — unimodality, bounds of the mode, and infinite divisibility.

If f is a constant function 1, then $T=\sigma^{mn}$. If $f(i)=1$ for $i=i_0$ and $f(i)=0$ for $i \neq i_0$, then $T=\tau_{i_0}^{mn}$. Hence our discussion includes passage times and sojourn times. Unimodality of passage times is proved by Rösler [17] and Keilson [8] and the class of passage time distributions is determined by Yamazato [23].

A birth-and-death process is important as a simple type of stochastic process in probability theory and as a stochastic population model in applications (see Ludwig [12]). It serves also as a discrete state analogue of a diffusion process. If we make smaller the distance of adjacent states and change the time scale appropriately, it approximates a diffusion process. Any diffusion process is a limit of a sequence of birth-and-death processes. The distributions of first passage times, sojourn times, and generalized sojourn times of the diffusion process are, if they are defined and finite almost surely, the limits of the distributions of the corresponding quantities of birth-and-death processes. Thus properties of these distributions are derived from those of birth-and-death process.

Diffusion processes appear in many places as biological models. They are especially important in population genetics and neurobiology (see Crow and Kimura [1], Maruyama [13], Holden [4], and Ricciardi [15]). Fixation time of a mutant gene and firing time of a single neuron are modeled by first passage times of diffusion. Generalized sojourn times of the type (1.2) appear in population genetics (see Nagylaki [14] and Maruyama [13]).

2. Unimodality.

Let μ be a distribution on the real line $\mathbb{R}$. Let $F(x)$ be its distribution function, that is, $F(x)=\mu((-\infty,x])$. The distribution μ is called unimodal if there exists a point M (called a mode) such that $F(x)$ is convex on $(-\infty,M)$ and concave on (M,∞). Equivalently, μ is unimodal if and only if there is a point M such that μ has nondecreasing density on $(-\infty,M)$ and nonincreasing density on (M,∞). The distribution μ is called strictly unimodal, if it is unimodal with a mode M and, for some $a \leqq b$, the density is increasing on (a,M), decreasing on (M,b), and zero outside of (a,b). Here we are using the words "increase" and "decrease" in the strict sense. The set of modes of a unimodal distribution is a one point set or a bounded closed interval; the mode of a strictly unimodal distribution is necessarily unique.

Let us present our result, using the notations introduced in the previous section.

Theorem 2.1. Assume $m < n$. The distribution of the generalized sojourn time T defined by (1.2) is unimodal. If $f(i)\neq 0$ for $0 \leqq i \leqq n-1$, then it is strictly unimodal. If $m=n-1$, then it is unimodal with a mode 0.

If $f(i)=1$ for $0 \leqq i \leqq n-1$, then Rösler [17] and Keilson [8] prove the unimodality and, in case $m=n-1$, the unimodality with a mode 0. If $f(i) > 0$ for $0 \leqq i \leqq n-1$, then the result reduces to the case $f(i)=1$ by a time change. But, if $f(i)$ takes positive and negative values, the distribution of T has support on the whole line and a new technique in needed for the proof.

3. Relations with exponential distributions.

The distribution of T has a close connection with exponential distributions. It is expressed by exponential distributions on the positive and the negative axis through mixing and convolution.

Theorem 2.1 on unimodality is a consequence of this expression.

Denote $\mathbb{R}_+=[0,\infty)$ and $\mathbb{R}_-=(-\infty,0]$. For a positive number a, the exponential distribution μ_a on $\mathbb{R}_+$ with parameter a is given by

$$\mu_a(dx) = \begin{cases} 0 & \text{on } (-\infty,0] \\ ae^{-ax}dx & \text{on } (0,\infty). \end{cases}$$

Similarly, for a negative number b, we define the expoential distribution μ_b on $\mathbb{R}_-$ with parameter b as

$$\mu_b(dx) = \begin{cases} -be^{-bx}dx & \text{on } (-\infty,0) \\ 0 & \text{on } [0,\infty). \end{cases}$$

Classes of mixtures of exponential distributions on $\mathbb{R}_+$ or $\mathbb{R}_-$ are defined as follows. The class ME_k^+ is the set of μ such that there exist positive numbers $p_1,\ldots,p_k$ and distinct positive numbers $a_1,\ldots,a_k$ satisfying

$$\mu = \sum_{i=1}^{k} p_i\mu_{a_i} \quad \text{and} \quad \sum_{i=1}^{k} p_i = 1. \tag{3.1}$$

The class ME_k^{0+} is the set of μ such that there are positive numbers $p_0,\ldots,p_k$ and distinct positive numbers $a_1,\ldots,a_k$ satisfying

$$\mu = p_0\delta_0 + \sum_{i=1}^{k} p_i\mu_{a_i} \quad \text{and} \quad \sum_{i=0}^{k} p_i = 1. \tag{3.2}$$

Here δ_0 denotes the probability measure concentrated at the origin. Similarly, ME_k^- is the set of μ such that there are positive numbers $p_1,\ldots,p_k$ and distinct negative numbers $b_1,\ldots,b_k$ that satisfy (3.1) with b_i in place of a_i. The class ME_k^{0-} is the set of μ satisfying (3.2) with some positive numbers $p_0,\ldots,p_k$ and some distinct negative numbers $b_1,\ldots,b_k$ replacing $a_1,\ldots,a_k$. We call the numbers $a_1,\ldots,a_k$ or $b_1,\ldots,b_k$ the parameters of μ. Further we denote by CE_k^+ the class of μ such that, for some (not necessarily distinct) positive numbers $a_1,\ldots,a_k$,

$$\mu = \mu_{a_1} * \cdots * \mu_{a_k}, \tag{3.3}$$

and by CE_k^- the class of μ such that (3.3) holds with some negative numbers $b_1,\ldots,b_k$ in place of $a_1,\ldots,a_k$. Again the numbers $a_1,\ldots,a_k$ or $b_1,\ldots,b_k$ are called the parameters of μ. We define the classes ME_0^{0+}, ME_0^{0-}, CE_0^+, and CE_0^- as the sets with a single element δ_0.

Theorem 3.1. Assume that $m < n$ and that $f(i) \neq 0$ for $0 \le i \le n-1$. Let μ be the distribution of the generalized sojourn time T of (1.2).

(i) If $f(m) > 0$, then

$$\mu = \mu^{(1)} * \mu^{(2)} * \mu^{(3)} * \mu^{(4)}, \tag{3.4}$$

where $\mu^{(1)} \in ME^{+}_{\ell_1+1}$, $\mu^{(2)} \in ME^{0-}_{\ell_2}$, $\mu^{(3)} \in CE^{+}_{\ell_3}$, $\mu^{(4)} \in CE^{-}_{\ell_4}$ for some nonnegative integers $\ell_1, \ell_2, \ell_3, \ell_4$.

(ii) If $f(m) < 0$, then (3.4) holds with $\mu^{(1)} \in ME^{0+}_{\ell_1}$, $\mu^{(2)} \in ME^{-}_{\ell_2+1}$, $\mu^{(3)} \in CE^{+}_{\ell_3}$, $\mu^{(4)} \in CE^{-}_{\ell_4}$ for some nonnegative integers $\ell_1, \ell_2, \ell_3, \ell_4$.

We do not know probabilistic meaning of the decompositions (3.4) of μ. But the numbers ℓ_j, $1 \le j \le 4$, have relations with the function $f(i)$. Given a nonvanishing f, let N^{+}_{k} be the number of i such that $0 \le i \le k-1$ and $f(i) > 0$, and let $N^{-}_{k} = k-N^{-}_{k}$, the number of i such that $0 \le i \le k-1$ and $f(i) < 0$. Then we can get a refinement of Theorem 3.1 by adding the following assertion.

Theorem 3.2. The factors $\mu^{(j)}$, $1 \le j \le 4$, can be chosen in such a way that $\ell_1 \le N^{+}_{m}$, $\ell_2 \le N^{-}_{m}$, and

$$\begin{cases} \ell_3 = N^{+}_{n} - N^{+}_{m} - 1, \quad \ell_4 = N^{-}_{n} - N^{-}_{m} & \text{in case } f(m) > 0, \\ \ell_3 = N^{+}_{n} - N^{+}_{m}, \quad \ell_4 = N^{-}_{n} - N^{-}_{m} - 1 & \text{in case } f(m) < 0, \end{cases}$$

and that all parameters of $\mu^{(j)}$, $1 \le j \le 4$, are different from each other.

4. Bounds of modes of distributions related to exponential distributions.

Let us consider distributions described in Theorem 3.1. More generally, let μ be a distribution admitting a decomposition

$$\mu = \mu^{(1)} * \mu^{(2)} * \mu^{(3)} * \mu^{(4)} \tag{4.1}$$

such that $\mu^{(1)} \in ME^{+}_{\ell_1+1}$ or $ME^{0+}_{\ell_1+1}$, $\mu^{(2)} \in ME^{-}_{\ell_2+1}$ or $ME^{0-}_{\ell_2+1}$, $\mu^{(3)} \in CE^{+}_{\ell_3}$, and $\mu^{(4)} \in CE^{-}_{\ell_4}$ for some nonnegative integers ℓ_j, $1 \le j \le 4$. The distributions $\mu^{(1)}$ and $\mu^{(3)}$ have positive parameters and are supported on $\mathbb{R}_+$, while $\mu^{(2)}$ and $\mu^{(4)}$ have negative parameters and are supported on $\mathbb{R}_-$. Let a be the minimum among the parameters of

$\mu^{(1)}$ and $\mu^{(3)}$, and let b be the maximum among the parameters of $\mu^{(2)}$ and $\mu^{(4)}$.

Theorem 4.1. Under the condition stated above, the distribution is strictly unimodal and the mode M satisfies

$$\ell_4/b \leq M \leq \ell_3/a. \tag{4.2}$$

If $\ell_3=\ell_4=0$ in particular, then (4.1) reduces to $\mu=\mu^{(1)}*\mu^{(2)}$ and (4.2) means M=0. Since $\mu^{(1)}$ and $\mu^{(2)}$ are unimodal with mode 0 and are concentrated on different sides, this result is a consequence of Lemma 7.1 given later.

If $\mu=\mu^{(1)}*\mu^{(3)}$ with $\mu^{(1)} \in ME^{+}_{\ell_1+1}$ or $ME^{0+}_{\ell_1+1}$ and $\mu^{(3)} \in CE^{+}_{\ell_3}$, then μ is strictly unimodal and $0 \leq M \leq \ell_3/a$. It is known that, if μ is the ℓ-th convolution power of μ_a, then the mode is $(\ell-1)/a$. In fact, this μ is a gamma distribution and the density is written explicitly.

5. Bounds of modes of general unimodal distributions.

Let μ be a unimodal distribution with a mode M. For $p > 0$ let

$$\beta_p = \int |x|^p \mu(dx),$$

the absolute moment of order p. If $\beta_1 < \infty$, then let m be the mean of μ and, for $p \geq 1$,

$$\gamma_p = \int |x-m|^p \mu(dx),$$

the central absolute moment of order p. Johnson and Rogers [7] show that

$$|M-m| \leq \sqrt{3}\,\gamma_2^{1/2}$$

and that $\sqrt{3}$ is the best constant. The following theorem of Sato [18] generalizes this result.

Theorem 5.1. If $\beta_1 < \infty$, then

$$|M-m| \leq (p+1)^{1/p}\gamma_p^{1/p}$$

for $p \geq 1$. The inequality is the best in the sense that the equality holds for some non-degenerate unimodal μ.

For $p > 0$ we have the following result [18].

Theorem 5.2. Let A_p be the unique solution of the equation

$$x^{p+1} - (p+1)x - p = 0$$

for $x > 1$. Then

$$|M| \leq A_p \beta_p^{1/p}$$

and A_p is the best constant for this inequality.

We see that $A_p > (p+1)^{1/p}$ for $p > 0$, $A_2=2$, $A_1=1+\sqrt{2}$, and, approximately, $A_{1/2}=2.81451$. As p increases, A_p decreases. We have

$$\lim_{p\downarrow 0} A_p = A \quad \text{and} \quad \lim_{p\uparrow\infty} A_p = 1,$$

where A is the unique positive solution of the equation

$$x \log x - x - 1 = 0.$$

An approximate value is $A=3.59112$.

It is to be noted that the bounds of modes given in Theorems 5.1 and 5.2 sometimes give better results than Theorem 4.1 for the distributions considered in Section 4.

6. Infinite divisibility.

A distribution μ is called infinitely divisible if, for each positive integer n, there is a distribution $\mu^{(n)}$ such that μ is the n-th convolution power of $\mu^{(n)}$. The class of infinitely divisible distributions plays a fundamental role in probability theory. A canonical representation of their characteristic functions is known and many properties are investigated (see Feller [2]).

Theorem 6.1. Assume $m < n$. The distribution of the generalized sojourn time T of (1.2) for a birth-and-death process is infinitely divisible.

This result is already proved by Kent [10]. We get this theorem as a consequence of Theorem 3.1.

There is a subclass of infinitely divisible distributions called the class L (see [2]). Infinitely divisible distributions are not always unimodal. However, by Yamazato's theorem [22], any distribution of class L is unimodal. The distribution of a first passage time does not necessarily belong to class L. Yamazato [23] describes their class as the set of convolutions of ME_k^+ and CE_ℓ^+ with $k \geq 0$, $\ell \geq 0$.

7. Method of proof of theorem.

We denote the moment generating function of a distribution μ by

$$\hat{\mu}(s) = \int e^{sx}\mu(dx). \tag{7.1}$$

For the exponential distribution on $\mathbb{R}_+$ with parameter a, we have

$$\hat{\mu}_a(s) = \frac{a}{a-s}.$$

A distribution μ is in ME_k^+ with parameters $0 < a_1 < \cdots < a_k$, if and only if

$$\hat{\mu}(s) = \text{const} \frac{(c_1-s)\dots(c_{k-1}-s)}{(a_1-s)\dots(a_k-s)}$$

with some $c_1,\dots,c_{k-1}$ such that $0 < a_1 < c_1 < a_2 < c_2 < \cdots < c_{k-1} < a_k$. Further, μ is in ME_k^{0+} with parameters $0 < a_1 < \cdots < a_k$, if and only if

$$\hat{\mu}(s) = \text{const} \frac{(c_1-s)\dots(c_k-s)}{(a_1-s)\dots(a_k-s)}$$

with $c_1,\dots,c_k$ satisfying $0 < a_1 < c_1 < \cdots < a_k < c_k$. Similar expressions are obtained for exponential distributions on $\mathbb{R}_-$ and distributions in ME_k^- and ME_k^{0+}. These moment generating functions are defined by (7.1) for s sufficiently close to 0 and extended to rational functions on the whole complex plane.

In order to prove Theorems 3.1 and 3.2, let $m < n$ and consider

$$\varphi_{mn}(\underline{s}) = E \exp \sum_{i=0}^{n-1} s_i \tau_i^{mn} \quad \text{for } \underline{s} = (s_0,\dots,s_{n-1}),$$

which is the generating function of the distribution (multivariate) of $(\tau_0^{mn},\dots,\tau_{n-1}^{mn})$. Introduce a system of polynomials $Q_i(\underline{s})$, $i \geq 0$, of $\underline{s}=(s_0,s_1,\dots)$ by

$$Q_0(\underline{s}) = 1, \quad Q_1(\underline{s}) = (\alpha_0 - s_0)/\alpha_0,$$

$$Q_{i+1}(\underline{s}) = \{(\alpha_i+\beta_i-s_i)Q_i(\underline{s}) - \beta_i Q_{i-1}(\underline{s})\}/\alpha_i \quad \text{for } i \geq 1.$$

This system is the infinite variables extension by Kent [10] of the polynomials of Ledermann, Reuter, Karlin, and McGregor. Then, by the strong Markov property and the induction, it is shown that

$$\varphi_{mn}(\underline{s}) = Q_m(\underline{s})/Q_n(\underline{s}).$$

This is Kent's result [10]. We get the moment generating function $\varphi(s)$ of the distribution of T of (1.2) by $\varphi(s)=\varphi_{mn}(\underline{s})$, letting

$\underline{s}$=(sf(0),sf(1),...). Thus $\varphi(s)$ is a rational function. Now we have to analyze the positions of the poles and zeros of this function, to obtain Theorems 3.1 and 3.2 by factorization. We need to introduce another auxiliary system of polynomials as in Yamazato [23] and to prove a sort of interlacing properties of the zeros of the polynomials. The procedure is complicated by the fact that our polynomials have not only positive zeros but also negative zeros and that the origin plays a special role. See [19] for details.

For the proof of Theorem 4.1, we use the following two lemmas. The first one is a special case of Lemma 6.1 of Sato and Yamazato [20]; the second one is a consequence of Ibragimov's theorem [5].

Lemma 7.1. If $\mu^{(1)}$ and $\mu^{(2)}$ are supported on $\mathbb{R}_+$ and $\mathbb{R}_-$, respectively, and if they are both unimodal with a mode 0, then their convolution $\mu^{(1)}*\mu^{(2)}$ is unimodal with a mode 0.

Lemma 7.2. If μ is an exponential distribution on $\mathbb{R}_+$ or $\mathbb{R}_-$, then, for every unimodal ν, the convolution $\mu * \nu$ is unimodal (in other words, μ is strongly unimodal).

These two lemmas show unimodality of μ in Theorem 4.1. Also its strict unimodality follows, since its density is real-analytic except at the origin. The bound (4.2) of the mode is derived from the partial fraction expansion of the moment generating function and some analytical device.

Now, under the condition that $f(i)\neq 0$ for $0 \leq i \leq n-1$, the assertions of Theorem 2.1 follow from Theorems 3.1, 3.2, and 4.1. Further, in general, the unimodality for $m < n$ and the unimodality with a mode 0 for $m=n-1$ follow from a limiting procedure.

Theorem 6.1 is proved as a consequence of Theorem 3.1. We note that exponential distributions are infinitely divisible, that any distribution in ME_k^+, ME_k^{0+}, ME_k^-, or ME_k^{0-} is infinitely divisible by Goldie's theorem [3], and that infinite divisibility is preserved under convolution and convergence.

8. Diffusion processes.

Let $X(t)$, $t \geq 0$, be a diffusion process on $\mathbb{R}_+$ with reflecting condition at 0. Let $x < y$ and let σ^{xy} be the first passage time to y for $X(t)$ starting at x. Given a continuous $f(x)$, define

$$(8.1) \qquad T = \int_0^{\sigma^{xy}} f(X(t))dt.$$

Since this process is obtained as the limit of a sequence of our birth-and-death processes in the sense of convergence of probability measures on the space of right-continuous paths with left-hand limits, unimodality and infinite divisibility of the distribution of T follow from Theorems 2.1 and 6.1. The result generalizes to the case where f is bounded and measurable. Note that unimodality and infinite divisibility are preserved in limiting procedure. Bound of the mode is obtained from the moments of T by Theorems 5.1 and 5.2. However, Theorem 4.1 does not seem to give any result on diffusion processes.

Consider a diffusion process on $\mathbb{R}$ which is the limit of reflecting diffusion processes on $[-n,\infty)$ as $n \to \infty$. Then the distribution of the first passage time conditioned to be finite is unimodal and infinitely divisible. If σ^{xy} is finite almost surely and f is bounded and measurable, then the same conclusion holds for the generalized sojourn time T defined by (8.1).

Infinite divisibility of the distribution of T is already noticed by Kent [10]. Of course the first passage time has been a a subject of many researches; see Itô and McKean [6] and Knight [11] for its infinite divisibility and its associated Lévy process. But we do not know how wide the class of the distributions of diffusion first passage times. Kent's problem raised in [9] when (or whether) they are of class L is not yet solved.

9. Concluding remarks.

We have assumed $\alpha_0 > 0$ for our birth-and-death process. This is a reflecting condition at the boundary. Also we have assumed $m < n$ for the starting point. If $\alpha_0=0$ (absorbing condition) or $m > n$, then finiteness of the first passage time σ^{mn} is not guaranteed. But the distribution of σ^{mn} conditioned to be finite is unimodal and infinitely divisible. If $\alpha_0=0$ and $m < n$, then, assuming $f(0)=0$, we can discuss the distribution of T.

Passage times, sojourn times, and generalized sojourn times are quantitites to be analyzed in many biological diffusion models. Especially, several methods are proposed for the study of first passage times; see Ricciardi, Sacerdote, and S. Sato [16] and references therein. It is desirable that bounds of their modes be given by intrinsic parameters of the diffusion. However, only bounds that we have so far are those given by absolute moments or central absolute moments (Theorems 5.1 and 5.2). In this connection we mention that S. Sato [21] and Nagylaki [14] discuss the moments of first passage times and generalized sojourn times, respectively.

References

[1] Crow, J.F., and Kimura, M., An introduction to population genetics theory. Harper and Row, New York, 1970.

[2] Feller, W., An introduction to probability theory and its applications. Vol.1, third ed., and Vol.2, second ed., Wiley, New York, 1968 and 1971.

[3] Goldie, C., A class of infinitely divisible random variables. Proc. Cambridge Phil. Soc. 63 (1967) 1141-1143.

[4] Holden, A.V., Models of the stochastic activity of neurons. Lecture Notes in Biomathematics, Vol.12, Springer, Berlin, 1976.

[5] Ibragimov, I.A., On the composition of unimodal distributions. Theor. Probab. Appl. 2 (1957) 117-119.

[6] Itô, K., and McKean, H.P., Jr., Diffusion processes and their sample paths. Springer, Berlin, 1965.

[7] Johnson, N.L., and Rogers, C., The moment problem for unimodal distributions. Ann. Math. Statist. 22 (1951) 433-439.

[8] Keilson, J., On the unimodality of passage time densities in birth-death processes. Statistica Neerlandica 35 (1981) 49-55.

[9] Kent, J.T., Discussion of F.W. Steutel's paper. Scand. J. Statist. 6 (1979) 62-63.

[10] Kent, J.T., The appearance of a multivariate exponential distribution in sojourn times for birth-death and diffusion processes, in Probability, Statistics and Analysis, ed. by J.F.C. Kingman et al. (London Math. Soc. Lecture Notes Series, No.79, 1983) 161-179.

[11] Knight, F.B., Characterization of the Lévy measures of inverse local times of gap diffusion, in Seminar on Stochastic Processes, 1981, ed. by E. Cinlar et al. (Birkhäuser, Boston, 1981) 53-78.

[12] Ludwig, D., Stochastic population theories. Lecture Notes in Biomathematics, Vol.3, Springer, Berlin, 1974.

[13] Maruyama, T., Stochastic problems in population genetics. Lecture Notes in Biomathematics, Vol.17, Springer, Berlin, 1977.

[14] Nagylaki, T., The moments of stochastic integrals and the distribtuion of sojourn times. Proc. Nat. Acad. Sci. U.S.A. 71 (1974) 746-749.

[15] Ricciardi, L.M., Diffusion processes and related topics in biology. Lecture Notes in Biomathematics, Vol.14, Springer, 1977.

[16] Ricciardi, L.M., Sacerdote, L., and Sato, S., On an integral equation for first-passage-time probability densities. J. Appl. Probab. 21 (1984) 302-314.

[17] Rösler, U., Unimodality of passage times for one-dimensional strong Markov processes. Ann. Probab. 8 (1980) 853-859.

[18] Sato, K., Modes and moments of unimodal distributions. To appear in Ann. Statist. Math.

[19] Sato, K., Extension of Yamazato's results on zeros of a system of polynomials and application to sojourn time distributions. In preparation.

[20] Sato, K., and Yamazato, M., On distribution functions of class L. Zeit. Wahrsch. Verw. Geb. 43 (1978) 273-308.

[21] Sato, S., On the moments of the firing interval of the diffusion approximated model neuron. Math. Biosc. 39 (1978) 53-70.

[22] Yamazato, M., Unimodality of infinitely divisible distribution functions of class L. Ann. Probab. 6 (1978) 523-531.

[23] Yamazato, M., Characterization of the class of upward first passage time distributions of nonnegative birth and death processes and its applications. To appear.

FLUCTUATION IN POPULATION DYNAMICS

Kōhei Uchiyama

Department of Mathematics
Nara Joshi Daigaku
Nara 630, Japan

Abstract. A dynamics for a large population of randomly mating individuals is formulated as a Markov process on a large product space which involves a pairwise interaction between components. Each individual in the population possesses a character (the state of individual). An individual undergoes Markovian change of its character during its life time. Two individuals may make random mating after which they die, leaving two children with new characters. Each individual is a unique member of a lineage at each time. We are interested in the number of lineages which comprise individuals possessing the character x_i at time t_i for $i = 1,\ldots,m$, where $x_1,\ldots,x_m$ and $t_1,\ldots,t_m$ are given in advance. If the initial distribution is i.i.d. and the size n of the population is very large, the proportion of this number to n is approximately computed by means of a joint distribution of a non-linear Markov process (for a single individual in a infinite population). We shall study the law of the error in this approximation and establish a limit theorem about it.

1. Introduction.

In this article we shall introduce a dynamics for a large system, modeling a population of randomly mating individuals, which will be formulated as a Markov process, and study asymptotic behavior of a typical sample path for a single lineage as the size of the population becomes large.

Each individual in the population possesses a character — an attribute which may comprise several factors hereditary or acquired, or physical states such as position or age. The character varies or is transformed into another randomly as time goes by in two manners. Firstly an individual changes his character during its life time, independently of the other individuals and its past history. Secondly the character is transformed into another through a pair-wise interaction: arbitrarily chosen two individulas simultaneously change their characters at random time according to a stochastic law which depends only on their present characters. This interaction may be taken as random mating after which parents die, leaving two children with new characters. (If two individuals mate only when they meet, then the character must include position.) A lineage is an ancestral line of consecutive individual every member of which is a child of its predecessor therein. Two new children born by a random mating are made to belong to lineages of the parents one to each at their birth. In this article we are interested in the stochastic law of the number of lineages which comprise indivisuals prossessing the character x_i at time t_i for $i=1,\dots,m$, where $x_1,\dots,x_m$ and $t_1,\dots,t_m$ are supposed to be specified in advance.

Denote the totality of characters by S. We assume S is at most countable. Let n be the total number of individuals in the population and $x_j^n(t)$ the character of the individual which constitutes the j-th lineage at time t. Set $X^n(t)=(X_1^n(t), X_2^n(t),\dots,X_n^n(t))$. Then $X^n(t)$ is described as a Markov process on S^n which is characterized by two sets of non-negative constants $L=\{L^x(y): x,y\in S,\ x\neq y\}$ and $K=\{K^{x,y}(x',y'):x,y,x',y'\in S,\ (x,y)\neq(x',y')\}$. We shall assume the symmetry $K^{x,y}(x',y')=K^{y,x}(y',x')$ and the bounds

$$(1)\qquad \sup_x \sum_{y\neq x} L^x(y)<\infty \quad\text{and}\quad \sup_{x,y} \sum_{(x',y')\neq(x,y)} K^{x,y}(x'y')<\infty.$$

L governs the Markovian motion of the character of each individual until the time when it interacts with another one and K devided by n represents the rate function of random mating so that the infinitesimal operator of the Markov process $X^n(t)$ on the product space S^n is given by

$$(2)\qquad G_n\phi(\underline{\underline{x}}) = \sum_{j=1}^{n} \sum_{x_j'\in S} [\phi(\underline{\underline{x}}_j')-\phi(\underline{\underline{x}})]\, L^{x_j}(x_j')$$
$$+ \sum_{j<k} \sum_{x_j'\in S} \sum_{x_k'\in S} [\phi(\underline{\underline{x}}_{j,k}')-\phi(\underline{\underline{x}})]\, K^{x_j,x_k}(x_j',x_k')$$

where $\underline{\underline{x}}=(x_1,\dots,x_n)\in S^n$, ϕ is a bounded function of S^n, $\underline{\underline{x}}_j'$ [resp. $\underline{\underline{x}}_{j,k}'$] is an element of S^n obtained from $\underline{\underline{x}}$ by replacing x_j [resp. x_j and x_k] with x_j' [resp. x_j' and x_k'], and the sum $\Sigma_{j<k}$ is taken over all pairs (j,k) such that $1\leq j<k\leq n$.

For $\underline{\underline{x}}=(x_1,\dots,x_m)\in S^m$ and $\underline{\underline{t}}=(t_1,\dots,t_m)$ with $0\leq t_1<t_2<\dots<t_m$ let $N^n(\underline{\underline{t}},\underline{\underline{x}})$ stand for the number of lineages which bear characters $x_1,\dots,x_m$ one after another along a sequence of times $t_1,\dots,t_m$, i.e.

$$N^n(t,x) = \#\{j;\ 1\leq j\leq n,\ x_j^n(t_k)=x_k \quad\text{for}\quad k=1,\dots,m\}.$$

As in [2], [5] etc. the propagation of chaos holds, which is paraphrased as follows: if there exists a probability measure μ on S such that

$$(3)\qquad \lim_{n\to\infty} \frac{1}{N} N^n(0,x) = \mu(x) \quad\text{in probability for all}\quad x\in S,$$

then $\lim_{n\to\infty}\frac{1}{n}N^n(\underline{\underline{t}},\underline{\underline{x}})=\mu(\underline{\underline{t}},\underline{\underline{x}})$ in probability for all admissible pairs of $\underline{\underline{t}}$ and $\underline{\underline{x}}$; moreover $\mu(\underline{\underline{t}},\cdot)$ is a joint distribution of a (non-linear) Markov process. This may be thought as a law of large numbers. The main objective of this note is to afford a corresponding centrallimit theorem, i.e., a convergence result for the fluctuation $[N^n(\underline{\underline{t}},\underline{\underline{x}})-n\mu(\underline{\underline{t}},\underline{\underline{x}})]/\sqrt{n}$.

2. Propagation of chaos. Let $D = D[0,1]$ denote the totality of (step) functions of the unit interval $[0,1]$ into S which are right-continuous and have limits from the left. $\mathcal{P}(D)$ and $\mathcal{P}(S)$ denote the spaces of all probability measures on D and on S, respectively. D and $\mathcal{P}(D)$ ($\mathcal{P}(S)$) are endowed, respectively, with the Skorohod topology and with the topology of the weak convergence. Let α^n be a $\mathcal{P}(D)$-valued random element which stands for the empirical distribution of orbits of $X_j^n(t)$, $0 \leq t \leq 1$ $(j=1,\ldots,n)$:

$$\alpha^n = \frac{1}{n}\sum_{j=1}^{n} \delta_{X_j^n(\cdot)}.$$

Let us denote generic elements of D by w, $\tilde{w}$ etc. For a (singed) measure ν on D and $0 \leq t \leq 1$ we define $\nu_t \in \mathcal{P}(S)$ by $\nu_t(\cdot)=\nu\{w:w(t) \in \cdot\}$. For $\mu \in \mathcal{P}(S)$ let $P^\mu \in \mathcal{P}(D)$ be a solution of the nonlinear martingale problem: for every $f \in C_b(S)$ (a bounded real function of S)

$$(4)\qquad \begin{cases} f(w(t)) - \displaystyle\int_0^t [Lf(w(s)) + \langle P_s^\mu, \Gamma f(w(s),\cdot)\rangle]ds \quad \text{is a } P^\mu\text{-martingale} \\ P_0^\mu = \mu, \end{cases}$$

where $\langle\nu,\phi\rangle$ expresses the integral of a function ϕ by a (singed) measure ν, $Lf(x)=\Sigma_y L^x(y)(f(y)-f(x))$ and

$$\Gamma f(x,y) = \sum_{x'} (f(x')-f(x))K_1^{x,y}(x') \quad \text{with} \quad K_1^{x,y}(x') = \sum_{y'} K^{x,y}(x',y').$$

Then the propagation of chaos in the path space may read as follows:

(5) <u>If</u> $\lim_{n\to\infty} \alpha_0^n = \mu$ <u>in probability for some</u> $\mu \in \mathcal{P}(S)$, <u>then</u> $\lim_{n\to\infty} \alpha^n = P^\mu$ <u>in probability.</u>

It is noted that we need not impose the symmetry on the distirbution of $X^n(0)$, since the symmetrization of it does not change the law of α^n; also that the premise of (5) is equivalent to the condition (3), so that the statement about $N^n(\underline{\underline{t}},\underline{\underline{x}})$ given there follows from (5), with $\mu(\underline{\underline{t}},\underline{\underline{x}}) = P^\mu\{w\colon w(t_k)=x_k,\ k=1,\ldots,m\}$.

A result such as (5) was first demonstrated by Kac [2]: essentially he deduced the convergence of α_t^n for every t from that of α_0^n for a model introduced by him. The formulation as in (4) first appeared in [8]. The limit theorem (4) is proved by Sznitman [5] in a mathematically interesting case. Here is outlined a proof of (4), which is an extension of arguments by Kac, somewhat different from Sznitman's, and partly included in the fluctuation result given in the next section.

For μ_n a finite measure on S^n, $\mu_{n|m}$, $m = 1,\dots,n$, denotes the marginal measure of μ_n for the first m coordinates: $\mu_{n|m}(x_1,\dots,x_m)=\Sigma_{x_{m+1}} \cdots \Sigma_{x_n} \mu_n(x_1,\dots,x_n)$. In below $\otimes$ indicates the direct product of measures.

<u>Lemma 1</u>. Let μ_n and $\mu_{n|m}$ be as above. Suppose that there exists a positive integer p and measures $\mu^{(1)},\dots,\mu^{(p)}$ and μ on S such that

(i) μ_n is symmetric with respect to the coordinates $x_{p+1},\dots,x_n$ $(n > p)$

(ii) $\mu_{n|m} \longrightarrow \mu^{(1)} \otimes \cdots \otimes \mu^{(p)} \otimes \mu^{(m-p)}$ as $n \to \infty$ $(m \geq p)$

(iii) $c: = \sup_n \mu_n(S^n) < \infty$.

Let $e^{tG_n^*}$ be the semi-group of operators generated by G_n^* the adjoint of G_n and set $u_n(t)=e^{tG_n^*}\mu_n$. Then, for each $t>0$ and $m \geq p$, $u_{n|m}(t)$ weakly converges to $u^{(1)}(t) \otimes \cdots \otimes u^{(p)}(t) \otimes u(t)^{(m-p)\otimes}$ where $u(t)=P_t^\mu$ and $u^{(j)}(t)$ is a solution of the linear problem

$$
(6) \qquad \begin{cases} \dfrac{d}{dt}\langle u^{(j)}(t),\phi\rangle = \langle u^{(j)}(t), L\phi + \sum\limits_y \Gamma\phi(\cdot,y)u(t,y)\rangle & \text{for} \quad \phi \in C_b(S) \\ u^{(j)}(0) = \mu^{(j)}. \end{cases}
$$

The proof of Lemma 1, essentially the same as in Kac [1], is based on the hierarchical equations

$$
(7) \qquad u_{n|m}(t) = e^{(m/n)tG_m^*}\mu_{n|m} + \left(1-\frac{m}{n}\right)\int_0^t e^{(m/n)(t-s)G_m^*} K^{m,m+1}\mu_{n|m+1}(s)ds
$$

where $K^{m,m+1}$ is an operator which transforms a summable function $\phi \in L_1(S^{m+1})$ into a function of $L_1(S^m)$ by

$$
K^{m,m+1}\phi(x_1,\dots,x_m) = \sum_{j=1}^m \sum_{x_j'} \sum_{x_{m+1}'} [\phi(\underline{\underline{x}}_{j,m+1}')K_1^{x_j',x_{m+1}'}(x_j)-\phi(\underline{\underline{x}}_{m+1}')K_1^{x_j,x_{m+1}'}(x_j')],
$$

where $x=(x_1,\dots,x_{m+1})$ and $\underline{\underline{x}}_j'$ and $\underline{\underline{x}}_{j,k}'$ are the same as in (2). The successive substitutions of relations in the hierarchy (7) one into its predecessor leads to an expansion of $u_{n|m}(t)$ in which the k-th term is a transform of $\mu_{n|m+k}$. It is easy to justify that one can take a limit term-wise in the expansion for $0 \leq t \leq 1/2c$ and to see that the resulting series expresses $u^{(1)}(t)\otimes\cdots\otimes u^{(p)}(t)\otimes u(t)^{(m-p)\otimes}$. The latter can be seen either directly through algebraic munipulations or by the uniqueness assertion for the Boltzmann hierarchy. Since $\tilde{\mu}_n=u_n(1/3c)$ satisfies the conditions (i) to (iii), one can repeat this procedure to extend the time interval as far as he needs.

Lemma 2. Let μ_n be a probability on S^n, $n=1,2,\ldots,$ and suppose the conditions (i) to (iii) in Lemma 1 are satisfied. Let $\mathbb{E}_{\mu_n}$ indicate the expectation by the probability $\mathbb{P}_{\mu_n}$ for the Markov process $X^n(t)$ with the initial law μ_n. If $0=t_0<t_1<\cdots<t_\ell$, $\phi_k^{(j)}\in C_b(S)$, $k=0,\ldots,\ell$, $j=1,\ldots,m$ and $f_k(\underline{x})=\Pi_{j=1}^m\phi_k^{(j)}(x_j)$ for $\underline{x}\in S^n$ $(n\geq m)$, then

$$(8)\qquad \lim_{n\to\infty}\mathbb{E}_{\mu_n}\Big[\prod_{k=0}^{\ell} f_k(X^n(t_k))\Big]=\prod_{j=1}^{m}\int_D\prod_{k=0}^{\ell}\phi_k^{(j)}(w(t_k))P^{\mu}(dw).$$

Proof. We can assume $\phi_k^{(j)}\geq 0$. The proof is carried out by induction on ℓ. Let (8) hold with $\ell-1$ in place of ℓ. Define a finite measure $\tilde{\mu}_n$ by

$$\langle\tilde{\mu}_n,f\rangle=\mathbb{E}_{\mu_n}[f_0(X^n(t_0))\cdots f_{\ell-1}(X^n(t_{\ell-1}))f(X^n(t_{\ell-1}))],\qquad f\in C_b(S^n).$$

Obviously $\tilde{\mu}_n$ satisfies the conditions (i) and (iii) in Lemma 1. Let the presumed condition (ii) for μ_n hold with $p=p_0$. Then by taking $m\geq p_0$ the induction hypothesis shows that the condition (ii) holds for $p=m$ also with $\tilde{\mu}^{(j)}$'s and $u(t_{\ell-1})$ in place of $\mu^{(j)}$'s and μ where $\langle\tilde{\mu}^{(j)},\phi\rangle$ equals the j-th factor of the right-hand side of (8) but with the last factor $\phi_\ell^{(j)}(w(t_\ell))$ of the integrand being replaced by $\phi(w(t_{\ell-1}))$. By applications of Lemma 1 and Markov property of X^n, the left-hand side of (8) equals $\Pi_{j=1}^m\langle\tilde{u}^{(j)}(t_\ell-t_{\ell-1}),\phi_\ell^{(j)}\rangle$ where $\tilde{u}^{(j)}(t)$ is a solution of (6) but with $u(t)$ and $\mu^{(j)}$ replaced by $u(t+t_{\ell-1})$ and $\tilde{\mu}^{(j)}$, respectively. By the uniquness of a solution of (6), $\langle\tilde{u}^{(j)}(t_\ell-t_{\ell-1}),\phi^{(j)}\rangle$ agrees with the j-th factor of the right-hand side of (8). This completes the proof of Lemma 2.

The proof of (5) now is ready. We can assume that the initial distributions μ_n of X^n are all symmetric as remarked just after (5). It suffices to prove that the law, say $P_{n|m}$, of S^m-valued process $(X_1^n(t),\ldots,X_m^n(t))$ converges to the m-fold direct product of P^μ. It is not hard to see that $\{P_{n|m}\}_{n=m}^\infty$ is pre-compact and that $\lim_{n\to\infty}\alpha_0^n=\mu$ implies that $\mu_{n|m}$ converges to the m-fold direct product of μ. From the latter the convergence of finite dimensional distributions of $P_{n|m}$ follows in view of Lemma 2. The proof is complete.

3. Fluctuation. The limit theorem expressed in (5) may be considered as a law of large numbers. The next stage is to study the corresponding central limit theorem, i.e., the asymptotic behavior of the fluctuation of α^n about P^μ which is defined by

$$\eta^n = \sqrt{n}(\alpha^n - P^\mu).$$

For the diffusion model introduced by McKean [3] in relation to a nonlinear diffusion equation the problem of the fluctuation η^n is studied in several papers [4] [6] [7] [8]. Shiga and Tanaka [6] treated the problem also for a class of pure jump type Markov processes, which however admit no simultaneous jumps of two individuals at a time. Methods which are employed in these papers, though elegant, do not seem to be applicable to the present model. A similar problem of the fluctuation in path space is studied by Dawson and Gorostiza [1] for an infinite system of independent branching processes of randomly moving particles.

To state our result we must introduce several notations. For $\phi \in C_b(S^{m+2})$, $0=t_0<t_1<\cdots<t_m<t\leq 1$ set

$$\begin{aligned}\mathcal{A}_{\underline{t},t}\phi(x_0,\dots,x_m,x) &= \sum_{x'} L^x(x')[\phi(x_0,\dots,x_m,x')-\phi(x_0,\dots,x_m,x)] \\ &+ \int_D^{\mu} P^\mu(dw) \sum_{x'}\sum_{y'} K^{x,w(t)}(x',y')[\phi(x_0,\dots,x_m,x')-\phi(x_0,\dots,x_m,x) \\ &\qquad + \phi(w(t_0),\dots,w(t_m),y')-\phi(w(t_0),\dots,w(t_m),w(t))]\end{aligned}$$

where $\underline{t}=(t_0,\dots,t_m)$ and the first and the second sums are taken over all x' from S and (x',y') from S^2, respectively. It is easy to see that the linear problem

$$\begin{cases} \frac{\partial}{\partial s}\phi_s^t(x_0,\dots,x_m,x) = -\mathcal{A}_{\underline{t},s}\phi_s^t(x_0,\dots,x_m,x) & \text{for} \quad t_m \leq s \leq t \\ \phi_t^t = \phi \end{cases}$$

is uniquely solved. Let ι be a contraction operator which transforms a function $\phi \in C_b(S^{m+1})$ into a functin $\iota\phi \in C_b(S^m)$ by equating the last two variables, i.e., $\iota\phi(x_1,\dots,x_m) = \phi(x_1,\dots,x_m,x_m)$. Starting from $\iota\phi_{t_m}^t$ afresh one extends ϕ_s^t for $t_{m-1} \leq s \leq t_m$, and step by step for $0 \leq s \leq t$. Next define a two-parameter family of operators $\mathcal{U}_s^t$, $0 \leq s \leq t$ acting on those functions F of $w \in D$ which are of the form

$$F(w) = F_t^\phi(w) := \phi(w(t_0),w(t_2),\dots,w(t_m),w(t))$$

with $\phi \in C_b(S^{m+2})$, by

$$\mathcal{U}_s^t F(w) = \phi_s^t(w(t_0),\dots,w(t_k),w(s)) \quad \begin{cases} \text{for} \quad t_m \leq s \leq t & \text{if} \quad k=m \\ \text{for} \quad t_k \leq s < t_{k+1} & \text{if} \quad k=0,\dots,m-1. \end{cases}$$

Finally set

$$\mathbb{L}_k F_t^{\phi}(w) = \sum_{x'} [\phi(w(t_0),\dots,w(t_m),x') - F_t^{\phi}(w)]^k L^{w(t)}(x')$$

$$\Lambda_k F_t^{\phi}(w,\tilde{w}) = \sum_{x'} \sum_{y'} [\phi(w(t_0),\dots,w(t_m),x') - F_t^{\phi}(w) + \phi(\tilde{w}(t_0),\dots,\tilde{w}(t_m),y') - F_t^{\phi}(\tilde{w})]^k K^{w(t),\tilde{w}(t)}(x',y')$$

$(k=1,2,3;\ w,\tilde{w}\in D)$ and

$$Q_t(F_t^{\phi}) = \langle P^{\mu}, \mathbb{L}_2 F_t^{\phi}\rangle + \frac{1}{2}\langle P^{\mu}\otimes P^{\mu}, \Lambda_2 F_t^{\phi}\rangle .$$

We shall need the following conditions on L and K

(9) $$\sup_x \sum_{x'\neq x} L^{x'}(x) < \infty,\quad \sup_x \sum_y K^{x,y}\{S^2\} < \infty,\quad \sup_{x'} \sum_{x\neq x'} \sup_y K_1^{x,y}(x') < \infty$$

where

$$K^{x,y}\{S^2\} = \sum_{(x',y')\neq(x,y)} K^{x,y}(x',y').$$

The second condition in (9) may be interpreted that two individuals whose characters are very much different from each other hardly mate and the third analogously.

Theorem. Suppose that L and K satisfy conditions in (9) and that the initial distributions μ_n of $X^n(t)$ satisfy

$$\sup_n \sup_x \mathbb{E}_{\mu_n} |\langle\phi_0^n, \chi_{\{x\}}\rangle|^2 < \infty,$$

$$\lim_{n\to\infty} \mathbb{E}_{\mu_n} [\exp(\sqrt{-1}\langle\eta_0^n,\phi\rangle)] = C(\phi) \quad \text{for} \quad \phi\in L_1(S)$$

where χ_B denotes the indicator function of B and $C(\phi)$ is a functional of $L_1(S)$. Let F_t^{ϕ} be defined as above. Then

$$\lim_{n\to\infty} \mathbb{E}_{\mu_n} [\exp(\sqrt{-1}\langle\eta^n,F_t^{\phi}\rangle)] = C(\phi_0^t)\exp\{-\frac{1}{2}\int_0^t Q_s(\mathcal{U}_s^t F_t^{\phi})ds\}.$$

Let f be a smooth function of the whole real line which together with all its derivatives is bounded. By Markov property of X^n and Taylor expansion of f one can easily see that

(10) $$f(\langle\eta^n,F_t^{\phi}\rangle) - \int_{t_m}^t \{\langle\eta^n,\mathbf{A}_s F_s\rangle f' + \frac{1}{2}Q_s(F_s^{\phi})f'' + R_{s,f,\phi}^n\}ds$$

$$= \text{a martingale} + O(1/\sqrt{n}) \quad \text{for} \quad t_m \le t \le 1$$

where $f^{(i)} = f^{(i)}(\langle\eta^n,F_s^{\phi}\rangle)$ $(i=1,2)$ and

$$\mathbf{A}_t F_t^{\phi}(w) = \mathbf{L}_1 F_t^{\phi}(w) + \int_D \Lambda_1 F_t^{\phi}(w,\tilde{w}) P^{\mu}(d\tilde{w})$$

$$R^n_{t,f,\phi} = \frac{1}{2\sqrt{n}} \langle \eta^n \otimes \eta^n, \Lambda_1 F_t^{\phi} \rangle f' + \frac{1}{2}\{\langle \alpha^n - P^{\mu}, \mathbf{L}_2 F_t^{\phi}\rangle + \frac{1}{2}\langle \alpha^n \otimes \alpha^n - P^{\mu} \otimes P^{\mu}, \Lambda_2 F_2^{\phi}\rangle\} f''.$$

The Theorem readily follows from (10) if one proves the following lemma.

Lemma 3. Under the assumption of Theorem there exists a constant C independent of $\underline{\underline{t}}$ and t such that for $\phi \in L_1(S^{m+2})$

$$\sup_n \mathbb{E}_{\mu_n} |\langle \eta^n, F_t^{\phi}\rangle|^2 \leq C\left(\sum_{\underline{\underline{x}} \in S^{m+2}} |\phi(\underline{\underline{x}})|\right)^2.$$

The details to the proof of Theorem and Lemma 3 will be given elsewhere.

References.

[1] D. A. Dawson an L. G. Gorostiza, Limit theorems for supercritical branching random fields, Math. Nachr., 118 (1984), 19-46.

[2] M. Kac, Foundation of kinetic theory, Proceedings of 3rd Berkley Symposium on Math. Stat. and Prob., Vol.3 (1956), 171-197.

[3] H. P. McKean, A class of Markov processes associated with nonlinear parabolic equations, Proc. Nat. Acad. Sci., 56 (1966), 1907-1911.

[4] A. S. Sznitman, Nonlinear reflecting diffusion process, and the propagation of chaos and fluctuations associated, J. Func. Anal., 56 (1984), 311-336.

[5] A. S. Sznitman, Equations de type de Boltzmann, spatialement homogenes, Z. Wahrscheinlichkeitstheorie verw. Geb., 66 (1984), 559-592.

[6] T. Shiga and H. Tanaka, Central limit theorem for a system of Markovian particles with mean field interactions, Z. Wahrscheinlichkeitstheorie verw. Geb., 69 (1985) 439-459.

[7] H. Tanaka, Limit theorems for certain diffusion processes with interaction, Proceedings of the Taniguchi International Symposium on Stochastic Analysis (K. Itō ed.), Katata and Kyoto (1982), 469-488.

[8] H. Tanaka and M. Hitsuda, Central limit theorem for a simple diffusion model of interacting particles, Hiroshima Math. J., 11 (1981), 415-423.

Bio-mathematics

Managing Editor: **S. A. Levin**

Volume 17

Mathematical Ecology

An Introduction

Editors: **Th. G. Hallam, S. A. Levin**

1986. 84 figures. XII, 457 pages. ISBN 3-540-13631-2

Contents: Introduction. - Physiological and Behavioral Ecology. - Population Ecology. - Communities and Ecosystems. - Applied Mathematical Ecology. - Author Index. - Subject Index.

Volume 16

Complexity, Language, and Life: Mathematical Approaches

Editors: **J. L. Casti, A. Karlqvist**

1986. XIII, 281 pages. ISBN 3-540-16180-5

Contents: Allowing, forbidding, but nor requiring: a mathematic for human world. - A theory of stars in complex systems. - Pictures as complex systems. - A survey of replicator equations. - Darwinian evolution in ecosystems: a survey of some ideas and difficulties together with some possible solutions. - On system complexity: identification, measurement, and management. - On information and complexity. - Organs and tools; a common theory of morphogenesis. - The language of life. - Universal principles of measurement and language functions in evolving systems.

Volume 15

D. L. DeAngelis, W. M. Post, C. C. Travis

Positive Feedback in Natural Systems

1986. 90 figures. XII, 290 pages. ISBN 3-540-15942-8

Contents: Introduction. - The Mathematics of Positive Feedback. - Physical Systems. - Evolutionary Processes. - Organisms Physiology and Behavior. - Resource Utilization by Organisms. - Social Behavior. - Mutualistic and Competitive Systems. - Age-Structured Populations. - Spatially Heterogeneous Systems: Islands and Patchy Regions. - Spatially Heterogeneous Ecosystems; Pattern Formation. - Disease and Pest Outbreaks. - The Ecosystem and Succession. - Appendices. - References. - Subject Index. - Author Index.

Springer-Verlag
Berlin Heidelberg New York
London Paris Tokyo

Springer

Lecture Notes in Biomathematics

Vol. 58: C.A. Macken, A.S. Perelson, Branching Processes Applied to Cell Surface Aggregation Phenomena. VIII, 122 pages. 1985.

Vol. 59: I. Nåsell, Hybrid Models of Tropical Infections. VI, 206 pages. 1985.

Vol. 60: Population Genetics in Forestry. Proceedings, 1984. Edited by H.-R. Gregorius. VI, 287 pages 1985.

Vol. 61: Resource Management. Proceedings, 1984. Edited by M. Mangel. V, 138 pages 1985.

Vol. 62: B. J. West, An Essay on the Importance of Being Nonlinear. VIII, 204 pages. 1985.

Vol. 63: Carme Torras i Genís, Temporal-Pattern Learning in Neural Models. VII, 227 pages, 1985.

Vol. 64: Peripheral Auditory Mechanisms. Proceedings, 1985. Edited by J.B. Allen, J.L. Hall, A. Hubbard, S. Neely and A. Tubis. VII, 400 pages. 1986.

Vol. 65: Immunology and Epidemiology. Proceedings, 1985. Edited by G.W. Hoffmann and T. Hraba. VIII, 242 pages. 1986.

Vol. 66: Nonlinear Oscillations in Biology and Chemistry. Proceedings, 1985. Edited by H.G. Othmer. VI, 289 pages. 1986.

Vol. 67: P.H. Todd, Intrinsic Geometry of Biological Surface Growth. IV, 128 pages. 1986.

Vol. 68: The Dynamics of Physiologically Structured Populations. Edited by J.A.J. Metz and O. Diekmann. XII, 511 pages. 1986.

Vol. 69: S.H. Strogatz, The Mathematical Structure of the Human Sleep-Wake Cycle. VIII, 239 pages. 1986.

Vol. 70: Stochastic Methods in Biology. Proceedings, 1985. Edited by M. Kimura, G. Kallianpur and T. Hida. VI, 229 pages. 1987.